The malleable body

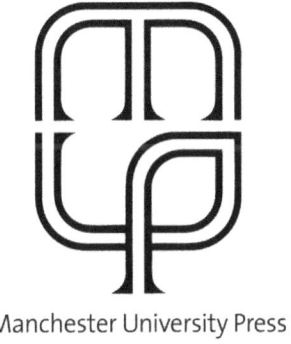

Manchester University Press

SOCIAL HISTORIES OF MEDICINE

Series editors: David Cantor, Anne Hanley and Elaine Leong

Social Histories of Medicine is concerned with all aspects of health, illness and medicine, from prehistory to the present, in every part of the world. The series covers the circumstances that promote health or illness, the ways in which people experience and explain such conditions, and what, practically, they do about them. Practitioners of all approaches to health and healing come within its scope, as do their ideas, beliefs, and practices, and the social, economic and cultural contexts in which they operate. Methodologically, the series welcomes relevant studies in social, economic, cultural, and intellectual history, as well as approaches derived from other disciplines in the arts, sciences, social sciences and humanities. The series is a collaboration between Manchester University Press and the Society for the Social History of Medicine.

To buy or to find out more about the books currently available in this series, please go to: https://manchesteruniversitypress.co.uk/series/social-histories-of-medicine/

The malleable body
Surgeons, artisans, and amputees in early modern Germany

HEIDI HAUSSE

Manchester University Press

Copyright © Heidi Hausse 2023

The right of Heidi Hausse to be identified as the author of this work has been asserted in accordance with the Copyright, Designs and Patents Act 1988.

Published by Manchester University Press
Oxford Road, Manchester M13 9PL

www.manchesteruniversitypress.co.uk

British Library Cataloguing-in-Publication Data
A catalogue record for this book is available from the British Library

ISBN 978 1 5261 6065 2 hardback
ISBN 978 1 5261 9083 3 paperback

First published 2023
Paperback published 2025

The publisher has no responsibility for the persistence or accuracy of URLs for any external or third-party internet websites referred to in this book, and does not guarantee that any content on such websites is, or will remain, accurate or appropriate.

EU authorised representative for GPSR:
Easy Access System Europe – Mustamäe tee 50, 10621 Tallinn, Estonia
gpsr.requests@easproject.com

Typeset
by Cheshire Typesetting Ltd, Cuddington, Cheshire

To Dave

Contents

List of figures	*page* viii
Acknowledgements	xi
List of abbreviations	xiv
Introduction	1
1 Writing the craft of surgery	19
2 Communities face the cold fire	51
3 Visions of the body	82
4 After the operation	119
5 Mechanical hands	155
6 Prosthetic technology on the move	210
Epilogue	238
Bibliography	245
Index	267

Figures

2.1	Leg amputation in Walther Hermann Ryff, *Die groß Chirurgei* (Frankfurt am Main, 1545), title page (detail). By kind permission of The College of Physicians of Philadelphia.	68
3.1	Hand amputations in Johannes Scultetus, *Wund-Artzneyisches Zeug-Hauß* (Frankfurt am Main, 1666), Tab. LIII. By kind permission of The College of Physicians of Philadelphia.	89
3.2	"Serratura" in Hans von Gersdorff, *Feldbuch der Wundarznei* (Strasbourg, 1517). By kind permission of The College of Physicians of Philadelphia.	95
3.3	St. Anthony's Fire in Hans von Gersdorff, *Feldbuch der Wundarznei* (Strasbourg, 1517), 65v. By kind permission of The College of Physicians of Philadelphia.	97
3.4	Patient with prosthetic leg in Pieter Adriaanszoon Verduyn, *Neue Methode, die Glieder abzunehmen* (Amsterdam, 1697), Tab. VII. Courtesy of SLUB Dresden. Public Domain Mark.	106
4.1	Practitioners in a hospital sickroom in Paracelsus, *Opus Chyrurgicum* (Frankfurt am Main, 1565), title page (detail). Courtesy of Wellcome Collection. Public Domain Mark.	120
4.2	Master of the legend scenes, *Wunderbare Beinheilung durch die Hll. Cosmas und Damian*, early sixteenth century. Inv.-Nr. 4968. Courtesy of Österreichische Galerie Belvedere (Vienna). CC BY-SA 4.0.	138
5.1	Ruppin Hand, left hand prosthesis with forearm casing, sixteenth century. Inv. Nr. V-2039-H. Sammlung Museum Neuruppin. Courtesy of Museum Neuruppin.	157
5.2	Ruppin Hand (detail), left hand prosthesis with forearm casing, sixteenth century. Inv. Nr. V-2039-H. Sammlung Museum Neuruppin. Photo by author.	158
5.3	Original fragments and reconstruction of Balbronn Hand. Inv. Nr. MH 4052 a–b; Inv. Nr. MH 4053. Museé Historique	

Figures

	(Strasbourg). Courtesy of Musées de la ville de Strasbourg, M. Bertola.	159
5.4	Grüningen Hand, right arm prosthesis, sixteenth century. Courtesy of bpk Bildagentur / Deutsches Historisches Museum (Berlin, Germany) / Sebastian Ahlers / Art Resource, NY.	161
5.5	Ersthand, right hand prosthesis, c. 1510. Schlossmuseum Götzenburg (Jagsthausen). Courtesy of Archiv der Freiherren von Berlichingen.	164
5.6	Zweithand, right hand prosthesis with forearm casing, c. 1530. Schlossmuseum Götzenburg (Jagsthausen). Courtesy of Archiv der Freiherren von Berlichingen.	165
5.7	Ingolstadt Hand, left hand prosthesis, c. 1520. Inv. Nr. 7924. Bayerisches Armeemuseum (Ingolstadt). Photo by author.	168
5.8	Zweithand mechanisms in Christian von Mechel, *Die eiserne Hand des tapfern deutschen Ritters Götz von Berlichingen* (Berlin: Decker, 1815), Tab. II. Courtesy of ETH-Bibliothek Zürich, Rar 2224, doi: 10.3931/e-rara-14841. Public Domain Mark.	172
5.9	Eisfeld Hand at partial flexion, left hand prosthesis, c. 1525–1550. Inv. Nr. 307. Museum Eisfeld. Photo by author.	174
5.10	Eisfeld Hand, left hand prosthesis, c. 1525–1550. Inv. Nr. 307. Museum Eisfeld. Photo by author.	175
5.11	Internal mechanisms of Eisfeld Hand, left hand prosthesis, c. 1525–1550. Inv. Nr. 307. Museum Eisfeld. Photo by author.	176
5.12	Braunschweig Hand, above-the-elbow arm prosthesis, seventeenth century. Inv. Nr. Waf 11. Courtesy of Herzog Anton Ulrich-Museum Braunschweig. Photo: Claus Cordes.	178
5.13	Wrist mechanisms of Braunschweig Hand with spanners placed on shafts. Drawing by Lauren Woods.	180
5.14	Darmstadt Hand, right hand prosthesis with forearm casing, c. 1650. Inv. Nr. W 61:24. Hessisches Landesmuseum Darmstadt. Photo by author.	182
5.15	Darmstadt Hand (detail), right hand prosthesis with forearm casing, c. 1650. Inv. Nr. W 61:24. Hessisches Landesmuseum Darmstadt. Photo by author.	183
5.16	Nuremberg Hand, right arm prosthesis, c. 1617. Inv. Nr. WI 448. Courtesy of Germanisches Nationalmuseum (Nuremberg).	186
5.17	Fingers of Nuremberg Hand (detail), right arm prosthesis, c. 1617. Inv. Nr. WI 448. Germanisches Nationalmuseum (Nuremberg). Photo by author.	187
6.1	Mechanical hand in Ambroise Paré, *Les Oeuvres* (Paris, 1614), 902 (detail). By kind permission of The College of Physicians of Philadelphia.	215

6.2	Artificial hand with strap fastenings in Ambroise Paré, *Les Oeuvres* (Paris, 1614), 902 (detail). By kind permission of The College of Physicians of Philadelphia.	216
6.3	Artificial arm in Ambroise Paré, *Les Oeuvres* (Paris, 1614), 903 (detail). By kind permission of The College of Physicians of Philadelphia.	217
6.4	Kassel Hand, right hand prosthesis, sixteenth century. Inv. Nr. KP B XIV.32. Courtesy of Museumslandschaft Hessen Kassel, Sammlung Angewandte Kunst. Photo: Mirja van IJken.	219
6.5	Internal mechanisms of Kassel Hand, right hand prosthesis, sixteenth century. Inv. Nr. KP B XIV.32. Courtesy of Museumslandschaft Hessen Kassel, Sammlung Angewandte Kunst. Photo: Mirja van IJken.	219
6.6	Diagram of Kassel Hand mechanisms. Drawing and 3D model by Ben Tulman.	220
6.7	Diagram of Kassel Hand thumb mechanism. Drawing and 3D model by Ben Tulman.	222
6.8	Mechanical hand in Ambroise Paré, *Wund-Artzney* (Frankfurt am Main, 1635), 749 (detail). Courtesy of Archives & Special Collections, Columbia University Health Sciences Library.	228
6.9	Artificial hand mechanisms in Ambroise Paré, *Les Oeuvres* (Paris, 1614), 902 (detail). By kind permission of The College of Physicians of Philadelphia.	229

Acknowledgements

Many institutions and individuals made this book possible. Its kernel formed from the insights of Anthony Grafton, William Chester Jordan, Pamela O. Long, Yair Mintzker, and Jennifer Rampling on my early notions of a long historical transformation in Western medicine. I especially thank Tony for his intellectual generosity and steadfast support through the years it took for that kernel to grow into a full manuscript.

Much of this work developed from the resources and support provided by the Society of Fellows in the Humanities at Columbia University and a Molina Fellowship in the History of Medicine and Allied Sciences at the Huntington Library. A College of Liberal Arts New Faculty Semester Release from Teaching Grant and a CLA–History Department Image Subvention from Auburn University were instrumental in the final push. This publication is made possible in part with support from the Barr Ferree Foundation Fund for Publications, Department of Art and Archaeology, Princeton University. For support during early research phases, I also thank the American Council of Learned Societies, the Consortium for History of Science, Technology and Medicine, the Herzog August Bibliothek, and Princeton University.

My exploration of rare books and archives over many years depended on the dedicated librarians and archivists who guided me through collections, including those of the Herzog August Bibliothek, the Bayerische Staatsbibliothek, the Stadtbibliothek Braunschweig, the Wellcome Library, the Historical Medical Library of The College of Physicians of Philadelphia, the Huntington Library, Firestone Library, Butler Library, Columbia University Health Sciences Library, Stadtarchiv München, Stadtarchiv Augsburg, Niedersächsisches Landesarchiv Wolfenbüttel, and Stadtarchiv Ulm.

Locating prosthetic artifacts and learning to read them was only possible because of a network of museums and private collections whose curators and staff offered generous access to examine them, shared documentation, and contributed invaluable expertise. Particular thanks goes to Konrad Freiherr von Berlichingen and Schlossmuseum Götzenburg; Tobias Schönauer and the Bayerisches Armeemuseum; Thomas Eser and the Germanisches

Nationalmuseum Nürnberg; Alfred Walz and the Herzog Anton Ulrich-Museum; Wolfgang Glüber and Hessisches Landesmuseum Darmstadt; Monique Fuchs and Museé Historique Strasbourg; Hansjörg Albrecht, Carola Zimmermann, and Museum Neuruppin; Heiko Haine and Museum Eisfeld; Antje Scherner and Museumslandschaft Hessen Kassel; Jürgen Schulte-Hobein and the Sauerland-Museum; and Hans-Christoph Freiherr von Hornstein and his family. I also thank Dirk H. Breiding and the Philadelphia Museum of Art.

I learned much from feedback I received presenting portions of this work in several venues, including the Sixteenth Century Society & Conference, the Renaissance Society of America, the Society for the History of Technology, the History of Science Society, the Society of Fellows Thursday Lecture Series, Yale University, New York University, University of Michigan, University of Minnesota, and the Huntington Library. There are too many individuals to name from the scholarly communities that were so vital to producing this book. For their insight and support during my time in the Society of Fellows I especially thank Donna Bilak, Emily Bloom, Benjamin Breen, Christopher L. Brown, Clarence Coaxum, Julie Crawford, Christopher Florio, Eileen Gillooly, María González Pendás, David Gutkin, Arden Hegele, Matthew L. Jones, Joel A. Klein, Lauren Kopajtic, Whitney Laemmli, Lan Li, Reinhold Martin, Max Mishler, Carmel Raz, Kavita Sivaramakrishnan, Pamela H. Smith, Tillman Taappe, and Kay Zhang. Of the many others who have touched this project in different ways through the years, from sharing practical advice to creating opportunities for dialogue, I particularly thank Babak Ashrafi, Adam Beaver, Paola Bertucci, Amanda Caspar, Frederic Clark, Maria Pia Donato, Susan Felch, Kristen Gaylord, Brian Hamilton, Mareike Heide, Jessica Keating, Meg Leja, Jebrŏ Lit, Noria Litaker, Melissa Lo, Valeria López Fadul, Howard Louthan, Carolina Malagon, Robyn Radway, Trish Ross, Margaret Schotte, Molly Taylor-Poleskey, Maarten Ultee, Mara R. Wade, Maura Whang, and Amanda Wunder. A special thanks to Ben Tulman and Lauren Woods for their wonderful drawings. My history colleagues at Auburn University provided great encouragement and advice, especially Kate Craig, Ralph Kingston, and Rupali Mishra. My biggest thanks go to Christopher Ferguson, who read chapters, talked through ideas, and provided a combination of intellectual creativity and compassion throughout the disruptions of the pandemic.

Portions of Chapters 2 and 6 first appeared in "Bones of Contention: The Decision to Amputate in Early Modern Germany," *The Sixteenth Century Journal* 47:2 (2016): 327–350 and "The Locksmith, the Surgeon, and the Mechanical Hand: Communicating Technical Knowledge in Early Modern Europe," *Technology and Culture* 60:1 (2019): 34–64. I thank these publishers for allowing their inclusion here. I also thank my editors at Manchester University Press, Meredith Carroll and Elaine Leong, for their guidance and support in bringing this book to print. This manuscript additionally benefited from the valuable feedback of the anonymous readers.

Above all, I am grateful for the encouragement of friends and family through many years and constant changes of address. I especially thank Glenn, Jan, and my LRs for their enduring friendship. For her enthusiasm, kindness, and wit in the best and worst of times, Louise will always have my heartfelt gratitude. I wish to give a special thanks for the support, patience, and tireless love of my family—the Georges, Hausses, and Kujawas. As the supreme cheerleaders of this book, my parents Les and Holly showed unwavering faith as it took shape over the years. My final thanks go to my husband, Dave Lucsko, who spent countless hours listening and talking through every idea expressed in these pages and pored over draft after draft with a keen editor's eye. He dedicated his time, intellect, and heart to the completion of this book; dedicating the result to him is the least I can do to show my gratitude and love.

Abbreviations

AHRG   Rudolf Wissell, *Des Alten Handwerks Recht und Gewohnheit*, 6 vols., 2nd ed., ed. Ernst Schraepler (Berlin: Colloquium Verlag, 1971–1988)
H   Handschriften
HAUM   Herzog Anton Ulrich-Museum, Braunschweig
KR   Kämmerei. Kammerechnung
NLA-WO   Niedersächsisches Landesarchiv Wolfenbüttel
StdAM   Stadtarchiv München
StdAU   Stadtarchiv Ulm

Introduction

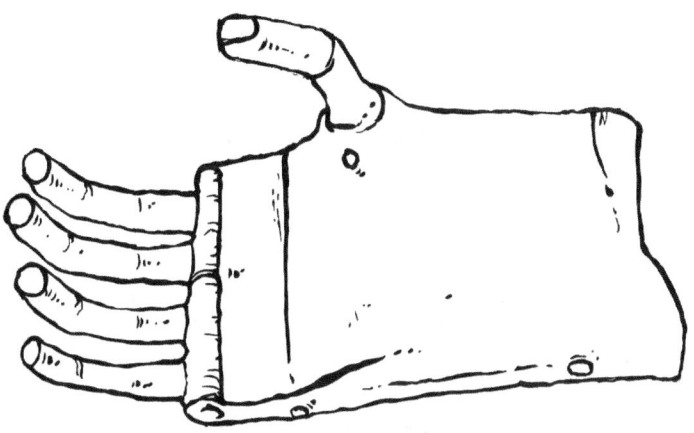

Götz von Berlichingen (1480–1562) lost his right hand in the dog days of summer in 1504.[1] In memoirs dictated to a scribe decades later, when he was elderly and blind, he reflected on that fateful event.[2] He had been an eager young knight in Albrecht IV of Bavaria-Munich's forces besieging the town of Landshut in southeast Germany. During a skirmish, "the Nurembergers directed the artillery toward us, and indeed, into friend and foe."[3] A blow from a culverin, a light piece of artillery, split the pommel of his sword hilt. "One half flew into my arm," Götz recalled, "and three plates of [forearm guard] with it."[4] Broken remains of the hilt wedged violently between gauntlet and forearm. His arm "was shattered in back and in front."[5] "And so as I look there," he recounted, "so the hand still hangs a little by the skin, and the lance lies under the horse's hooves."[6] He managed to reach his camp and the field-surgeon, who sliced through the remaining bit of skin near the wrist, severing the hand completely.

The account of his long convalescence describes not only his physical and emotional anguish, but also a crucial turning point in his life. For months he stayed at the lodgings of a good friend (who was fighting on the other side of the conflict) in the still-besieged town of Landshut. "What pains I suffered at that time," Götz remembered, "anyone can well understand."[7] Despondency soon spiraled into deep despair. "It was my plea to God, which I made: if ever I were in His godly mercy," he prayed, "then in God's name He should let me die;

I would certainly be ruined—a poor soldier."[8] Comrades visited to keep him company, assuring him of his heroism in battle and bringing news. Perhaps it was during these conversations, or in the lonely hours he lay awake, that Götz recalled Kochle, a knight of whom he had heard from his late father and other old knights. Kochle had only one hand yet was "able to accomplish a thing against enemies in the field, just as another."[9] The story of this one-handed fighter gave Götz hope. After all, he reasoned, without God's grace it would not matter if he had twelve hands. "And I thought therefore," he explained, "if I had nothing more than a little aid—an iron hand, or some such—so I would wish, with God's grace and assistance, to still be as good on the battlefield as any healthy man."[10] In his retelling, the traumatic loss of his hand becomes a triumph of his faith in God. He concludes the episode by declaring that for the next sixty years he warred and feuded "with one fist."[11]

The oldest manuscript of Götz's narrative, which dates to no later than 1567, resides in the Berlichingen family archive in Jagsthausen, a small town in southwest Germany. Also in the Berlichingen collection are two mechanical right hands made of iron and purported to have belonged to Götz (figures 5.5–5.6).[12] The knight only mentioned in passing his artificial hand—that "little aid" he first envisioned while in his sickbed.[13] A rare print edition of his autobiography appears alongside the sixteenth-century prostheses when they are displayed in the small museum of the Götzenburg, the Renaissance castle overlooking the town. The larger and more mechanically complex of the two has an iron casing that extends up the wearer's forearm near the elbow. The simpler one is lightweight and small, less than twenty centimeters in length at full extension. Perforated holes at the hand's base presumably enabled it to be attached to the wrist with cord or fabric. Its spindly fingers, which curve toward their ends, seem too narrow for the squat, square body of the hand. The thumb is stiff, but the wearer could use a natural hand to passively operate the other four fingers. When pressed, these move at the base of the knuckles, where the fingers meet the hand, locking at increments to curl closer and closer to the thumb, until the thumb and fingers form a circle. Those fingers, at once peculiar and plain, contain surprising details. Engraved lines create the effect of wrinkles at the knuckles, and impressions in the wrought iron make fingernails. The body of the hand is rough and half-covered in the remnants of a coat of paint, damaged and ranging from beige to brown—shades reminiscent of human skin.

The objects on display today in Jagsthausen form a written and physical record of traumatic bodily change and adaptation, one that points to a larger story about early modern medicine. The expansion of gunpowder warfare in the sixteenth century caused grisly contused injuries, which required amputation on a scale Europeans had never before seen. Destructive military technologies strained a tradition of non-invasive therapies, pushing medical practices to the breaking point. The challenges of amputation sparked new discussions about the body among surgeons, which grew over the following century. Meanwhile, efforts to treat the loss of limbs drew on skills from different parts of the community. Amputees turned not to surgeons, but to artisans. Locksmiths, clockmakers, and armorers began to fashion devices to artificially replace natural limbs. Change came slowly. In 1500, surgeons and artisans were hesitant to manipulate the body's shape. By 1700, a large and more complex pool of practices and techniques existed for doing just that. Medical practitioners taught and debated many different amputation methods, inside and outside of a battlefield context, and social elites could obtain sophisticated mechanical limbs made of iron, brass, and wood. Götz's experience with injury and those two iron hands in Jagsthausen mark the early stages of a gradual yet profound transformation. But what was this transformation exactly? How did it happen? And what meanings might it hold for historians of medicine and technology, scholars of disability and the body, and those studying practical knowledge and material culture? These are the questions *The Malleable Body* sets out to answer.

This book contends that out of two centuries of surgical and artisanal intervention in the shapes and textures of arms and legs arose a vision of the malleable body: a growing perception, fundamental to biomedicine today, of the human body as an entity that could be artificially altered under certain circumstances. This was not a stable or monolithic idea, but rather a change in expectations among surgeons and their patients, and artisans and their amputee-patrons, about the number and degree of interventions possible.

Early moderns began to discern this malleability in different ways. For surgeons, the practices and discussions surrounding operations and the resulting architectures of stumps formed the locus of the shift. Where and how to cut soft and hard tissues, whether to cauterize or ligate blood vessels—these thoughts increasingly imbued the body with latent possibilities of what could be and what the surgeon could choose to create. Patients and their families, meanwhile, saw parts of the body die when limbs were afflicted with a condition surgeons called the "cold fire." They witnessed traumatic bodily change in an amputation. It was traumatic in its suddenness and extent, the physical pain it caused, its danger to one's life, and the uncertainty of convalescence, when some patients felt phantom sensations of the very body parts that had been removed. For the amputees who survived, malleability in a basic sense was conceived as a response to this bodily change. Iron arms show us this was much more complicated than an attempt to return to a sense of "wholeness." In a world in which artificial limbs had yet to be medicalized, amputees with the desire and means to obtain prostheses made individual decisions about the forms these objects would take. The artisans they charged with making them approached malleability from their material experience, applying techniques and tools in new ways to create singular objects.

The malleable body, then, was one that reflected different degrees of perceived ability for surgical and artisanal intervention in the lengths, textures, shapes, and even materials of human arms and legs. It applied to many ways of approaching the body at once. Its creation and development were nonlinear: one major way of thinking did not give way to another, then another, in neat succession. This body had the element of the potential—of what could be—when surgeons considered which procedure to perform or amputees and artisans discussed the commission of a mechanical limb. Perhaps most essential to our definition is the possibility for change to occur multiple times. Surgeons, artisans, and amputees *shaped* and *reshaped* a body when they removed a natural limb and obtained an artificial one.

The nature of Hippocratic-Galenic surgery was non-invasive, but this did not mean that medieval and early modern bodies were perceived as solid, static entities. On the contrary, historians of medicine and the body have established that early modern bodies, composed of humors, were porous and in constant flux as they interacted with their environment.[14] The "malleable body" this book introduces concerns a different kind of perceived fluidity, one intimately tied to medical and artificial interventionism in the body's limbs.

Early modern Europeans did not invent surgical dismemberment or prostheses, of course. Rather, the shift this book uncovers is about a multiplicity of amputation methods, a need and willingness among surgeons to perform these procedures, and the development of intricate mechanical hands and arms. A hallmark of early modern medicine was its conservative approach to invasive procedures, and amputation was the most invasive of all. This book shows that early moderns were *less* conservative by the end of the period than at its beginning precisely because by then they could imagine and carry out far *more* options for treating limbs that required removal, and the resulting stumps. They came to perceive the body in a way their predecessors had not.

Change came from people *doing* and then discussing, and the influence of those discussions on developing thought and practice. The process was long, spanning four or five generations. This book examines evidence of this gradual shift in early modern Germany on two major fronts: surgery and prosthetic limb production. Surgeons and artisans created new possibilities for injured patients and elite amputees. They were entangled in different ways in the challenges of bodily loss and efforts to manage it. Beneath the surgeon's scalpel, amputated limbs and the resulting stumps could be shortened or lengthened, the textures of their edges worked and reworked with thread, cautery irons, and caustic medicines. Surgeons recorded and debated their techniques in treatises, developing passionate schools of thought about where and how to remove a limb. Amputees who survived such procedures sought out their own artificial aids. Wearers of elaborate prostheses commissioned artisans to employ art, craft, and innovative technology to reshape the contours of their bodies yet again. In so doing, they blurred the lines between nature and artifice, creating unique objects from a tradition of artisanal production that was adaptive, creative, and almost never written down. Technology became intertwined with the very shape of the human body, both in the ways surgeons cut gangrenous bodies apart and in the imaginative devices artisans designed.

Echoes of practice provide evidence of the way this transformation unfolded. Surgical treatises recorded techniques which authors had either already attempted or knew of from other sources. Many works recorded firsthand perspectives on practices, but some borrowed so extensively from their predecessors that scholars consider them more representative of late medieval surgery than early modern.[15] All surgical treatises are filtered for publication and layered with discussions of other practitioners and a rich body of surgical literature. Yet they also offer windows into scenes of people processing intense emotional and physical pain, into relationships between people in moments of extreme emergency. This is all the more significant because firsthand accounts from amputees, such as Götz von Berlichingen, are exceedingly rare. With their publications, surgeons also provide one of the few written sources about early modern mechanical limbs. But they wrote as outsiders looking in; the fabrication of artful prosthetic hands was the domain of locksmiths, woodworkers, clockmakers, and other artisans. Most surviving examples of their work are anonymous—we do not know who made them or who wore them. Yet the techniques and materials evident in them reveal much about their makers and wearers. Both kinds of sources, surgical treatises and prosthetic artifacts, are essential for uncovering the different forms of practical intervention that early moderns developed in response to grievous injury and the loss of limbs.

The broader shift this book explores has gone unnoticed for so long in the history of medicine in large part because of how these two bodies of evidence have been treated. There is, on the one side, the way the existing literature approaches amputation. Historical monographs on early modern Europe treat this surgical procedure only superficially, while voluminous medical surveys and reference works provide detailed lists of techniques and authors without deeper historical analysis.[16] On the other side is the absence of surviving mechanical hands and arms in historical monographs. These artifacts are discussed in museum exhibition catalogs and medical articles, but almost never in the work of early modern historians.[17] The paucity of written sources about artificial limbs has led scholars to do brilliant work on literary and artistic portrayals, but this does not allow detailed insight into hands-on practices.

By drawing together surgical treatises and prosthetic artifacts for historical analysis, this book puts together two halves of a single story. It provides a close analysis of amputation techniques in surgical treatises in order to follow discussions among surgeons, to find evidence of the social world in which they practiced, and to uncover ideas about the body embedded in surgical techniques and debates about them. It also turns to new sources, bringing surviving artificial limbs into critical historical study to shed new light on our understanding of medicine, culture, and technology in the early modern period. This book is about the body taken apart, put back together, and augmented. Only through the full arc of this story does the rise of the malleable body become apparent.

Setting the stage

Götz von Berlichingen's experience of amputation began with the roar of artillery fire, and it is on the Renaissance battlefield that our larger story begins. For hundreds of years, the Hippocratic-Galenic tradition of medicine in Europe had advocated non-invasive surgical therapies whenever possible. By the turn of the sixteenth century, the pressures of gunpowder warfare were creating new kinds of injuries in great numbers. In his *Speculum chirurgicum*, the barber-surgeon Joseph Schmid (1600–1667) discussed leg injuries through a series of brief case histories about soldiers with gunshot wounds. Many of these featured patients who required an immediate amputation or developed complications during treatment that led to the procedure. Janus Abraham à Gehema (1647–1715) later described the putrefaction caused by the contused wounds of bullets in depth in his *Krancke Soldat*.[18] The influence of gunpowder warfare on a wider textual dialogue about amputation was not immediate. After all, written records of practices usually lagged behind the practices themselves, from building a canal to mining for silver.[19] The stirrings of a new kind of amputation debate did not appear in surgical treatises until the second half of the sixteenth century. The process it initiated had the slow but inexorable power of a sea change rather than the rush of a flood, and it was contingent on and linked to several other concurrent developments.

The increasing scale on which warfare was waged during the early modern period compounded the dangers of new military technologies. Surgeons had followed armies between the twelfth and fifteenth centuries; however, medieval campaigns were often short and rarely featured large pitched battles, and it is unclear whether surgeons treated common soldiers.[20] The growing sizes of early modern armies and the sustained nature of warfare created larger populations of soldiers in need of more field-surgeons for greater lengths of time.[21] In early modern Germany, surgeons played official and prominent roles in the new fighting forces of *Landsknechte*, mercenaries raised and recruited from within the Holy Roman Empire.[22] Both princes and cities contracted surgeons in preparation for war, and more surgeons were needed to care for the growing numbers of common soldiers serving in the infantry and artillery.[23] In the seventeenth century, warfare reached a calamitous new pitch. The Thirty Years' War, the most devastating military conflict of the period, drew Catholic and Protestant powers from across Europe into an escalating contest on German soil. In this long struggle, armies of over a hundred thousand marched into battle, ravaged the countryside, and destroyed cities.[24] The careers of a generation of surgeons bore the indelible marks of this period of sustained warfare.

The role of surgeons in armies and navies contributed to their growing visibility in early modern Germany. Trained in a master–apprentice system, many were members of guilds or confraternities.[25] They took on vital functions in flourishing urban institutions, including hospitals and specialized houses for pox and plague.[26] Another significant factor in their increased prominence involved the printing press. Surgeons composed works in the vernacular to convey operative techniques, advertise their profession, and argue for the value and antiquity of their craft. As part of this conscious attempt to advance their status, they drew on intellectual and cultural trends that emphasized the importance of firsthand experience. Increased focus on anatomy and human dissection in university medical education in particular lent prestige to hands-on work with the body.[27] While Renaissance anatomy was slow to make its way into German universities, German-speaking students attended institutions such as Padua and returned to the empire to practice as physicians. Through their treatises, master–apprentice-trained surgeons and barber-surgeons also emphasized the importance of anatomy to medical instruction and the craft of surgery. Within this broad professional, intellectual, and cultural milieu, surgeons claimed and won a higher status.

German surgeons were well positioned to engage with the printing press as authors and readers because the Holy Roman Empire remained a major crossroads for printing throughout the sixteenth and seventeenth centuries. Print shops in urban centers like Frankfurt am Main, Nuremberg, and Augsburg published works from all over Europe in Latin or German translation. Like artists and engineers, surgeons sought to enhance their social position by giving their tacit knowledge formal written form. Print culture enabled an outpouring of works that discussed hands-on practices in different ways. Already in the fifteenth century, manuscript books on military technology, engineering, painting, and sculpture circulated in south Germany and parts of Italy. These works advanced the antiquity, nobility, and even rational character of the practices they described.[28] With the rapid spread of print came a proliferation of technical treatises and how-to manuals claiming to provide details on the practical arts. Technical recipe books such as the enormously popular *Kunstbüchlein* presented everything from metallurgy to methods for removing stubborn stains from clothing.[29] Thus, surgeons who published did so in an environment of expanding markets for medical works, how-to manuals, and artisans' technical treatises.[30] Surgical texts took many different forms and contained both craft and academic currents: their authors engaged with a learned body of medical literature while also emphasizing the importance of firsthand experience. Some also wrote with audiences for how-to manuals in mind. There were treatises for the sick soldier or the sick patient more generally, and treatises written in a question-and-answer format to prepare young surgeons to take the examinations most German towns required. The printing press and the voracious print culture that grew steadily through the period propelled the wide circulation of medical texts new and old, in Latin and the vernacular, written by learned and unlearned authors and practitioners.

The weapons that injured men and women, the publications that discussed amputation, and the artificial limbs that replaced natural ones were all produced within a diverse artisanal marketplace. Early modern Germany was a center for skilled artisans and craft production. For over a century, a number of imperial cities in southern Germany dominated the market for spring-driven clocks. Armor-makers also flourished in centers like Innsbruck, Augsburg, and Nuremberg. Craft trades in early modern Germany experienced increasing specialization and heavy regulation in most urban centers. Yet the fluidity of the craft market also provided ample opportunity for craftspeople to execute unique orders. Metalworkers devised a variety of custom instruments and machines. Clockmakers, for example, made automata, luxury items often created in coordination with goldsmiths.[31] Some unique orders were made for display in art cabinets (*die Kunstkammern*) and cabinets of curiosities (*die Wunderkammern*).[32] Such collections might hold a miniature palace made of seashells, paper-thin shapes of turned ivory, or a celestial globe with clockwork—all objects of wondrous design that obscured the boundaries between art and nature. The crafting of mechanical limbs took place in this vibrant context of skilled artisanal production and the culture of the *Kunstkammer*.

The confluence of these developments helped create among surgeons, amputees, and artisans an environment for a more intensive focus on limb loss, and for ways to manage it. Amputation remained an extraordinary and high-risk procedure throughout the early modern period. Of those who survived it, only amputees belonging to the upper circles of society possessed the means to commission mechanical prostheses. The experiences of the group of patrons explored in this book did not reflect those of the majority who came from more humble circumstances. Their efforts, however, were a vital part of the practical endeavors that gradually transformed the early modern body. Expectations about the abilities of surgeons and artisans to reshape limbs shifted as practices surrounding this task diversified and grew.

Craft, healing, and bodywork

The relationship between surgeons and artisans—between craft and healing—is a recurring theme throughout this book. Surgeons belonged to a craft group comparable to smiths, engineers, furniture-makers, and others. In recent years, some have explored these important craft connections, particularly by emphasizing social and economic links to adjacent occupational groups concerned with the body.[33] I build on this developing thread of the literature by drawing even more explicitly from the methodologies of historians of science and technology to examine tacit and vernacular bodies of knowledge and the creation, codification, and transfer of practical knowledge.[34] I examine surgical treatises as both evidence of practical knowledge-making and complex sites of knowledge-making in their own right. Likewise, I study surgeons as makers of practical knowledge, but also, through the printing press, as participants in a larger medical conversation that involved learned physicians and anatomists.[35]

This framework shapes my analytic perspective on surgical treatises as technical literature. I use them to learn about social interactions and moments of emotional crisis. In surgical operations, knowledge-making practices intersected directly with extreme experiences and sensations. Descriptions of these are embedded in what may seem at first to be dry, technical instructions. I use these instructions to uncover surgeons' ideas about the body, their profession, and the lessons gleaned from their previous experience. The rise of the malleable body was not simply a byproduct of barber-surgeons codifying practical knowledge or of learned physicians circulating their Latin works in vernacular translation. I therefore look for signs of a dialogue—a conversation of many voices both learned and unlearned, of works by authors from German-speaking lands and outside them—taking place in surgical literature printed and/or circulated in the Holy Roman Empire. By focusing on works that appeared in German, either originally or in translation, I examine a body of literature that was accessible to most German-speaking surgeons, and to which they contributed as authors. I reconstruct dialogues that put barber-surgeons and surgeons from master–apprentice backgrounds in conversation with university-educated physicians and anatomists. This book, then, is concerned with practices and ideas about practices. In *Body of the Artisan*, Pamela Smith argues that artisans gained knowledge from hands-on experience with natural materials and the ways those materials interacted with their own bodies. In this period, the patient's body became the natural material with which surgeons learned. Their treatises offer glimpses into how they made knowledge and drew meaning from these encounters.

Surgeons were not the only ones crafting bodies. This book also considers how surgeons interacted with artisans and how knowledge of the prosthetic technology they devised could move through surgical literature. I use artifacts—surviving mechanical arms and hands—to study the movement of technical knowledge in print. Here again, the methodologies that historians of science and technology have created to examine technical treatises, which involved manual instructions for an endless array of activities, provide important points of approach for surgical treatises.[36] What is the relationship of these written works, which attempt to convey hands-on techniques, to craft knowledge and practices? I reexamine and reinterpret written discussions and illustrations of mechanical limb technology in surgical treatises through a side-by-side comparison with surviving examples of the objects they purportedly describe. Material and textual cultures shed light on one another. Rather than the invention of surgeons, as is commonly suggested, these written instructions and images were the byproducts of ongoing craft practices among locksmiths, clockmakers, and other artisans. Surviving prostheses have broad implications for our understanding of how technical knowledge traveled back and forth between oral workshop and print cultures.

As it is crucial to understand surgeons as a craft group, so it is vital to consider the medical role of artisans who created artificial limbs. Doing so expands our view of early modern medicine. Scholars such as Nancy Siraisi have demonstrated that medicine was a capacious category, containing a broad collection of skills, intellectual interests, and institutions.[37] Recent work in early modern healing emphasizes that the boundaries of medicine and the identities of medical practitioners were labile.[38] I push this point further. This book shows that artisans who would not have considered themselves medical practitioners were nonetheless doing work of a medical kind. Mechanical limbs exhibit the techniques of locksmiths, clockmakers, armorers, woodworkers, and other skilled craftspeople. Neither surgeons nor physicians were involved in their creation, yet they were made to address medical challenges. With these objects, this book makes room for artisans as healers. The efforts of historians of medicine to situate surgeons within wider networks and to broaden our definition of practitioner have laid the groundwork for this next step. Sandra Cavallo coined the term "artisans of the body" to draw out the interconnections among barbers, surgeons, jewelers, tailors, wigmakers, perfumers, and upholsterers as actors with a common concern for the care, health, and beauty of the body.[39] Makers of prostheses pushed that enterprise to its limits.

This book brings surviving mechanical limbs from the sixteenth and seventeenth centuries into a critical historical analysis, treating them as primary sources to examine a larger story and to probe broad questions. Extant prostheses, such as the two in Jagsthausen (figures 5.5–5.6), reveal an area of medicine that was not quite medical for most of the sixteenth and seventeenth centuries. They place amputees into a larger social and economic context in which former patients became artisanal patrons. And they show us important and unexpected intersections of technology and culture in fashioning mechanical limbs using the latest craft techniques.

This book provides a corrective to the way the objects themselves are presented to the public in museums and exhibition catalogs, where they are frequently described as the possessions of wounded knights. To be sure, Götz von Berlichingen provides a compelling example of the impact of military technology and warfare on early modern surgery. The battlefield was not the only setting for severe injury or disease, however, and there is not strong material evidence to support a de facto connection between anonymous prosthetic artifacts and male warriors. Indeed, romanticized accounts of most of them originated in the eighteenth and nineteenth centuries.

My approach to the artifacts builds upon recent efforts in the history of science, technology, and medicine to engage with objects and their circulation.[40] Following the interdisciplinary methods of material culture studies and disability history, I examine the objects themselves to rewrite what we know about their creation and use.[41] As the artifacts in my source base are largely anonymous, each of them acts as a starting point from which I build outward.[42] I study them for signs of how they were made, using the skills they exhibit to link them to production processes, places, and—most importantly—groups of people. Following the evidence, I recast the cultural context for understanding these objects as the art cabinet and craft workshop, rather than the battlefield.

Artisans crafted artificial limbs for those who commissioned them. This book uses material culture to uncover the existence of a small group of individuals who responded creatively to the loss of a limb, broadening our understanding of early modern amputees and providing new insights into their contributions to the development of prosthetic technology and early modern surgical knowledge. In recent years, scholars of disability in the premodern past have employed a myriad of social, cultural, and intellectual approaches to uncover the so-called lived experience as well as the mentalities of mental and physical difference.[43] This book's approach reflects the influence of this scholarship, drawing on several threads concerning the body, material culture, and early modern notions of infirmity. It attempts in part to answer the calls of scholars such as Michael Rembis, Catherine Kudlick, and Kim E. Nielsen to bring disability "closer to the center" of scholarly discussions.[44] The result is not simply a more nuanced grasp of changing attitudes and practices surrounding surgical and artificial intervention in the human body, but rather the uncovering of sources and directions of influence, indeed of whole portions of our story that would otherwise be (and previously have been) misconstrued or remain invisible.

Two interrelated models of disability have been particularly fruitful in formulating my account. The social model—which distinguishes between physical impairment and disability—is fundamental to this book's discussion of those who survived an amputation procedure.[45] "Amputee" is a twentieth-century term, but it has recognizable conceptual parallels in early modern Germany for those whose arms or legs were surgically removed. By contrast, the modern category of disability and its connotations do not map neatly onto early modern European notions. I therefore only refer to actors as "disabled" in specific moments when I am applying an analytic interpretation, and in those instances, I define what the term means in those particular contexts. The cultural model, which builds on the social model to suggest that impairment as well as disability is historically constructed, also provides a valuable lens of analysis. It posits the body as "changeable [and] unperfectable" and considers the term "disability" as "inherently unclear" and "categorically unstable."[46] While this offers a useful analytic device for premodern scholars interested in the history of the body more generally, it is particularly evocative for the subject of this book—a transformation in perceptions of the body's ability to change and adapt, and of human ability to guide such change, in Western medicine.

Mechanical limbs offer evidence of the efforts of amputees to reshape their own bodies in the sixteenth and seventeenth centuries. The relationship between artisans and those unidentified individuals I refer to as amputee-patrons could aptly be described as "bodywork."[47] This notion attempts to make the study of medicine a broader and more inclusive enterprise. It is a category that keeps the multiple roles of patients from disappearing from the story: they were sufferers, clients, and (self-)healers. "Patient," however, is not the appropriate identifier in this context. In the United States today, one needs a medical prescription to obtain an artificial limb.[48] Not so in early modern Germany, where the design and creation of mechanical arms and hands developed from a collaborative relationship between amputees and artisans.

Amputee-patrons played active roles in creating new bodies. By describing their commissions for prostheses as acts of self-healing, I do not suggest that they required "fixing."[49] Rather, I am locating and identifying *their* actions as crucial evidence of practical responses early moderns undertook when a limb required surgical removal. Studying the objects they commissioned allows us to explore their perspectives and the ways in which they actively shaped how others perceived them. These figures sponsored material practices that eventually influenced the medical discussions appearing in surgical treatises. The expansion of possibilities in surgical and artisanal intervention, evident by the close of the seventeenth century, occurred because surgeons, artisans, *and* amputees experimented. Over two centuries, they retained and adapted well-tried techniques while adding new ones, resourcefully responding to individual cases in ways that, bit by bit, made the body's form more flexible and its parts more fungible.

The body taken apart and put back together

The rise of the malleable body in early modern medicine is a story of people and practices, of ideas and discussions, of pain and perseverance. Until now, the history of amputation and artificial limbs in early modern Europe has been most closely tied to that of military surgery, with an emphasis on identifying medical innovation.[50] Scholars traditionally point to the reintroduction of ligature—tying blood vessels with thread—to prevent hemorrhaging as crucial to the creation of stumps capable of bearing prostheses.[51] It is from this vantage point that Bernard J. Ficarra began his essay, "Amputations and Prostheses through the Centuries," with the triumphant claim that "a narrative on amputations is of necessity a reiteration of surgical progress."[52] Ficarra's optimism mirrored that of medical scholarship in the mid-twentieth century, as well as the continued interest among practicing and retired surgeons in contributing to our historical knowledge of this topic. This book is not a story of progress. It is, however, one of transformation. It suggests a profound change in early modern perceptions of the body caused by and reflected in the practices of surgeons and artisans. It is written from the perspective of a cultural historian interested in the intersections between medicine, technology, culture, and the body.

In order to tell this story, this book creates a narrative of the body taken apart and put back together. The first half examines the putrefying and dismembered body. The second half turns to the convalescence and management of the body after amputation, highlighting the roles of amputees and artisans.

Chapter 1, "Writing the craft of surgery," sets out connections between surgeons and other craft groups by examining how they learned and how they wrote. To embark on a more nuanced exploration of printed surgical discourse circulating in early modern Germany, I introduce the term "vernacular surgeons" to describe one category of author. These were practitioners, primarily trained by apprenticeship rather than at university, who used the printing press to publish. The chapter explores how they describe, compare, and differentiate forms of surgical work. It identifies and articulates the various positions of these authors in contrast to university-educated physicians and anatomists whose Latin treatises were translated into German. As subsequent chapters demonstrate, attuning to the different voices in early modern conversations about surgery allows us to follow the interchange of techniques and ideas among learned and craft spheres of medicine.

Chapter 2, "Communities face the cold fire," explores the diagnosis and prognosis of a putrefying limb. In order to understand the process of diagnosis, it examines early modern medical concepts of putrefaction called *der heisse Brand* and *der kalte Brand*—the hot and cold fires. A close reading of surgical treatises reveals that formulating a prognosis was a group activity. The more serious a patient's condition, the more the surgeon drew learned colleagues, family members, and spiritual advisors into a series of negotiations to decide if amputation was necessary. These exchanges converted members of the patient's circle from bystanders into assistants.

The next chapter also deals with community, albeit of a different type. "Visions of the body" investigates a series of passionate debates within surgeons' technical instructions for performing amputation procedures. In contrast to their medieval counterparts, early modern surgeons systematically recorded an increasing number of experimental amputation techniques and trained others to perform them. These techniques, practiced alongside traditional methods, point to influences from inside and outside Germany, including France, Italy, and the Dutch Republic. By the seventeenth century, surgeons learned multiple ways to perform amputations. This signaled a new kind of experimentation with the body's shape, and it generated heated disputes. At the root of the fight were competing visions of the body: was it a material entity to be preserved at all costs, or a machine to be reshaped at the surgeon's discretion?

Chapter 4, "After the operation," examines how surgeons thought through questions about the body in light of their experiences with and observations of amputees. It explores two issues. The first is documented in an exchange of letters between a surgeon and a physician about patients who experienced sensations in amputated limbs—early modern "phantom limbs." The second focuses on the formulation of surgeons' more abstract ideas about amputees after convalescence through "false restorations"—the artificial replacement of what the surgeon had removed. Each case reveals a distinct dynamic between surgeons' practical experiences with bodies and a corpus of textual knowledge.

Chapter 5, "Mechanical hands," uses artifacts to tease out the existence of amputees who commissioned prostheses as an act of social and economic power. The chapter scrutinizes these prosthetic artifacts individually to build production narratives, recreating the networks of craft groups involved. This reveals a diverse range of artisans working in collaboration, and drawing on the latest technology in their trades, to answer a customer's unique and urgent need. Amputee-patrons used these objects to shape others' perceptions—and were so successful at doing so that their material practices eventually appeared in surgical literature and influenced medical thought.

Chapter 5 discusses how to read a prosthesis; Chapter 6 looks at how to read *about* a prosthesis. "Prosthetic technology on the move" shows that artifacts can transform our knowledge of written sources. It uses an obscure sixteenth-century artifact to reexamine a famous sixteenth-century woodcut of a mechanical hand. The image, published in the work of the French surgeon Ambroise Paré, circulated widely in early modern Germany. The chapter reinterprets the woodcut's design, usually seen as the invention of a surgeon, as a byproduct of ongoing craft activity. While the technology depicted in it was too complex for most general readers to comprehend, the image was not simply a curious illustration.

It offered layers of coded information that other master artisans could adapt. The chapter therefore works in two ways. First, it examines the relationship between surgeons and artisans in the design and creation of mechanical limbs, bringing us full circle from Chapter 1 to consider surgery and craft. Second, it explores the broader implications of artifacts for our understanding of tacit knowledge and the transmission of craft knowledge through print. The book closes with a brief consideration of the significance of the malleable body for modern notions of medical intervention in biomedicine today.

In its focus on amputation and artificial limbs, surgeons and artisans, texts and artifacts, this book is a thematic case study built around the changing shape of the human body, from the putrefaction of a natural limb to the polishing of a mechanical one. Surgical treatises and objects not only take us into different spaces, but they reveal and clarify connections among the different groups of actors who inhabited them. The study of these sources also contributes to larger discourses concerning the exchanges between learned and vernacular knowledge, practical knowledge and its making, the relationship between text and object, and the role of technology and culture in medical practice. Throughout this story, I have aimed both to recover intimate scenes and to explore broad issues. Between 1500 and 1700, something changed in the way early moderns cut apart the body and worked to put it back together. This book explores the mechanisms and meanings of that change.

Notes

1 Berlichingen, *Mein Fehd und Handlungen* (hereafter, *MFH*), 75: "in den Hundβtagen." Unless otherwise noted, all citations of the autobiography refer to this edition, which transcribes the earliest known sixteenth-century manuscript.
2 Stuart, Introduction, xi. For discussion of the autobiography: Cohn, "Götz von Berlichingen"; Frohne, "Performing Dis/ability?" 57–62. For a modern biography: Ulmschneider, *Götz von Berlichingen*.
3 *MFH*, 76: "so habenn die Nurnnbergischenn das geschutz inn unns gericht, inn feindt unnd freundt." All translations are mine.
4 Ibid.: "mir das halbtheil inn arm gienng, unnd drey armschinenn darmit."
5 Ibid.: "der arm hindenn und vornn zerschmettert wahr."
6 Ibid.: "Unnd wie ich so dar siehe, so hanngtt die hanndt noch ein wenig ann der hautt, unnd leitt der spieβ dem gaull unnder denn fuessenn."
7 Ibid., 77: "Was ich die zeitt fur schmertzenn erlittenn habe, das khann ain jeglicher woll erachtenn."
8 Ibid.: "unnd wahr das mein bitt zu gott, die ich thet, wann ich inn seiner gottlichenn gnadt wer, so solt er im namen gottes mit mir hinfarenn, ich wehr doch verderbtt zu einem kriegsman."
9 Ibid.: "hett ebenn alβbaldt ein ding im feldt gegenn feindenn auβrichtenn khonnen, als ein annderer."

10 Ibid.: "Unnd vermeint dernnhalbenn, wann ich doch nit mehr dann ein wenig ein behelff hett, es wehr gleich ein eisenne hanndt oder wie es wehr, so wollt ich demnach mit gottes gnadt unnd hilff im feldt noch irgenndt alls gutt sein, alls sonnst ein heiloss mensch." *Heiloss* appears in the oldest manuscripts, but scholars suggest the writer to whom Götz dictated the autobiography made an error, and that Götz likely meant *ein heiles mensch*: Ibid., 77n144.
11 Ibid., 77: "mit einer faust."
12 See chap. 5.
13 *MFH*, 118.
14 Of course, alternative and modified theories of humoralism did arise in this period. On the fluidity of the "inner" body: Duden, *Woman Beneath the Skin*; Pomata, "Menstruating Men"; Rublack and Selwyn, "Fluxes."
15 E.g., Ralf Vollmuth interprets the works of Walther Ryff (1500–1548), who was not a surgeon, as evidence of late medieval surgery: *Traumatologie*.
16 Gurlt, *Geschichte*, 3 vols.; Sachs, *Geschichte*, 5 vols.
17 E.g., Burhenne, *Prothesen*; Knoche, *Prothesen der unteren Extremität*. Notable exceptions include Heide, "Arbeitsarm und Sonntagshand" and *Holzbein und Eisenhand*. See also Gagné, "Emotional Attachments." By contrast, there are fascinating monographs on artificial limbs from the nineteenth century onward: Linker, *War's Waste*; Hasegawa, *Mending Broken Soldiers*; Crawford, *Phantom Limb*.
18 Schmid, *Speculum chirurgicum*, 154–160; Gehema, *Der krancke Soldat*, sig. F2r.
19 Mukerji, *Impossible Engineering*; Smith, "Codification of Vernacular Theories."
20 Mitchell, *Medicine in the Crusades*; Siraisi, *Medieval and Early Renaissance Medicine*, 182–183; DeVries, "Military Surgical Practice," 134–139.
21 Hale, *War and Society*, 47; Nimwegen, "Transformation of Army Organisation"; DeVries, "Sites of Military Science," 316; Reddig, *Bader*, 116. For a broader discussion of military changes in early modern Europe: Parker, *Military Revolution*; Rogers, *Military Revolution Debate*.
22 On the *Landsknechte*: Baumann, *Landsknechte*; Nimwegen, "Transformation of Army Organisation," 162–167. On the roles of surgeons: Garrison, *Military Medicine*, 102–104.
23 DeVries, "Sites of Military Science," 316; Reddig, *Bader*, 116.
24 For an overview: Wilson, *Thirty Years War*.
25 Chap. 1 discusses the complex range of surgical practices and practitioners in-depth. For an overview: Jütte, *Ärzte, Heiler und Patienten*, 17–29; Lindemann, *Medicine and Society*, 128–136. For surgical practitioners in early modern Germany: Jütte, "Seventeenth-Century German Barber-Surgeon"; Sander, *Handwerkschirurgen*; Kinzelbach, *Chirurgen und Chirurgie-Praktiken*, "Erudite and Honoured Artisans?" and "Zur Sozial- und Alltagsgeschichte."
26 Jütte, *Ärzte, Heiler und Patienten*; Stein, *Negotiating the French Pox*; Kinzelbach, *Gesundbleiben, Krankwerden, Armsein*.
27 Klestinec, *Theaters of Anatomy*; Nutton, "Humanist Surgery"; Gadebusch Bondio, "Anatomie der Hand"; Stolberg, "Bedside Teaching"; French, *Dissection and Vivisection*.
28 Long, "Power, Patronage, and the Authorship of *Ars*."

29 Eamon, *Science and the Secrets of Nature*, 112–133. On the genre of recipes: Leong and Rankin, *Secrets and Knowledge*; DiMeo and Pennell, *Recipe Books*.
30 Kinzelbach, "Erudite and Honoured Artisans?" 677–678.
31 *AHRG*, 6 vols.; Mayr, *Automatic Machinery*, 6, 8–9, 13–14; Farr, "Shop Floor," 27; Keating, *Animating Empire*, 10–11, 41, 98; Voskuhl, *Androids*, 29.
32 See Bredekamp, *Lure of Antiquity*; Schlosser, *Art and Curiosity Cabinets*.
33 E.g., Stolz, *Die Handwerke des Körpers*; Cavallo, *Artisans of the Body*; Kinzelbach, "Erudite and Honoured Artisans?"; Chamberland, "Corporate Ethos"; Valeriani, "Grasping the Body."
34 E.g., Smith, *Body of the Artisan*; Long, *Artisan/Practitioners*.
35 Domenico Bertoloni Meli and Cynthia Klestinec emphasize that early modern surgery lends itself well to explorations of the nature of practice, learning, and knowledge-making in "Renaissance Surgery," 1–5. On knowledge-making and the developing field of the history of knowledge: Daston, "History of Science and the History of Knowledge"; Östling et al., "History of Knowledge." On practical knowledge and its role in developing more abstract systems of knowledge, see the essays in Valleriani, *Structures of Practical Knowledge*; and Grafton, "Philological and Artisanal Knowledge Making."
36 E.g., Ash, *Power, Knowledge, and Expertise*; Schotte, *Sailing School*.
37 Siraisi, "Medicine, 1450–1620."
38 E.g., Rankin, *Panaceia's Daughters*; Leong, *Recipes and Everyday Knowledge*.
39 Cavallo, *Artisans of the Body*, 1. Kinzelbach, "Erudite and Honoured Artisans?" applies this concept to early modern Germany.
40 Dacome, *Malleable Anatomies*; Daston, *Biographies of Scientific Objects* and *Things that Talk*; Findlen, "Early Modern Things."
41 Mihm, Ott, and Serlin, *Artificial Parts, Practical Lives*; Ott, "Disability Things"; Gerritsen and Riello, "Introduction."
42 This approach is similar in spirit to what the authors of *Tangible Things* describe as "a method of investigation that begins with a specific artwork, artifact, or specimen and then moves outward in an ever-widening circle." See Ulrich et al., *Tangible Things*, 2.
43 Much of this work focuses on the Middle Ages and antiquity or appears in collected volumes on premodern history: Metzler, *Disability in Medieval Europe* and *Social History of Disability*; Turner and Vandeventer Pearman, *Treatment of Disabled Persons*; Eyler, *Disability in the Middle Ages*; Frohne, *Leben mit "kranckhait"*; Krötzl et al., *Infirmity in Antiquity*; Nolte, *Phänomene der "Behinderung" im Alltag*; Nolte et al., *Dis/ability History*. For a recent work focused on early modern representations of disability: Bearden, *Monstrous Kinds*.
44 Rembis, Kudlick, and Nielsen, "Introduction," 11.
45 Metzler, *Disability in Medieval Europe*, 1–5, 9; Metzler, "Social Model," 59–61.
46 Frohne, "Cultural Model," 61–63.
47 Fissell, "Introduction," 10–14; Cabré, "From a Master to a Laywoman." "Bodywork" reflects a broader interest in investigating patient experience, a trend discussed at length in Stolberg, *Experiencing Illness*, 1–18.
48 The medicalization of prosthetic limbs did not occur in the United States until the First World War: Linker, *War's Waste*, 102.

49 For a related discussion: Kudlick, "Social History of Medicine and Disability History."
50 This emphasis on medical innovation reflects the contributions of modern practicing surgeons: e.g., Ficarra, *Essays*; Wangensteen and Wangensteen, *Rise of Surgery*, 16–52; Kirkup, *Limb Amputation*. For recent work by early modern historians with different emphases: Hausse, "The Locksmith, the Surgeon, and the Mechanical Hand" and "Bones of Contention"; Heide, "Arbeitsarm und Sonntagshand"; Gagné, "Emotional Attachments"; Benhamou, "Artificial Limb in Preindustrial France." Medieval historians have broken ground here too: Ferragud, "Wounds, Amputations, and Expert Procedures"; Van Cant, "Surviving Amputations."
51 E.g., Lindemann, *Medicine and Society*, 132; Wear, "Medicine in Early Modern Europe," 297.
52 Ficarra, *Essays*, 51.

1

Writing the craft of surgery

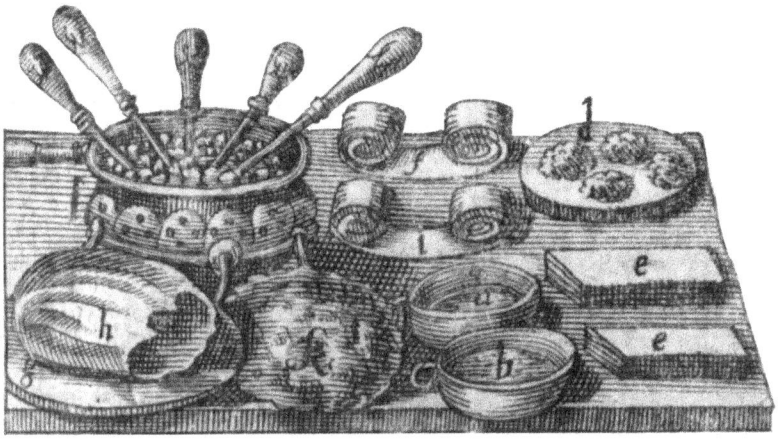

Matthäus Purmann (1649–1711) considered surgery's preeminence among the healing arts an unequivocable truth. The preface of his *Wund-Artzney*, first published in 1684, made a bold case. Purmann divided medicine into three parts: diet, pharmacy, and surgery. "Surgery and wound medicine," he explained, "is the very oldest, first, and most splendid."[1] A series of biblical references establish the antiquity of this craft, beginning with the prophet Isaiah's use of a fig plaster to heal King Hezekiah. The obvious effects of surgery, so readily apparent to the naked eye, place it above the uncertainties of diet and pharmacy. The latter two might be efficacious, but how could anyone *really* know if Nature would not have produced the same outcomes without prescribing food and drink, or ingesting internal medicines?[2] Surgeons, by contrast, gave clear results. For "who does not see with eyes full of amazement," Purmann declared, how the surgeon's efforts cure "injured and wounded limbs (be they struck, beaten, shot, cut or stabbed), fractured bones, dislocated joints, putrefaction, all manners of boils, tumors, and ulcers, lithotomy in the bladder, [and] all manners of ruptures."[3] The visibility of surgery also kept its practitioners accountable: a surgeon's mistakes were immediately evident and set aright. The workings of inner medicines and prescriptions could be "more hidden," and a practitioner's faults quickly attributed to any number of unknowable causes.[4] Here Purmann flipped a long-held argument for the superiority of physicians—the theoretical basis of their branch of medicine—on its head. "In sum," he concluded, "who can say enough of the necessity and utility of this noble art, which every virtuous physician, if he wants to be a fully accomplished doctor of medicine and successful practitioner, should know and understand."[5]

Purmann's encomium exhibits some of the rhetorical strategies employed by surgeons who published about their craft in the sixteenth and seventeenth centuries. They were one of many groups of hands-on practitioners who did this to enhance their social status. Like artists and engineers, surgeons sought to give their tacit knowledge formal written form.[6] With the works of Hieronymous Brunschwig (c. 1450–c. 1512) and Hans von Gersdorff (1455–1529), printed surgical treatises began circulating in German.[7] These took several forms, from brief treatments of specific topics to lengthy textbooks.

We could describe many of their authors as "vernacular surgeons"—a type of writer that contributed to early modern print discourse. They often published in vernacular languages, though their works could appear in Latin translation. There were two interrelated reasons for this. First, they published in the languages they learned and worked within. Some author-practitioners, such as Purmann, showed familiarity with the academic Latin used by learned physicians, but many were not fluent in it. That is because they largely came from a tradition of vernacular knowledge shared by day-to-day surgical practitioners. Like Purmann, they learned as apprentices and journeymen working with master surgeons, and many gained experience as field-surgeons. This form of training was their most salient attribute. Second, publishing in German rather than Latin made their works accessible to a wider audience of common surgical practitioners and general readers. Vernacular surgeons, their works diverse in substance, style, and personal experience, brought the perspectives of day-to-day surgical practitioners into a larger textual dialogue.

The practice of surgery, as patients experienced it in German cities, was a craft.[8] Surgeons' qualifications came from years of hands-on work as apprentices and journeymen rather than university degrees. They performed operations not only in their shops, but also in the homes of patients, in the marketplace, in hospitals, lazarettes, and other urban institutions, on ships, in fields and in tents. Many practitioners moved in and out of these different spaces on a regular basis. Surgery was loud and physical, since patients frequently endured procedures while fully conscious. Bones cracked. Flesh tore. Bodies bled. Surgeons *hurt* patients to help them, and this set them apart from physicians and apothecaries.

Surgery was a technical art, but it was also an area of academic learning closely tied to anatomical study. It encompassed a corpus of theoretical knowledge about the body and its structures, transmitted through university lectures and in treatises. Dedicating specialized textbooks to surgery, rather than including surgery within larger works of medicine, was an innovation of the twelfth and thirteenth centuries among learned authors drawing on

Hippocratic-Galenic texts and Arabic works in Latin translation.[9] Particularly in the period between 1240 and 1320, a series of authors were concerned with formulating, as Michael McVaugh has coined it, a "rational surgery."[10] These were works that came from a learned tradition and emphasized that surgery had a place in university medical education, but were also intended to be of practical use. Producing learned works with practical dimensions continued into the early modern period, especially with the influence of Renaissance humanism on medical education in the sixteenth century. In "humanist surgery," the high-minded ideals of humanist physicians and academic surgeons to use classical texts to improve surgical knowledge and instruments seeped into a broader medical literature.[11] This was connected to a new emphasis on anatomical study in university medical education,[12] an emphasis that quickly appeared in the treatises of vernacular surgeons. As historians have suggested, early modern surgery lay somewhere "between learning and craft."[13]

Surgical treatises provided a space in which many different voices, craft and academic, came together to reflect on the relationship among skills, practice, and theory. In his *Wund-Artzney*, Purmann did not dismiss theoretical knowledge, nor suggest that surgery was a self-sufficient branch of medicine. Instead, his closing entreaty to physicians to learn operative surgery rested on a view of internal and external medicines as entwined. "Internal and external medicine are so closely joined with one another," he argued, "that neither can exist without the other."[14] Even as he touted the superiority of surgery, Purmann sought to engage with a larger conversation that included learned physicians. His efforts point to the significant role of the printing press in the creation and circulation of medical knowledge during the early modern period.

This chapter carves out a space to discuss the vernacular surgeon as a category of author contributing to a complex printed surgical discourse that circulated in German during the early modern period. In doing so, it presents an analytic tool for examining surgical treatises. Much has been written about learned medicine and authors who published in the academic tradition. Far less systematic attention has been paid to practicing surgeons who published about their activities. Studies of early modern surgery have always drawn on their treatises, of course. Scholars have even devoted entire books or articles to some of the most well-known authors and their works.[15] What they have not yet done is take careful stock of vernacular surgeons as a *group* to consider how they engaged with and influenced a body of written knowledge that was previously the domain of the learned.[16] Exploring that relationship teaches us not only about surgery as a set of ideas and practices "between learning and craft," but also touches on fundamental questions about knowledge-making more broadly. Crucial to such investigations is discerning how early modern authors of surgical treatises related in various ways to hands-on practice, reading, and writing.

Considering vernacular surgeons as a group focuses attention on authors trained by apprenticeship to become surgeons and who had experience practicing surgery. Even though they were exceptional for publishing, as voices in a larger textual dialogue, theirs is closest to the majority of everyday practitioners.

Using publications circulating in early modern Germany, this chapter offers one model to locate vernacular surgeons as a group, moving step by step from the realm of everyday practice to an analysis of how these authors understood their work within a craft context. After first considering how surgeons learned and practiced their art, attention turns to the growing body of surgical literature with which German-speakers engaged as readers and writers. This exploration points to different ways print linked the local world of everyday practice in the German-speaking lands to a wider medical world in the mediated forms of translated, edited, and annotated editions. With that dynamic established, focus narrows to one group of authors—those who learned surgery by apprenticeship—to explore how they wrote about their profession. Our final discussion of vernacular surgeons, then, is not limited to individuals who practiced surgery in the German-speaking lands. Rather, it examines a category of author for texts that circulated in German and were accessible to German-speaking practitioners. It yields a perspective that was both localized and connected to a wider medical world.

The advantage of this approach is twofold. It requires us to constantly acknowledge that there was no one-to-one correlation between text and practice, keeping the layers of mediation involved in these written sources at the forefront of our minds. At the same time, it empowers us to consider everyday practitioners as part of a larger network of ideas and practices. We have a natural inclination to think of learned authors in this way: they wrote in Latin, a universal language for the educated across Europe, participated in epistolary exchanges, rubbed shoulders at universities, and collected books for their private libraries. But vernacular surgeons did not read, write, and think about surgery in isolated bubbles; nor were everyday practitioners who consumed printed works without publishing their own limited to reading local authors. The model here, while not intended to be all-encompassing, suggests a way forward for listening to the voices of vernacular surgeons as a group, seeking a balance between local contexts of practice and a broader network of ideas with which practitioners engaged.

This chapter explores the language—in particular, the craft metaphors—vernacular surgeons used to tease out how they understood their work. Practitioners viewed surgery as a form of craft, but the singular qualities of the human body as its natural materials made it a craft of a unique kind. Sandra Cavallo has pointed to the close social, cultural, and economic connections between Italian barber-surgeons and other craft groups concerned with the care of the body.[17] This chapter builds on her work, taking this emphasis on craft north to the German-speaking lands, and earlier in time. The language of vernacular surgeons reveals how their self-conceptions as practitioners and their strategies to connect to readers were deeply embedded in a craft framework. It suggests that while the relationship between text and practice was complex, there were integral links between the nature of day-to-day surgical practice and the perspectives evident in what vernacular surgeons wrote.

Surgeons as practitioners

How did one become a surgeon in early modern Germany? In theory, one could train as an apprentice to a master surgeon, or one could earn a university degree. In practice, learned doctors of surgery were rare. One could take courses in surgery and anatomy at German universities, but students had to venture outside the Holy Roman Empire to obtain a degree in them.[18] Those who did so and returned to the German-speaking lands could use the combined title of physician and surgeon (*Physicus & Chirurgus*). They might become personal physicians attached to a princely court, or professors of anatomy and surgery at the few German universities with such a position.[19] They could join a local body of physicians and oversee the examinations of surgeons, and even perform complex procedures in severe cases. They could and did author learned surgical treatises for Latin and vernacular audiences alike. But these figures did not typically perform surgery in their day-to-day practice. One became a *practicing* surgeon, then, through some form of training in a master–apprentice system.

There were many kinds of surgical practitioners who made their livings entirely or in large part from performing major or minor procedures. The terminology can be slippery in the sources, as early moderns could use titles such as "barber-surgeon" (*Balbierer*) and "surgeon" (*Wundartzt*) interchangeably in different contexts.[20] But there were crucial distinctions. In general, surgeons or master surgeons could perform all major procedures. Barber-surgeons could also perform a wide variety of major and minor procedures, but—unlike master surgeons—they regularly cut hair, shaved beards, and performed bloodletting.[21] Some were more experienced at surgery than others, and practitioners could move up the hierarchy over time.[22] Both a surgeon and a barber-surgeon could serve as a field-surgeon (*ein Feldscherer*), whether with a mercenary army or a local town regiment. There were also others who provided minor services. The bath master (*der Bader*), for instance, performed cupping, leeching, and the like.

Surgeons, barber-surgeons, barbers, and bath masters could belong to related guilds or confraternities, but during the early modern period they increasingly organized into separate groups.[23] Surgeons and barber-surgeons in particular sought to distinguish themselves as members of a more prestigious profession with links to academic medicine. Like other craft groups, these guilds had regulations stipulating rules for members, from the criteria to become an apprentice to qualifications for mastership. They had elected offices and could designate forms of oversight beyond those required by the local government. Such organizations created an internal hierarchy by designating levels of aptitude and experience among their members. Crucially, they provided status in the wider community, performed for all to see when they appeared in civic and religious processions.

Guilds could attempt to create monopolies on different services, but in reality practitioners competed for patients in a diverse medical marketplace that adapted to consumer demand. Early modern men and women had many options for medical care, starting at home with family members and household recipe books. Itinerant practitioners offered specific surgical services, including the tooth-puller (*der Zahnbrecher*) and specialists in bladder stones and hernias (*der Stein- und Bruchschneider*). Villagers and townspeople alike trekked many miles to visit local cunning folk, men and women who practiced folk medicine and magic. Midwives treated pregnant women and small children. Noblewomen distilled tonics for the poor and the wealthy. The injured and afflicted consulted with executioners, trained to heal the bodies they tortured. Surgeons operated within this wider context of medical practice.[24]

They also belonged to a larger hierarchy of practitioners with different legal rights and privileges. The higher one's status, the more services one was qualified—or locally licensed—to provide or oversee. Physicians, specializing in internal medicine, sat at the top of the professional hierarchy because they held university degrees.[25] While notions about the superiority of their education reached back to the thirteenth century, it was in the sixteenth that their authority took organized form and increasingly influenced civic life in German communities.[26] In most cities physicians belonged to a *Collegium medicum*, a body that granted licenses to physicians and oversaw other practitioners, including surgeons. The annual salaries of municipally appointed offices clearly reflect these degrees of status in a civic context, with town surgeons often earning a fraction of what town physicians received.[27]

While colleges of physicians and surgeons' guilds were shared features of medical practice in Germany, France, Italy, England, and the Netherlands, German towns tended to more rigidly maintain divisions among branches of medicine than other parts of Europe.[28] In Cologne, for instance, physicians needed to swear they had never practiced surgery in order to maintain their status.[29] Barber-surgeons attended to patients in the pox hospitals of Augsburg only under the supervision of a physician, and surgeons also made daily rounds in Vienna hospitals together with physicians.[30]

The master–apprentice system in which surgeons and barber-surgeons trained unfolded in three distinct stages, comparable to other craft groups.[31] First was an apprenticeship with a master surgeon for two to four years. For a fee, the master provided room, board, and instruction on dressing wounds, setting broken bones, performing bloodletting, and other essential tasks. In the second stage, lasting several years, the novice became a journeyman. He could not open his own practice and, during this uncertain period, usually did not marry. Journeymen were expected to spend part of this time traveling to learn from different masters.[32] They found opportunities for learning in both civilian and military settings.[33] Indeed, the battlefield became a major school for surgery in the early modern period.[34]

Traveling was such a crucial component of surgeons' educations because it exposed them to different techniques and a wider variety of contexts of practice. These experiences could impact their approaches profoundly. Fabry von Hilden (1560–1634) provides one example. His time as a journeyman began in Düsseldorf assisting Cosmas Slot, personal surgeon to a local duke. Slot was a former pupil of the famed anatomist Andreas Vesalius and an enthusiastic proponent of the "new anatomy" connected to changes in anatomical education in Renaissance universities. After Slot died in 1585, Fabry traveled to Geneva to work with the surgeon Jean Griffon, another advocate of the new anatomy. Fabry was trained in a craft tradition, but his experiences as a wandering journeyman cultivated interests that shaped his career as a master surgeon who engaged with academic medicine. When he relocated to Lausanne in 1586 to open his own practice, he held anatomical demonstrations. In 1611, he even visited Leiden to study with the renowned anatomist Peter Pauw.[35] Fabry's case demonstrates an important aspect of itinerant training: journeymen absorbed the techniques and examples set by multiple masters.

Once a journeyman gained enough years of experience, he qualified for his mastership exam, the last stage of his training. The examination itself evaluated a practitioner's skills and theoretical knowledge through a series of questions that probed the examinee's competence. It also required demonstrations in surgical technique and the making of plasters and ointments.[36] Those who administered the exam included master surgeons as well as physicians and members of the city government, who together formed a local board of health that controlled licensing. Once he passed his examination, the new master surgeon could open his own practice. If later he wished to relocate to a different town, he had to seek local approval to practice there.

Most surgical practitioners in early modern Germany did not attend university and receive a degree. But master–apprentice training and university study were not mutually exclusive. Surgeons trained by apprenticeship could attend university lectures, and medical students could board with master surgeons to learn from them. Fabry's career reflected both: he listened to commentaries on Hippocrates's *Aphorisms* in Cologne and boarded and trained a number of academic pupils.[37] Surgeons and barber-surgeons could also attend and assist anatomical dissections. In addition, they learned from technical treatises that both discussed operative techniques and transmitted knowledge of human anatomy and more abstract explanations of health and illness grounded in humoralism.[38] For example, in his *Examen chirurgicum*, the Augsburg barber-surgeon Joseph Schmid (1600–1667) explained the relationship between the seasons and the four humors. Blood increases in the spring, yellow bile (or choler) in the summer, black bile (or melancholia) in the autumn, and phlegm in the winter.[39] The 1649 edition of this treatise sold for a little less than 1.5 Gulden, relatively expensive given that one could purchase over eighteen pounds of good quality meat for about the same price, yet still a fraction of the cost of a surgeon's services for treating a fractured leg or dislocated shoulder.[40] Buying such works was an investment. Obtaining some theoretical knowledge as well as practical instruction from printed literature could help the journeyman become a master surgeon and allow a master surgeon to present himself as more learned than his competitors. Indeed, over time education gained increasing importance among surgeons in some communities.[41]

Still, they used their *hands* to treat bodies. Day-to-day practicing surgeons belonged to a craft group whose trade involved physical tasks and was learned by doing.[42] The business of running a surgical practice had many features of a craft workshop: once they became masters, surgeons opened shops and took on apprentices and journeymen. Barber-surgeons lived in their shops, and while medical treatises rarely mention surgeons' wives, there is evidence that they sometimes fit within a wider craft dynamic in which they, like other master craftsmen's wives, played active roles in workshop production.[43] The *Hausfrau* could assist the surgeon in carrying out major procedures: in 1551, for instance, the city council of Munich paid the barber-surgeon Ulrich Welser for performing two amputations and gave his wife (*Hausfrau*) one Gulden for her assistance. She received the same amount given to three barbers and an assistant who also participated in the operations.[44] In his writings, Fabry von Hilden made clear that he consulted his wife, Marie Colinet, about cases, and that she occasionally visited patients as his proxy. She also set fractures and dislocated bones in his absence.[45]

The family lives of surgeons were also intertwined with other craft groups. For some practitioners, as in other crafts, pursuing surgery meant taking up the family trade. Joseph Schmid's father was the barber-surgeon Balthasar Schmid,[46] whom he claimed taught him and his brothers the fundamentals of anatomy and surgery from childhood. He followed his father's example, explaining that one of his goals in composing his *Spiegel der Anatomiae* was to instruct his own sons.[47] Surgeons' apprentices could also come from families linked to other crafts. The barber-surgeon Johann Dietz (1665–1738) described his father as a rope-maker, alderman, and beer inspector in Halle. Another barber-surgeon, Georg Händel (1622–1697), was the son of a coppersmith. Surgeons could marry into a broad social spectrum of families, from academics to goldsmiths.[48] Those recorded as witnesses to Joseph Schmid's marriage in 1626—including his brother (also a barber-surgeon), a weaver, a tailor, and a goldsmith—underscore the many kinds of connections surgeons could have with other craftspeople.[49]

Just as in weaving, tailoring, and metalwork, surgical practice involved tacit knowledge. There were procedures that had to be learned by performing them, and afflictions that had to be seen to be recognized and understood. Early modern authors increasingly provided firsthand observations intended to share sensory details of encounters with readers to assist them in interpreting patients' conditions. But these same writers pressed surgeons to build their own repertoires of firsthand experiences. In his *Speculum chirurgicum*, Joseph Schmid argued that one "must not stay sitting at home by the fire, but rather travel to foreign lands, and converse with learned people without timidity, visit poor houses and hospitals where all sorts of sick and injured people lie."[50] Even the most learned made terrible mistakes when they lacked experience, and surgeons would encounter many things in practice that were not in their books. The surgeon must integrate reading and practice: "it costs not merely silver or gold, but rather life itself."[51]

Surgeons as authors

Though Schmid reiterated that "reading alone does not make a practitioner," his own career as a barber-surgeon and author demonstrates that the printed word still held an important place in the development and circulation of surgical knowledge.[52] He published several works, including treatises on instruments, anatomy, and field surgery; a work on the surgeon's field chest; a general textbook; and an examination guide.[53] The latter presented information in a question-and-answer format, covering theoretical and practical knowledge. It prepared journeymen to take their mastership examinations and aimed to educate young and inexperienced surgeons in general. Schmid's *Examen chirurgicum* promised that each "young aspiring field-surgeon or surgeon" would learn:

> how he should behave with all wounds (be they cut, punctured, shot, thrown, poisoned or not), to recognize symptoms of them, respond to them, and make provisions, likewise to learn manual operations: how to set all dislocated limbs, to straighten and heal fractured bones, also what generally to direct against diseases in an encampment, and how to manage medical consultation and aid in the absence of a physician.[54]

Schmid not only discussed how surgeons should treat the living, but also how to handle the dead. In one example, he asked the reader what to do if called upon to examine a child for signs that it had been choked or smothered by its mother. In another, he discussed how to determine if a person had been wounded while he or she was still alive, or if an injury had occurred postmortem.[55] All of these topics appeared in a work printed small enough for convenient travel. Schmid and his publisher expected that surgeons might bring it with them as wandering journeymen or field-surgeons moving with armies. It suggests a vision of young surgeons learning through a combination of firsthand experience and reading.

Surgical treatises were a fluid medium. They could facilitate the exchange of practices and ideas between university anatomists and common barber-surgeons. Whether heavy tomes or thin field manuals, these works circulated across social, geographic, and linguistic barriers. Especially when published in the vernacular, they connected the local world of day-to-day activities we have been describing—Joseph Schmid's world of practice—to a wider medical world. This book's discussion of surgical literature in early modern Germany must therefore extend beyond the works of those who practiced there. German-speaking audiences consumed a vast body of medical literature originating all over Europe, including works by Italian, Spanish, French, and Dutch authors.[56] These publications could circulate in Latin or the vernacular. Figures like Peter Uffenbach (1566–1635), who translated treatises by the widely influential French surgeon Ambroise Paré and the Italian anatomist Girolamo Fabrizi d'Acquapendente, among others, worked diligently to render works into German. Print shops in Frankfurt am Main and Nuremberg were perhaps the most productive at issuing works from authors outside of the empire, particularly in the vernacular.[57] German translations also came from Leipzig, Ulm, Hamburg, Hannover, Wittenberg, and Berlin.[58] In addition, through compilations, translated excerpts of authors from across Europe could circulate in one volume. Uffenbach, for example, compiled and edited excerpts from nine German, French, Italian, and Swiss authors in his *Thesaurus chirurgiae*. These contributors were nearly all contemporary—only one dated prior to the sixteenth century.[59] Joseph Schmid, Matthäus Purmann, and other surgeons conceived of their writings within this broader context of medical publishing.

A diverse body of surgical literature circulated in early modern Germany. General surgeries were hefty volumes covering theory and practice in depth. The 1635 German translation of Paré, for instance, numbers nearly a thousand pages, each thirty-five centimeters in height.[60] By contrast, field manuals were meant to be small so they could be carried around and consulted more easily. Their size and purpose made them less comprehensive and more concise. Some targeted military surgeons, such as Schmid's *Kriegs-Arzney* (1664) and Purmann's *Feldscher* (1680).[61] Examination guides could be extensive in the number of topics they covered, but succinct and accessible for the advanced journeyman. Recipe books for wound medicine could also be brief, like the collection of Lorenz Burres (sixteenth century).[62] Authors could also dedicate their works to specific topics, such as instruments, or specific injuries, illnesses, and treatments, including gunshot wounds, pestilential boils, and scurvy.[63] Fabry von Hilden published numerous works addressing particular topics, including burn wounds and bladder stones, whereas Franz Renner, the town surgeon of Nuremberg, published exclusively on the French Disease, revising and expanding his handbook over several years.[64] Treatises could be particular in another way by focusing on a series of case histories, discussing the diagnosis and treatment of individual patients. Books of surgical observations, a sub-genre of a new kind of medical literature in early modern Europe, illustrated a growing esteem for firsthand observation and experience.[65] These could serve as standalone publications or form substantial sections of multi-part works.[66] Finally, surgical treatises also appeared as collected volumes—either compilations of a single author's works, or collections of excerpts from different authors.

Surgical treatises mediated the exchange of ideas not only across long distances, but also across vast temporal spaces. In addition to composing new works, authors preserved, recycled, expanded, and modified. For example, ancient and medieval authors influenced early modern readers both through references made by contemporary writers and through various edited Latin and German print editions.[67] Once published, a treatise became an ongoing project. The work of Sebastian Greiff vividly illustrates this. Greiff, an obscure medical practitioner in Erfurt in central Germany, published a defense of Paracelsus in 1589 as well as a couple of minor works in the 1590s.[68] His approach to surgical practice was of interest to Johann Mercker, a physician in Schleusingen, a town eighty kilometers south of Erfurt, who edited Greiff's surviving work into a treatise published posthumously in Greiff's name in 1622 and 1630.[69] The title page of both editions declared that it was drawn from Paracelsus and from Greiff's own twenty-eight years of experience. Decades later, Mercker's publication of Greiff caught the attention of Laurentius Lose, the town and countryside physician of Heldburg, approximately forty kilometers north of Schleusingen. Lose edited and annotated Greiff's work in 1679. In his annotation to the first chapter, he apologized to readers for Greiff's poor organization and style.[70] The work, he explained, was based more on the author's "practice and experience" than on "theory."[71] Significantly, though, he defended the value of Greiff's knowledge, however unsophisticated its presentation. Lose's annotated edition reveals layer upon layer of reading, thinking, and practice, and he took pride in its composite character. Surgical writing was a multifaceted and multilayered enterprise.

These projects could incorporate learned Latin works and works by non-German-speakers into a corpus of German vernacular literature. Consider the 1676 German translation of the learned Italian surgeon Leonardo Botallo (1530–1587). It appeared in a decade in which Johann Tauber's Nuremberg printshop issued a spate of translations of surgical treatises from outside the empire, including those by the Italian anatomist Pietro de Marchetti, the French army physician Leonard Tassin, and the Spanish surgeon Francisco de Arce.[72] The 1676 Botallo edition, entitled *Zwey Chirurgische Bücher*, translated a 1660 Latin edition from Leiden featuring the annotations of the Dutch anatomist Johannes Van Horne (1621–1670). Van Horne's detailed marginalia and commentary include references and remarks about other authors, including German writers like Fabry von Hilden and the Ulm physician Johannes Scultetus (1595–1645). He even engages in lengthy responses to them regarding their methods or their discussions of Botallo.[73] Translating this edition not only brought a learned sixteenth-century work into the German vernacular, but also placed it—through Van Horne's seventeenth-century annotations—helpfully in conversation with authors already well known to German readers. Through this long process, Botallo became part of a surgical dialogue circulating in German and accessible to barber-surgeons.

These writers represented a wide variety of social backgrounds and contexts of practice. Johannes Scultetus and Fabry von Hilden, who were both orphaned fairly young, had relatives or benefactors to support their attendance at local Gymnasiums. Only after this period of schooling did both embark on a surgical profession, one as an apprentice and the other as a medical student. Scultetus attended the University of Padua, a leading center of medical learning in Europe, and graduated with honors as a doctor of philosophy, medicine, and surgery.[74] Joseph Schmid, by contrast, was raised in a barber-surgeon's shop, where he learned the fundamentals of the profession as a child.

Their careers as medical practitioners and authors were equally diverse. Matthäus Purmann served as a field-surgeon for several years before setting up a successful practice in the towns of Halberstadt and Breslau.[75] Johann von Jessen, a Hungarian nobleman who studied at Leipzig, multiple Italian universities, and ultimately earned a degree from Wittenberg, published the first edition of his *Institutiones chirurgicae* (1601) in Wittenberg while he was a professor of medicine there.[76] Theophrastus von Hohenheim (1493/4–1541), better known as Paracelsus, was a self-proclaimed empiric and philosopher who stirred controversy wherever he went.[77] Walther Ryff was not a surgical practitioner at all. While he had some medical training, he earned a living by publishing a vast amount of literature, consulting practitioners and drawing from existing texts to inform his writing.[78] Some authors, such as Ryff or Joseph Schmid, published multiple works during their lifetimes. Fabry von Hilden's authorship spanned several decades as he published numerous works from the

1590s onward.[79] Others, such as Sebastian Greiff or Franz Renner, published only minor works, a single large work, or had works appear posthumously. Johannes Scultetus died while the manuscript for his single work, the voluminous *Armamentarium Chirurgicum* (1655), was still in preparation. His nephew fulfilled his publishing ambitions ten years after his death.[80]

Authors drew from their different backgrounds, pedagogical formations, and experiences to strategically present themselves to readers as reliable authorities and skillful practitioners. Fabry von Hilden often recalled his time assisting Cosmas Slot and Jean Griffon as a journeyman.[81] Johannes Scultetus cited university lectures and referred to cases of Adriaan van den Spiegel (1578–1625) and even Girolamo Fabrizi d'Acquapendente (1533–1619), both renowned anatomists, that he witnessed during his student days at Padua.[82] Joseph Schmid, who could not claim a particularly famous mentor, spoke of his voracious appetite for medical literature both ancient and contemporary.[83] Paracelsus, of course, argued against the folly of ancient teachings and declared that his practice was not based on written knowledge.[84]

A rhetorical strategy of growing importance for all of these authors was to emphasize their firsthand experience. They recounted the number of years they had practiced, the numbers of patients they had treated, and any positions of significance they held in civilian or military practice. In his *Speculum chirurgicum*, for example, Schmid informed readers that his knowledge was based on his twenty-seven years observing and practicing surgery. He also claimed that during his field experience he cured over two thousand soldiers from Sweden alone.[85] Learned authors also emphasized their firsthand experience. The Dutch physician Paul Barbette (1620–c. 1666) claimed to share only the techniques described by ancient and contemporary writers that he had proven to be effective in practice by observing numerous operations.[86] Like Schmid, Barbette acknowledged that reading alone could not equip a practitioner with enough knowledge to understand a technique. At one point, he explained that he did not include instructions on the way to perform a particularly difficult limb extension "because such can be learned much better through observation than by reading."[87] Admissions of this kind reflected the complex relationship between practice and theory, but they also served as a rhetorical device to reinforce claims to authoritative knowledge based upon firsthand observation.

In their dedications and prefaces, these authors framed their treatises as ways to share their skills, learning, and experience for the betterment of surgical knowledge, practice, or both.[88] Many alluded to their intentions to benefit the wider community, or even humankind. Felix Würtz (c. 1500–c. 1590), surgeon of Basel, claimed in his dedication to the emperor that his book would serve "the human race."[89] Though authors' self-professed intentions could be universal in scope, the language in which they published made an important statement about their intended audience. Those who positioned their work within a learned tradition tended to write in Latin. Johannes Scultetus, for example, composed his manuscript in Latin and described himself as following in the footsteps of Girolamo Fabrizi.[90] When the work appeared (posthumously) in German translation, the greatest substantive change the translator made was to frame its purpose as benefiting humble practitioners unlearned in Latin.[91] While this declaration would have been out of place in Scultetus's original manuscript, most authors or translators who published in the vernacular explicitly aimed to educate barber-surgeons. Würtz, writing about the need to address poor surgical practices, declared that his instructions would help prospective surgeons.[92] He emphasized that his work applied as much to German practitioners as it did to "the Italian, French, Dutch and others."[93]

Authors positioned their instructions as essential to combatting weaknesses in surgical training. Purmann, for one, lamented that too many who called themselves surgeons had learned little more than to cut, clean, powder, and perfume hair, perhaps let blood, and heal a fresh wound.[94] One of the most caustic critiques came from the field-physician Janus Abraham à Gehema (1647–1715), who characterized apprenticeship as a farcical arrangement that created a self-perpetuating cycle of poorly trained practitioners. Observing the state of military surgery, Gehema wrote that the field-surgeon was as capable "as a donkey is at dancing."[95] In his *Feld-Medicus*, he laid the blame for widespread incompetence almost entirely on the master–apprentice relationship that formed the cornerstone of the guild system. He wrote that instead of learning the fundamentals of surgery, an apprentice performed domestic tasks like polishing shoes and bringing water to the kitchen.[96] His derisive description contrasts sharply with the autobiographical accounts of figures like Fabry von Hilden, Joseph Schmid, and Felix Würtz.[97]

To improve education, vernacular editions could include additional aids to further assist surgeons and barber-surgeons in engaging with a sprawling and complex medical corpus. The inclusion of a full Latin–German vocabulary in Hans von Gersdorff's *Feldbuch der Wundarznei* (1517), one of the earliest printed surgical treatises, particularly reflects the broader accessibility and ownership of textual surgical knowledge that the printing press enabled. This vocabulary tract lists Latin terms alphabetically (divided into the categories of anatomy, infirmities, and herbs) and translates them into German. These kinds of reading aids could be quite useful because treatises were often peppered with words from other languages. It was not uncommon for vernacular treatises to carry over Latin medical terminology, or even to present whole recipes in Latin.[98] Treatises with dictionaries or vocabulary tracts equipped everyday practitioners with a vital tool to decipher these directions, evidence of the larger effort to bridge the distance between the learned and craft traditions of surgical knowledge.

Publications could link the local world of everyday practice in the German-speaking lands to a larger medical world in several ways, some more directly than others. One kind of connection appeared when a work's *author* was also a practicing surgeon. Another kind formed when a work's *readers* included practitioners. These different types of links also raise different sets of questions. Firsthand observations of *others* performing techniques, for example, draw our attention to witnessing as both a way to learn about practical skills and a literary convention. A work's claims about improving surgical training can point to a number of things, from a trite formula to a set of earnest critiques made more revealing by reading them against the grain. Some treatises, of course, had very little to do with practicing surgeons as authors, readers, or subject matter. But there were others with links as numerous and complex as an intricately woven spiderweb: the works of vernacular surgeons.

The language of vernacular surgeons

We have up to this point discussed the authors of surgical treatises broadly. Now it is time to focus on the voices of vernacular surgeons. As we have already seen, it is no simple task to categorize and sort these actors or their works. Further complicating matters, our period stretches across nearly two centuries and includes writers from different geographic regions whose work circulated in the Holy Roman Empire. Nonetheless, "vernacular surgeons" is a worthwhile construct to explore and a useful category for examining surgical treatises—as long as we are not too rigid in our characterizations, and we always consider their connections with the broader body of surgical literature to which they belonged. I propose the following definition: vernacular surgeons were author-practitioners who primarily trained in a master–apprentice system, rather than primarily at university, and who possessed some years of firsthand experience practicing surgery. These authors encompass a wide assortment of backgrounds and publishing careers, and their treatises present a range of content and styles. As they published overwhelmingly in the vernacular and came from a vernacular tradition of surgical knowledge, however, "vernacular surgeons" serves as a meaningful shorthand. This terminology does not imply a single or unchanging perspective. Instead it is a tool of analysis intended to aid the historian in drawing out the nuances of a complex textual dialogue.

Why discuss vernacular surgeons as a category at all? The majority of practitioners, whether young barber-surgeons or master surgeons, did not compose treatises about their work. Vernacular surgeons were exceptional because they engaged in publishing, and some enjoyed extraordinary success as authors. Yet their perspectives were shaped by master–apprentice backgrounds familiar to most German-speaking practitioners. They can give us a sense of practice on the ground, as well as ideas about their profession and how they were attempting to shape it. As historians of medicine continue to examine early modern surgeons and the relationship between craft and learning, it will be important to account for the voices of craft practitioners in the development of textual surgical knowledge, and the relationships among different kinds of practitioners in shaping ideas about surgery. Attuning to different voices in a textual debate, as I argue in Chapter 3, may present patterns in surgical techniques, reasoning, or rhetoric that allow us to identify directions of influence in changing ideas. But first, let us begin identifying these voices and how they discussed surgery. The printing press enabled textual discussions to develop among surgeons, learned physicians, and anatomists during the early modern period. How did craft practitioners position themselves in this dialogue? What rhetorical strategies did they use? How did they frame their profession and the nature of surgical work for their readers? Many of these issues were directly tied to the perceived gap between craft surgery and academic medicine. Some sought to bridge the distance, while others embraced it.

Vernacular surgeons deployed learned conventions when it suited them. For instance, they expounded on the antiquity and nobility of their craft. This chapter began with the words of Matthäus Purmann, who turned to biblical sources to establish surgery's ancient lineage. The dedication of Franz Renner's *Handtbüchlein* (1557) used a similar strategy, situating the origins of medicine within the biblical story of Creation and the Fall. After the serpent tempted Adam and Eve, God cast them out of Paradise. No longer immortal, they suffered the weight of "several illnesses." But human beings were made in the image of God as "a rational creature." They could use the things God made in different ways to preserve the body in good health. To this end, God mercifully endowed many learned and clever philosophers and medical practitioners with a special quality in their nature that spurred them to work day and night to learn and to write of their experience, giving an order to their knowledge of medicine. In this way, all medicine "comes from God."[99] Renner framed the origins of medicine as a combination of God's mercy and the blossoming of human rationality. In his account, his endeavor to write about and share his experience connected to a tradition of "learned" and "clever" authors, both Christian and pagan, whose inspiration ultimately came from God. The use of biblical references, and the discussion of the human body's transformation in the aftermath of the Fall, formed an established trope in medical literature. Johannes Scultetus, an example of a learned author and a rare doctor of medicine and surgery, began his preface with the same narrative, contrasting the immortality and unending health of the human body before the Fall to its diseased and shortened state in the generations that followed.[100]

Classical references also provided evidence of surgery's long and noble history. The preface of Joseph Schmid's *Speculum chirurgicum* took readers on a journey back to the era of Tiberius and the reign of Nero.[101] "So we see that the art of surgery is not new," he declared, "but rather, as it were, the oldest among the healers' arts."[102] The first to practice medicine, according to Schmid, were surgeons with knowledge of herbs. "As we then read in Homer," he explained, "that Podalirius and Machaon, the sons of Asclepius, who in the Trojan War followed the Greek prince Agamemnon from Crete, did nothing other than extract arrows and weapons and apply mild medicines."[103] Podalirius and Machaon proved powerful figures for early modern writers claiming a classical lineage for surgery and anatomy. The surgeon Rudolph Würtz added them as a learned garnish in a dedication appearing in later editions of his brother Felix's *Practica*.[104] While Felix originally dedicated the work to the Holy Roman emperor and spoke of its immediate utility, Rudolph's dedication to the Margrave of Brandenburg framed the treatise more broadly. It begins by tracing the art of surgery from biblical sources to pagan ones. Rudolph explained that, according to "the excellent Greek poet Homer in the second book of the Trojan War," the two sons of Asclepius accompanied King Agamemnon to aid "in the binding and healing of dangerous wounds."[105] The language employed is more flowery than Schmid's, and it is also more precise. Schmid refers to Homer; Rudolph references a specific book by Homer. Likewise, Schmid names Asclepius, whereas Rudolph identifies him as the Greek god of medicine. Despite differences in style, the writers' goals are the same. And in both cases, references to Podalirius and Machaon echo the arguments of the influential anatomist Andreas Vesalius in his dedication to the emperor Charles V in *De humani corporis fabrica* (Basel, 1543).

The appearance of the Homeric surgeons as a common trope is a striking example of the diffusion of learned ideas and rhetorical strategies through print. The question of how clearly or deeply vernacular surgeons comprehended the classical references they employed reminds us that transmission of such knowledge is not a straightforward phenomenon. For instance, the barber-surgeon turned court oculist Georg Bartisch (1535–1607) paid a theology student to insert quotations into his influential treatise on ophthalmology.[106] Others, like Schmid, did so themselves, with mixed results. The historical narrative of his *Speculum chirurgicum*, which interweaves details of his career with the story of ancient surgery, can be dizzying at times. At certain points it is clear that the author did not have a firm grasp of the chronology of the ancient practitioners he extolled. Galen appears as a world-renowned practitioner in the time of "king Xerxes of Persia," who traveled to Troy, Athens, and finally to Rome.[107] It is as if Schmid conflated Hippocrates and Galen, and then threw in the Homeric city of Troy for good measure. Still, his preface made a concerted effort to ennoble the practice of surgery by gesturing to its illustrious past. Schmid's meaning, if not his chronology, is clear. The treatise's title follows the same strategy, blending academic conventions into a vernacular work: *Speculum chirurgicum, oder Spiegel der Artzney*. The Latin short title shows

Schmid's conscious participation in and appropriation of a learned medical tradition. Whether he was aware of the long history of the speculum ("mirror") genre is, perhaps, beside the point.

Vernacular surgeons could also play with the conventions of scholarly works. Whereas Schmid incorporated learned elements into his *Speculum chirurgicum*, the Dutch naval surgeon Cornelis Solingen (1641–1687) defiantly thumbed his nose at them all in his *Hand-Griffe der Wund-Artzney*. In his preface, Solingen wrote that he would not spend time arguing that surgery was "the eldest, noblest, surest, most arduous, and most necessary branch of medicine."[108] Neither would he explain "who the first inventor or patron of surgery [was], or what renowned persons" had practiced it.[109] Ancient names for surgical operations and parts of the body likewise held no interest for him. And he would not clarify "what *Synthesis, Diaeresis, Exaeresis, Aphaeresis, Prothesis* and *Diorthosis*" were.[110] Here Solingen referred to the way authors often divided surgery into categories, as the physician Paul Barbette did at the beginning of his general surgery. According to Barbette, manual operations fell into four categories: *Exaeresis* (the removal of something superfluous), *Diaeresis* (the separation of what is joined), *Anaplerosis* (the reconstitution of what is lacking by birth, disease, or an unfortunate accident), and *Synthesis* (the assembly of what is disjoined).[111] Solingen rejected such an approach. At the same time, he acknowledged and participated in the very traditions he dismissed. The off-handed way in which he strategically cites authors who do all of the things he has no interest in discussing suggests to readers that he is so familiar with the corpus of surgical literature it wearies him. In contrast to Schmid, whose wobbly historical narrative reveals errors in his understanding of the parts of learned tradition he drew upon, Solingen's confidence was genuine. After training as an apprentice, working as a ship's surgeon, and practicing for ten years as a master surgeon in the Hague, he attended university—first at Leiden and then Utrecht—and became a doctor of medicine.[112] The title page of his treatise proudly identified him as "Doctor of Medicine and Surgery" ("Medicinae & Chirurgiae Doctoris"). His preface deftly used this university education to present himself as authoritative to academic readers while dismissing its relevance to the practicing surgeon.

Discussions of the ideal surgeon provided another avenue for vernacular surgeons to consciously build on a long-established tradition in medical writing.[113] Addressing aspiring practitioners in his *Examen chirurgicum*, Schmid expounded on the qualities a surgeon should have. He should, first of all, be "a righteous Christian" who loves God and humankind.[114] This distinguished the contemporary surgeon from the ancient heathen physicians who "knew nothing of belief."[115] Gambling, blaspheming, committing adultery, and brawling—all signs of moral weakness—were unfitting pastimes for this Christian surgeon. Positive character traits were important, too. In addition to possessing "an intrepid mind," he should be truthful and courageous.[116] Yet the surgeon must also have a shrewd sense of when to act, being bold but not reckless. He is both worldly and physically attractive. Schmid described a man "of well-formed body, delicate limbs, sharp face, [and] well-experienced in travel and books."[117] A certain finesse is also essential. The surgeon should "have his exercise with string music in order that he have a light arm, and nimble hands and fingers, which has nothing to do with chopping wood and other crude, hard labor, as Galen and others write thereof."[118] Here Schmid distinguished between fine and crude forms of physical work, like the Italian *paragone* in which painters and sculptors each tried to show that their work was more sophisticated than that of the others.[119] Descriptions of the ideal surgeon were a strategy for self-fashioning: they painted a portrait of the profession. In Schmid's example, the surgeon is not only a virtuous Christian, but also one who travels and reads extensively. His physical attributes emphasize that his work requires dexterity and skill, for surgical operations demanded a deft touch.

The distinction between the skillful surgeon's work and crude labor is a recurring theme in surgical treatises. Authors particularly called upon it in their attacks on empirics—often simply referred to as quacks—and unskilled practitioners. Fabry von Hilden bemoaned that every day one could see how empirics and the inexperienced "plunge so many patients into the deepest wretchedness."[120] These practitioners, according to Fabry, "seek their own advantage much more than their patients', and cannot make a distinction between the human body and stone and wood."[121] The heavy moral and medical failings charged against empirics and itinerant market criers, who competed with surgeons for patients, were economically motivated to some extent, but these critiques extended to inexperienced and unskilled surgeons, too.

Negative depictions of bad practitioners, like the reversal of light and dark in a photographic negative, actually point to strong positive assertions about what surgery is or should be. In Fabry's critique, not only is the nature of the surgeon's hands-on work sophisticated, but also the material with which he works—the human body—is distinctly delicate and complex. Practitioners who do not observe this distinction and treat their materials roughly damage the body and inflict unnecessary pain. "*In all of his operations and healing methods,*" Fabry admonished, "*the surgeon should strive to cause no pain,* but rather instead to attempt to prevent this and avert it."[122] Skillful surgeons perform operations with gentle dexterity and careful discernment. Deficient practitioners, according to Fabry, are those "who like cruel and tyrannical hangman's assistants—entirely unworthy of this ancient, noble art—only for their pleasure and without necessity most brutally torment and distress the sick and wounded to obtain a greater fee."[123] Physicians characterized bad practitioners as executioners, too.[124] In surgery, crude work was not simply unrefined. It was violent.

This brief look at the rhetorical strategies of vernacular surgeons already shows signs of how everyday practitioners were connected to a larger network of ideas. These authors sought to appropriate or subvert elements of the learned medical tradition precisely because they were forging a place for themselves—for those trained by apprenticeship—as creators and authorities in a body of textual knowledge previously controlled by the university-educated. In doing so, they drew at times intentionally and at others unconsciously on themes widespread in early modern intellectual and cultural spheres, from a profuse admiration for classical antiquity to the *paragone*. Still other, even more ubiquitous themes in early modern society provided additional ways to establish the practicing surgeon's place in the written corpus of medical learning, such as the story of Adam and Eve or the dishonorable status of the hangman. These strategies are significant because they reveal how vernacular surgeons entered the publishing fray, engaging in different ways with an established tradition to become part of it. Their strategies signal a long and multifaceted process through which the space between learned surgical publications and vernacular ones became smaller. In Schmid's wobbly recounting of ancient history and Renner's description of the Fall, we witness everyday practitioners working out how to talk to learned and unlearned readers simultaneously. While it might be tempting to dismiss their rhetoric as mere trimming, to do so would overlook an important way vernacular surgeons found their voices—how a written body of medical knowledge that included their perspective came to be.

Crafting the body

Like other craftspeople, surgeons used their hands and learned from firsthand experience. It was a challenge to try to convey their skills through text. Take the way Felix Würtz described a technique for treating a contused fracture that, without the surgeon's intervention, would shorten the length of the limb as it healed. He told the reader to "clench it then with both hands together, like a snowball, and press it to your liking."[125] Making a snowball may not present the most obvious parallel to "stretching" out a contused fracture, as Würtz put it, by applying pressure. But consider what Würtz was attempting to do. One technical act is explained by comparing it to another, in this case a mundane one that someone of almost any age might know (Würtz practiced in the Swiss cantons, after all). We can try it ourselves as a speculative exercise. Forget the cold and playful atmosphere of a snowball fight and concentrate on the shapes your hands make when forming a snowball. If you have ever done so, you immediately have a sense of what your hands should be doing. Or, to be more precise, you have a sense of how *you* would perform the activity. Some of us may even feel confident we understand the technique Würtz was trying to describe through this analogy. But there is an inherent limitation.

Is snowball-making a uniform practice? Do your hands make the same motions as mine? Do our hands make the same motions Würtz's did? Or, we might wonder, is the universality of this parallel not in the exactness of shapes and motions, but in signaling an objective all readers might understand? There is meaning in Würtz's choice of snow: it is a natural material that can be shaped and molded *up to a point* before it disintegrates in a puff or transforms into dense ice. The fractured limb of the surgeon's patient likewise could be shaped *up to a point* with the judicious application of pressure. Both involve shaping matter with one's hands while being sensitive to the pressure applied.

Würtz chose a commonplace activity for his analogy of a technique. More commonly, vernacular surgeons used other professions to define their own more clearly. Perhaps the most powerful and complex analogies they developed concerned craft and craft groups. In his discussion of treating wounds of the bowel lining, Hans von Gersdorff advised the surgeon to close the wounds "with a *nodt* like a furrier makes."[126] The term *nodt* (archaic for *die Naht*) referred to a suture in medicine and a seam in textiles. Gersdorff drew on both contexts to convey a technical skill—suture and seam here are one and the same. His approach effectively communicated a physical experience, likening the surgeon's encounter with human flesh to a furrier sewing pelts. The analogy was not an idle one. Different kinds of wounds located in different places on the body required different kinds of sutures. The furrier's stitch was tight and close. By contrast, "the common suture" (*die gemeinen Hafften*), considered particularly suitable for deep flesh wounds, called for larger stitches to allow putrid matter to flow out. A leaky intestine was not the ideal outcome when treating the bowel lining. The surgeon needed to seal it, and references to the furrier's tight seam indicated the appropriate technique.

Authors used the language of craft in many different ways. Some used it to describe the ideal surgeon as a craftsman (*einem handtwircker*), as Brunschwig did in the very first chapter of his surgical treatise.[127] They could draw on it to deride unskilled surgical work, such as Fabry's critique of practitioners who could not distinguish between the body and stone or wood. Their technical descriptions at times explicitly referred to the closeness of surgery to other crafts, as Gersdorff's *nodt*. Some authors went a step further to discuss not just surgical techniques, but also the instruments used to perform them. Solingen, whose younger brother was a smith, argued that the surgeon should be able to forge his own instruments, or at least design them. "Like a carpenter must have, at the very least, knowledge of his wood along with the art and matter of his cutting [and] other instruments," Solingen declared, "so I hold that a surgeon along with the knowledge of our most marvelous subject of man or of his body must also know at least the fundamentals of draughtsmanship."[128] Some skill with drawing was necessary for the surgeon to "share his opinions and inventions with a smith or another craftsman."[129] His argument reflects a major shift in early modern surgical treatises. Authors gave increasingly detailed attention to instruments, providing meticulous illustrations and descriptions and even devoting whole works to them.[130] Solingen's own treatise included a large folding plate of illustrated instruments. An important dimension of this increased emphasis was the self-fashioning of authors as innovators who claimed to have devised new instruments and improved old ones.[131] By singling out drawing as an essential skill, Solingen invoked a vision of the surgeon actively designing his tools and engaging with other craftspeople who could make them.

This understanding of instruments extended to their care and maintenance. The surgeon "must have knowledge of iron and steel and the art to govern, file, harden, and sharpen" them accordingly.[132] Some familiarity with metallurgy was essential to detect and fix flaws before they turned fatal. "When an instrument is made badly, so that it bends or breaks before one can carry out the operation with it," he explained, the surgeon should artfully repair it so that the patient must not wait in agony until he acquires another.[133] Patients of those who could not act quickly could become weak "and [wind] up dead in the surgeon's hands."[134] Knowledge of an operative technique should dovetail with knowledge of instruments.

Surgeons also used craft language to differentiate their work, exploring the limits of comparison between surgeons and other craft groups. Indeed, authors attended as much to the limits of the comparison as to the comparison itself. They clarified that, unlike other masters, surgeons could never exert total command over their craft, for they could never have mastery over the entire human body. In his *Examen chirurgicum*, Schmid explained to young barber-surgeons that "in my understanding a surgeon is the servant of Nature, so that he might be called a defender or helper of Nature."[135] The surgeon, he elaborated, performs operations and ameliorates symptoms, but "Nature is itself the practitioner in the bodies of the living."[136] Schmid conjured the image of an assistant who could do no more than come to nature's aid with medicine to offset symptoms. "[H]e is not a master," Schmid wrote, "like a smith, locksmith, tailor, carpenter, etc., whose craft is completely subject to him, since here it is not, for the medical practitioner can [do] nothing further than what Nature wishes."[137] In his *Wund-Artzney*, Fabry von Hilden explained that it was not in the surgeon's power to govern afflictions of the body in the way that "a goldsmith handles his gold and silver, or the locksmith his iron."[138] This was an important qualification to what surgeons could accomplish with their therapies. It echoes authors' advice to be circumspect in what one promises to a patient in order to avoid accusations of malpractice.[139] Authors used the limits of the craft analogy to articulate the limits of medicine.

Craft language played a crucial role in discussions of anatomy and its utility to surgical practice. Early modern authors built on a long tradition of describing anatomical parts using craft metaphors. In the medieval author Henri de

Mondeville's work, parts of the body appear as winnowing fans (lungs), tunics (various membranes), helmets (bones), wood (bones), and wax (flesh).[140] The importance of anatomy was also a point of concern in medieval texts. Guy de Chauliac used a metaphor of a blind man pruning a tree to explain the danger of the surgeon who operated without a firm understanding of anatomy. The earliest vernacular surgeons to publish picked up on the metaphor of the blind woodcarver to discuss anatomy.[141] Gersdorff, for instance, framed his tract on anatomy around the body as a tree.[142]

Early modern authors developed elaborate craft analogies to explain the importance of anatomy. Ignorance of the body's composition and its structures led to mistakes when surgeons cut, pulled, burned, stitched, and performed other operations. "In all arts, even common handicrafts," Fabry von Hilden wrote, "this is an incontrovertible rule: that each craftsman who desires to live by his art to his honor and the good of his neighbor, should know first and foremost the properties and nature of his subject—that is, the matter with which he works."[143] Fabry appealed to a set of basic criteria for skillful work shared among craftspeople. "When a goldsmith does not have the proper knowledge of gold and silver," he pressed, "which [is] malleable or unmalleable, pure or mixed with other metals—how will he fare, or how will he be able to make good work?"[144] High-quality results required knowledge of materials. One must know matter before one can "make good work" with it. While Fabry's analogy begins with a figure from the pinnacle of the guild hierarchy working with the most coveted of precious metals, it goes on to explain that this lesson applied to other craftspeople, too. Carpenters, cabinetmakers or joiners, stonemasons, and smiths had to know the nature and properties of wood, stone, and iron. Those who did not could never achieve a perfect knowledge of their craft. True masters who understood the art would always hold such flawed practitioners as "bunglers."[145] In this analogy, the human body is the surgeon's material just as metal is the goldsmith's.

Fabry proceeded with the analogy to formulate the special importance of surgical work:

> As now man, the most noble creation of God, is indeed the image of God himself, all those who handle [the body] should not cut it like a carpenter and stonemason does in wood and stone: but rather have precise knowledge of their subject, that is the human body, and especially of the location in which they wish to work. Because if some mistake should be made here, it is much different than with [wood and stone].[146]

The human body was the surgeon's material, but this was a uniquely precious material because of humanity's unrivaled position in the hierarchy of God's creation. The surgeon could not treat the image of God in the same way he might stone or wood. With this, Fabry established the limits of the comparison.

He then explored those limits to further explain what made surgical work unique. Considering the special nature of the surgeon's material, the stakes of his hands-on practices were overwhelmingly higher than those of any other craftsperson. If a goldsmith made a mistake in his work, he could simply toss the metal back into the crucible without losing anything except his time and effort. Likewise, Fabry continued, "a carpenter, builder and smith also lose nothing that one has cause to lament about, [still] less to weep for."[147] The surgeon, by contrast, "has the human body as his subject, therein he must work, and perform his activities."[148] The argument works on two levels. The first is the ability to "undo" a mistake by either converting the matter back to an unformed state (the goldsmith throwing metal back into the crucible) or by replacing it with fresh material (obtaining new wood) to begin again. Once surgically altered, the human body cannot be returned to its prior state. The body of one human being, moreover, is not interchangeable with another person's body in the way that one might replace wood or stone.

On a second level, the argument turns on emotion. The material difference between metal, wood, stone, and human flesh is also a *moral* one. A poorly crafted piece of wood or stone does not usually bring a person to tears. But one does weep at the loss of an arm or leg that could have been preserved, unnecessary pain experienced at the hands of an inexperienced practitioner, the frustrations of a limp created by a poorly set fracture, or even the death of a loved one from an incompetently performed procedure. The damage the surgeon could inflict on the body caused *suffering*. His errors hurt the patient (and possibly the patient's family and friends) in incalculable ways. Here the limits of the comparison among crafts again point to the singularity of the surgeon's craft. The human body is the surgeon's material, and he must understand its "marvelous and divine structures."[149]

It is no coincidence that this particular articulation of what was unique to the surgeon appeared most frequently in discussions of anatomy. Schmid, for instance, employed a similar craft analogy about the goldsmith in his *Spiegel der Anatomiae*, and he cited Fabry's treatise directly to support his defense of anatomy's utility.[150] Surgeons made this argument—one that likens their work to that of craftspeople while at the same time distinguishing it from all other crafts—at the very interstice at which academic medicine and craft surgery met in the early modern period. Vernacular surgeons were pitching the value of what was perceived to be a facet of learned medical education to barber-surgeons and surgeons from the craft tradition. At the same time, they were imbuing craft surgery with a distinct and solemn responsibility that emphasized its singular value to academic audiences. Schmid wrote that "the art of medicine demands a great diligence and ceaseless work, like other arts, since to work in the human body is a difficult and dangerous thing—[it] touches not stone or wood that is soon replaced again, but rather the image of God."[151] There was a sacred quality to the surgeon's work that no goldsmith or carpenter could claim.

During the early modern period, academic medicine and craft surgery converged in a more intense and dynamic way than had been possible in previous centuries. The printing press and the print culture that grew steadily through the sixteenth and seventeenth centuries propelled the wide circulation of texts new and old, in Latin and the vernacular, written by learned and unlearned authors and practitioners. Vernacular surgeons entered the fray with several strategies for establishing themselves as professionals, appealing to readers, and describing surgical work. In their treatises, they defended the technical arts in the same manner as other craft groups. They also had a complicated way of defining themselves along craft lines. Vernacular surgeons argued for the nobility of their hands-on practice and compared their work to that of craftspeople. On occasion they even called for better communication and collaboration with other craft groups. But they also argued that their work was special and unlike any other craft because they dealt with the most precious of all materials—the human body. And because their efforts could not be undone, nor their materials replaced, the surgeon's work was of the highest importance.

The remainder of this book considers the ways surgeons worked with and thought about this most precious material in moments when patients, fellow practitioners, artisans, and amputees revealed its many shifting shapes.

Notes

1 Purmann, *Wund-Artzney* (1684), sig. b3r: "Die Chirurgi und Wund-Artzney-Kunst aber ist die aller älteste/ erste und scheinbareste."
2 Ibid., sig. b2v–b3r.
3 Ibid., sig. b3v: "Denn wer siehet nicht mit Augen voller Verwunderung," "die verletzten und verwundeten Glieder/ Sie seyn gestossen/ geschlagen/ geschossen/ gehauen oder gestochen/ zerbrochne Beiner/ verrenckten Gelencke/ der Brand/ alle Arten der Beulen/ Geschwülste und Geschwäre/ der Steinschnitt in der Blasen/ alle Arten der Brüche Cur."
4 Ibid.: "mehr verborgen."
5 Ibid., sig. b3v–b4r: "In Summa/ Wer kan genugsam Worte machen von der Nothwendigkeit und Nutzen dieser edlen Kunst/ welche ein jeder rechtschaffener Medicus, wo er ein vollkommener Doctor Medicinae und glücklicher Practicus seyn wil/ wissen und verstehen soll."
6 E.g., Dürer, *Opera*; Furttenbach, *Architectura Recreationis*; Alberti, *De re aedificatoria*; Ramelli, *Le diverse et artificiose machine*. See also Long, "Power, Patronage, and the Authorship of *Ars*."
7 Brunschwig, *Buch der Cirurgia*; Gersdorff, *Feldbuch*. On vernacular medical texts before the printing press: Nutton, "Medicine in Medieval Western Europe," 145–146.

8 See Stolz, *Die Handwerke des Körpers*; Cavallo, *Artisans of the Body*; Kinzelbach, "Erudite and Honoured Artisans?"
9 Siraisi, "How to Write a Latin Book on Surgery," 91–92.
10 McVaugh, *Rational Surgery*, 11.
11 Nutton, "Humanist Surgery."
12 Wear, "Medicine in Early Modern Europe," 264–292.
13 Bertolini Meli and Klestinec, "Renaissance Surgery."
14 Purmann, *Wund-Artzney* (1684), sig. b4r: "die inner-und eusserliche Artzney-Kunst/ ist so genau mit ein ander verbunden/ das keines ohne des andern seyn und bestehen kann."
15 E.g., Berriot-Salvadore and Mironneau, *Ambroise Paré*; Panse, *Feldbuch der Wundarznei*; Bertolini Meli, "'Ex Museolo Nostro Machaonico.'"
16 A notable exception, localized to the Italian context and ideas of beauty surrounding a rhinoplasty procedure, is Paolo Savoia's comparisons between the writings of physicians and barber-surgeons in *Tagliacozzi*.
17 Cavallo, *Artisans of the Body*.
18 Reaching back to the Middle Ages, Italian universities in particular taught surgery to northern European students: Nutton, "Medicine in Medieval Western Europe," 162–163. Seventy-seven German professors of medicine were students at the University of Padua, an influential center of early modern medical education, between 1553 and 1673: Schadewaldt, "Padua und die Medizin," 251; Sachs, *Geschichte*, 4:216.
19 E.g., Murphy, *New Order of Medicine*, 68–69; Sachs, *Geschichte*, 4:12–13.
20 E.g., municipal employment records of Ulrich Welser in Munich: StdAM, KR 1540, 76r–KR 1556, 77v.
21 Jütte, "Seventeenth-Century German Barber-Surgeon," 187.
22 E.g., municipal employment records of the Munich specialized surgeon (*Schnidtartzt*) Tobias Zieger show his elevation over time: StdAM, KR 1610, 108v; KR 1623, 96v; KR 1624, 101v, 105r.
23 Kinzelbach, "Erudite and Honoured Artisans?" 674; Sander, *Handwerkschirurgen*, 201–203; Scheutz and Weiss, *Das Spital*, 349; *AHRG*, 6:66–68.
24 Lindemann, *Medicine and Society*, 235–280; Wear, "Medicine in Early Modern Europe," 232–241; Jütte, *Ärzte, Heiler und Patienten*, 22; Stolberg, *Experiencing Illness*, 58–64; Kinzelbach, "Women and Healthcare"; Hauri, *Die Steinschneider*; Whaley, *Women and the Practice of Medical Care*; Rankin, *Panaceia's Daughters*; Harrington, *Faithful Executioner*, 185–225.
25 On degrees and licensing: Jütte, *Ärzte, Heiler und Patienten*, 19–20.
26 Siraisi, *Medieval and Early Renaissance Medicine*, 48; Grob and Winckelmann, "Das Collegium Medicum zu Ulm"; Murphy, *New Order of Medicine*.
27 E.g., StdAM, KR 1568, 73r, 77v; KR 1569, 73r, 77v.
28 Wear, "Medicine in Early Modern Europe," 235. Stretching back to the Middle Ages, the gap between physicians and surgeons was more pronounced in northern than southern Europe, and Italy in particular: Nutton, "Medicine in Medieval Western Europe," 163; Wear, "Medicine in Early Modern Europe," 293. On surgical practice outside of early modern Germany: Pelling, *Common Lot* and

Medical Conflicts; Cavallo, *Artisans of the Body*; Savoia, *Tagliacozzi*; Gelfand, *Professionalizing Modern Medicine*; Brockliss and Jones, *Medical World*; De Moulin, *History of Surgery*.
29 Stuart, *Defiled Trades*, 151.
30 Stein, *Negotiating the French Pox*, 154; Scheutz and Weiss, *Das Spital*, 349.
31 *AHRG*, 1:274–358, 2:1–11; Sander, *Handwerkschirurgen*, 135–175; Lindemann, *Medicine and Society*, 129–130.
32 E.g., Jütte, *Ärzte, Heiler und Patienten*, 20.
33 E.g., Ecker-Offenhäußer, "Joseph Schmid," 121.
34 E.g., one could even apprentice to a master field-surgeon by Matthäus Purmann's time: Garrison, *Military Medicine*, 124. For more on Purmann's military experience: Sachs, *Geschichte*, 1:29, and "Matthäus Gottfried Purmann."
35 Hintzsche, Introduction, 7–19; Hirsch, *Biographisches Lexikon*, 2:462–463; Gurlt, *Geschichte*, 3:107–113; Hintzsche, *Guilelmus Fabricius Hildanus*, 9–16, 25.
36 See Ecker-Offenhäußer, "Joseph Schmid," 120, 122; Jütte, *Ärzte, Heiler und Patienten*, 20; Kinzelbach, "Zur Sozial- und Alltagsgeschichte," 126; Stein, *Negotiating the French Pox*, 118; Lindemann, *Medicine and Society*, 130.
37 Hirsch, *Biographisches Lexikon*, 2:462–463; Gurlt, *Geschichte*, 3:108; Hintzsche, Introduction, 11–12, 16; Hintzsche, *Guilelmus Fabricius Hildanus*, 16.
38 On literacy among surgeons: Sander, *Handwerkschirurgen*, 123–125; Kinzelbach, "Zur Sozial- und Alltagsgeschichte," 121; Scheutz and Weiss, *Das Spital*, 348.
39 Schmid, *Examen chirurgicum*, 6–8.
40 Ecker-Offenhäußer, "Volkssprachlich-medizinischer Buchdruck," 959–960; Kinzelbach, "Zur Sozial- und Alltagsgeschichte," 139–142, 139n114.
41 E.g., Kinzelbach, "Erudite and Honoured Artisans?" 688.
42 For a succinct definition of craft practice: Long, *Artisan/Practitioners*, 4.
43 Farr, *Artisans in Europe*, 108.
44 StdAM, KR 1551/52, 91r.
45 E.g., Hintzsche, Introduction, 10; Hirsch, *Biographisches Lexikon*, 2:464; Gurlt, *Geschichte*, 3:108; Hildanus, *Wund-Artzney*, 216, 765.
46 Ecker-Offenhäußer, "Joseph Schmid," 119–120, 120n14.
47 Schmid, *Spiegel der Anatomiae*, sig.):(9v–):(10r.
48 Dietz, *Meister Johann Dietz*, 14; Sachs, *Geschichte*, 5:71, 3:283; Oettinger, *German Barber-Surgeon*; Kinzelbach, "Zur Sozial- und Alltagsgeschichte," 117.
49 Stadtarchiv Augsburg, Bestand Reichsstadt, Hochzeitsamtsprotokolle 7, 1624–1629, p. 115.
50 Schmid, *Speculum chirurgicum*, 14: "müsse nicht daheim hinder dem Ofen sitzen bleiben/ sondern in frembde Länder reisen/ und mit gelehrten Leuten zu conversiren keinen Scheu tragen/ Arme Häuser und Spittäler/ allda allerhand krancke unnd schadhaffte Leut ligen/ zubesuchen."
51 Ibid.: "es kostet nicht allein Silber oder Gold/ sondern das Leben selbst."
52 Ibid., 23: "Das Lesen allein macht keinen Arzt."
53 Ecker-Offenhäußer, "Volkssprachlich-medizinischer Buchdruck," 947–962.
54 Schmid, *Examen chirurgicum*, sig. A6r: "jeder junger angehende Feldscherer oder Wundarzt," "wie er sich bey allen Verwundungen (sie seyen gleich

gehawen/ gestochen/ geschossen/ geworffen/ vergifft oder nit) verhalten soll/ deren Zufäll zu erkennen/ denselbigen begegnen/ und vorzubawen/ ingleichem die Handgriff zu erlernen/ wie alle außgehende Glieder einzurichten/ die gebrochne Beiner zu schlichten und zu heylen/ auch was gemeiniglich/ in einem Feldläger/ vor Kranckheiten regieren/ und wie denselbigen/ in Mangel eines Medici, Rath und Hülff zu schaffen seye."

55 Ibid., 397, 399.
56 Rarely did surgical works by English practitioner-authors appear in German translation before 1700: e.g., Brugis, *Vade Mecum Chirurgicum*.
57 A few examples: Arcaeus, *Fraxinalensis*; Fabricius ab Aquapendente, *Pentateuchos Chirurgicum* and *Wund-Artznei*; Paré, *Opera Chirurgica* (1594) and *Wundt-Artzney* (1601); Barbette, *Schrifften*; Herls, *Examen*; Muys, *Praxis*.
58 E.g., Barbette, *Chirurgische und Medicinische Wercke*; Blankaart, *Chirurgische Abhandlung*; Bontekoe, *Newes Gebäw*; Munnicks, *Praxis Cheirurgica*; Overcamp, *Neues Gebäude der Chirurgie*.
59 Uffenbach, *Thesaurus chirurgiae*. The authors are Fabry von Hilden (1560–1634), Jacques Houllier (c. 1498–1562), Jean Tagault (d. 1545), Ambroise Paré (1516–1590), Alfonso Ferri (1515–1595), Michelangelo Biondo (1497–1565), Angelo Bolognini (sixteenth century), Conrad Gesner (1516–1565), and Jacobus de Dondis (1298–1359).
60 Paré, *Wund-Artzney* (1635).
61 E.g., Hildanus, *New Feldt-Artzney-Buch*; Schmid, *Kriegs-Arzney*; Purmann, *Feldscher*.
62 Burres, *Ein new Wund Arzney Büchlein*.
63 E.g., Purmann, *Schuß-Wunden Curen*; Ferri, *De Sclopetorum sive archibusorum vulneribus*; Schmid, *Etliche kurtze und wohlbewehrte Artzneyen* and *Bericht*; Purmann, *Kurtze, doch gründliche Anweisung*.
64 Hildanus, *De combustionibus* and *Lithotomia Vesicae* (1626); Renner, *Handtbüchlein* (1557) and *Handtbüchlein* (1559).
65 Bertolini Meli, "'Ex Museolo Nostro Machaonico'"; Pomata, "Sharing Cases." On the importance of medical observations for the rise of empiricism: Pomata, "*Praxis Historialis*"; Mendelsohn, "The World on a Page."
66 E.g., Gehema, *Observationes*; Scultetus, *Wund-Artzneyisches Zeug-Hauß* (1666).
67 E.g., Galen, *De sanitate tuenda libri sex*; Lanfrancus, *Kleine Wundarzney*.
68 Little is known about Greiff. His posthumous publications refer to him as "Hospital-und Stadtartzt," but the use of *Arzt* here is likely meant in the general sense of a medical specialist holding a town office rather than a university-educated physician. The 1622 dedication of *Wundartzeney* refers to him as "Herr Sebastian Greiff" without indicating a medical degree. He was practicing surgery when he published works on Paracelsus in the 1580s and 1590s: Greiff, *Apologia und Refutation* and *Vom Cometen Anno 1596*.
69 Greiff, *Wundartzeney* and *Wolbewärte Wundarzney*.
70 Lose and Greiff, *Hand-Büchlein*, 3.
71 Ibid.: "praxin und experienz," "die Theoriam."
72 Marchetti, *Observationes*; Tassin, *Kurtze Kriegs-Wund-Artzney*; Arcaeus, *Fraxinalensis*.

73 E.g., Botallo, *Opera omnia medica & chirurgica*, annot. Johannes van Horne, 790–791, and *Zwey Chirurgische Bücher*, 2:299–300.
74 StdAU, H Leopold 2, Johann Dieterich Leopold, *Memoria Physicorum Ulmanorum seu Biographia Medicorum ordinariorum*, 128–132.
75 Sachs, *Geschichte*, 3:319–321.
76 Hirsch, *Biographisches Lexikon*, 3:431.
77 On Paracelsus's medicine: Pagel, *Paracelsus*; Webster, *Paracelsus*.
78 On Ryff's career: Eamon, *Science and the Secrets of Nature*, 96–105; Vollmuth, *Traumatologie*, 25–37.
79 On Fabry von Hilden's career as an author: Hintzsche, Introduction, 11–17.
80 Scultetus, *Armamentarium Chirurgicum* (1656), sig.)(3r–v [hereafter, *AC* (1656)].
81 E.g., Hildanus, *Gründlicher Bericht*, 9–11, 40, 43, 47, 57, 81, 106, 171.
82 E.g., Scultetus, *Wund-Artzneyisches Zeug-Hauß* (1666), 1:8–9, 99, 101, 178, 220, 228; and 2:8, 57, 80, 143, 187, 211–212.
83 E.g., Schmid, *Spiegel der Anatomiae*, sig.):(9v.
84 E.g., Paracelsus, *Der grossen wundartzney*, sig. A2v–A3v.
85 Schmid, *Speculum chirurgicum*, 11. These would have been a combination of soldiers fighting for the Crown of Sweden and Swedish mercenaries.
86 Barbette, *Schrifften*, sig.)(2v.
87 Ibid., 4: "weil solches viel besser durch den Augenschein selbsten/ als durch das Lesen kan erlernet werden."
88 E.g., Gehema, *Observationes*, sig. A2r.
89 Würtz, *Practica* (1596), sig. a2v: "allgemeinem Menschlichem Geschlecht."
90 *AC* (1656), sig.)(5v.
91 Amadeus Megerlin, Vorrede, in Scultetus, *Wund-Artzneyisches Zeug-Hauß* (1666), unpaginated.
92 Würtz, *Practica* (1596), 4.
93 Ibid., sig. a6v.
94 Purmann, *Wund-Artzney* (1692), sig. b3v.
95 Gehema, *Der krancke Soldat*, sig. A9r: "als ein Esel zu tantzen."
96 Gehema, *Feld-Medicus*, 29.
97 E.g., Würtz, *Practica* (1596), sig. a5r–a6r.
98 E.g., Hildanus, *Gründlicher Bericht*, 84.
99 Renner, *Handtbüchlein* (1557), sig. *2r–v: "mancherley kranckheit," "ein vernünfftige Creatur," "von Got kompt."
100 *AC* (1656), sig.)(5r.
101 Schmid, *Speculum chirurgicum*, 7.
102 Ibid., 7–8: "Also sehen wir ja/ daß solche Kunst der Wundartzney kein newe/ sondern gleichsam die Elteste ist unter den Aertzten."
103 Ibid.: "Wie wir dann bey dem Homero lesen/ daß Podalirius und Machaon, deß Aesculapii Söhne/ welche im Trojanischen Kriege/ der Griechen Fürsten Agamemnoni auß Creta gefolget/ nichts anders gethan/ als Pfeyl und Waffen außgezogen/ und gelinde Artzneyen darauff gelegt."

104 The earliest edition with this preface I have identified is Würtz, *Practica* (1612). The title page clarifies the work was revised and expanded by Rudolph Würtz, surgeon of Strasbourg, using his brother's handwritten books.
105 Rudolph Würtz, preface to Würtz, *Practica* (1639), sig.)(3v–)(4r: "der fürtreffliche Griechische Poet Homerus in dem andern Buch des Trojanischen Kriegs," "in Verbindung und Heylung der gefährlichen Wunden."
106 Wear, "Medicine in Early Modern Europe," 297.
107 Schmid, *Speculum chirurgicum*, 13: "Königs Xerxis in Persia."
108 Solingen, *Hand-Griffe*, sig. a2r: "das älteste/ edelste/ sicherste/ mühsamste und nothwendigste Theil der Artzeney-Kunst."
109 Ibid.: "wer der erste Erfinder oder Patron derselben ist/ oder was für Durchlauchtigste Personen ... dieselbe exerciret haben."
110 Ibid., sig. a2v: "Ich werde auch nicht weitläuftig erklähren/ was *Synthesis, Diaeresis, Exaeresis, Aphaeresis, Prothesis* und *Diorthosis* sey."
111 Barbette, *Schrifften*, 1. See also Jessen, *Wund-Artznei*, 191.
112 Grooss, *Cornelis Solingen*, 6; De Moulin, *History of Surgery*, 134.
113 E.g., Celsus, *De Medicina*, 3:297; Jessen, *Wund-Artznei*, sig. a4v.
114 Schmid, *Examen chirurgicum*, 5–6: "ein rechtschaffner Christ."
115 Ibid.: "die Alten Arzt/ als Heyden/ nichts von dem Glauben unnd der Liebe Gottes gewust."
116 Ibid.: "eines redlichen Gemüts."
117 Ibid.: "wolgeformiretes Leibs/ subtiler Glieder/ scharpffes Gesichts/ in Reysen unnd Büchern wol erfahren."
118 Ibid.: "mit Saitenspil sein Ubung habe/ damit er leichter Armb/ ringe Händ und Finger habe/ welche von Holtzhacken/ und anderer grober harter Arbeit ist nit gethon/ wie Galenus und andere darvon schreiben."
119 Cynthia Klestinec connects the *paragone* debates with the language of surgeons in Italy: "Renaissance Surgeons," 52–55.
120 Hildanus, *Wund-Artzney*, 1054: "so viel Krancke in das höchste Elend stürtzen."
121 Ibid.: "sie viel mehr ihren eignen als der krancken Nutzen suchen/ und nicht wol zwischen deß Menschen Leib und zwischen Stein und Holtz einen underscheid machen können."
122 Hildanus, *Gründlicher Bericht*, 157: "*Bei all seinen Operationen und Heilmaßnahmen soll der Wundarzt danach trachten, keinen Schmerz zu verursachen*, sondern vielmehr suchen, diesem vorzubeugen und ihn abzuwehren."
123 Ibid.: "die als unmenschliche und tyrannische (dieser uralten edlen Kunst ganz unwüridge) Henkersknechte darauf aus sind, nur zu ihrer Lust und ohne Notwendigkeit die Verwundeten und Kranken aufs allergrausamste zu plagen und zu peinigen, damit sie um so größeren Lohn erhalten."
124 E.g., Gehema, *Observationes*, sig. A7r.
125 Würtz, *Practica* (1639), 361: "balle ihn dann mit beyden Händen zusammen/ wie ein schneeballen/ und drucke ihn eben nach deinem gefallen."
126 Gersdorff, *Feldbuch*, 31r: "mit einer nodt als ein Kürßner macht." For a fuller description of this suture, see Walther Ryff, whose work draws extensively from medieval authors like Mondeville: Ryff, *Die groß Chirurgei*, 9v.

127 Brunschwig, *Buch der Cirurgia*, fol. 9v. Compare Jessen's discussion of surgery as a handicraft: *Wund-Artznei*, sig. a5v.
128 Solingen, *Hand-Griffe*, sig. a3v: "gleich wie ein Zimmermann/ zum wenigsten von seinen Holtze/ nebst der Art und Materie/ seines so schneidenden/ als andern Werckzeuges/ muß Käntniß haben; So halte ich dafür/ daß ein Chirurgus nechst der Wissenschafft/ dieses unsers herrlichsten Subjects des Menschen/ oder desselben leib/ auch zum wenigsten die Fundamenta der Zeichen-Kunst müsse wissen."
129 Ibid.: "damit er einem Schmiede oder andern Handwercksmann seine Meynung und Erfindung könne zu verstehen geben."
130 E.g., Schmid, *Instrumenta chirurgica*.
131 E.g., many treatises devoted attention to instruments that extracted bullets from gunshot wounds: Gersdorff, *Feldbuch*, 39r; Paré, *Wundt-Artzney* (1601), 483.
132 Solingen, *Hand-Griffe*, sig. a3v: "muß er Wissenschaft haben von Eisen und Stahl/ und der Art dieselben zu regieren/ zu feilen/ härten und schleiffen."
133 Ibid.: "wann ein Instrument übel gemachet ist/ so daß/ ehe man mit denselben die Operation vollführen kan/ es sich beuget oder bricht."
134 Ibid.: "ja wol gar drüber schwach werde/ und unter den Händen todt bleibe."
135 Schmid, *Examen chirurgicum*, 1–2: "Nach meinem Verstand ist ein Wundarzt der Natur Diener oder Knecht/ also daß er wol ein Defensor oder Auxiliarius Naturae mag genennet werden."
136 Ibid., 2: "die Natur ist selbst der Arzt in den Cörpern der Lebendigen."
137 Ibid., 3: "ist er kein Meister/ als ein Schmid/ Schlosser/ Schneider/ Zimmermann/ zc. dem ist sein Handwerck gäntzlich unterworffen/ das dann hier nit ist/ dann der Arzt kan nit weiter/ als die Natur auch will."
138 Hildanus, *Wund-Artzney*, 943: "wie ein Goldschmied mit Gold und Silber/ oder ein Schlosser mit dem Eysen umbgehet."
139 Barbette, *Schrifften*, 221.
140 Pouchelle, *Body and Surgery*, 106–108.
141 De Moulin, *History of Surgery*, 78.
142 Gersdorff, *Feldbuch*, 1r. For more on plant metaphors: Savoia, *Tagliacozzi*, 152.
143 Hildanus, *Wund-Artzney*, 937: "In allen Künsten/ ja gemeinen Handwercken ist diese eine unwidersprechliche Regel/ daß ein jeder Handwercksmann/ der zu seinen Ehren und Nutz deß Nechsten/ seiner Kunst begehrt zu leben/ am allerersten die Eygenschafft und Natur seines subjecti, das ist materi darinn er arbeitet/ soll erkennen."
144 Ibid.: "wann ein Goldschmidt nicht hat die rechte Erkantnuß deß Golds und Silbers/ welches geschmeydig oder ungeschmeydig/ lauter oder mit anderen Metallen vermischt ist; wie wird er bestehen/ oder wie wird er gute Arbeit machen können?"
145 Ibid.: "Stümpler."
146 Ibid.: "Wann nun der Mensch das alleredelste Geschöpff Gottes/ ja das Ebenbild GOTTEs selber ist/ solten billich alle die/ so mit demselben umbgehen/ nicht hinein hawen/ wie ein Zimmerman/ und Steinhawer in Holtz und Stein: sondern/ ihres subjecti, das ist deß Menschen Leib/ und sonderlich deß Orts/ darinn sie

arbeiten wöllen/ rechte Erkantnuß haben. Dann wo fern allhier etwas solte versehen werden/ ist es viel einanders/ als mit dem obgedachten."
147 Ibid.: "Ein Zimmermann/ Mäwrer unnd Schmid verlieren auch weiters nichts/ daß man Ursach habe zu beklagen/ weniger zu beweinen."
148 Ibid., 937–938: "hat deß Menschen Leib zu seinem subjecto, darinn er muß arbeiten/ und seine Würckungen verrichten."
149 Ibid., 938: "die überauß wunderbarliche und Göttliche Zusamensetzungen."
150 Schmid, *Spiegel der Anatomiae*, sig.):(8v–):(9v.
151 Schmid, *Speculum chirurgicum*, 29: "die Kunst der Artzney einen grossen Fleiß und unablässige Arbeit/ wie andere Künste/ erfordert und haben will/ dann in deß Menschen Leib zu arbeiten/ ist ein schwer und gefährlich Ding/ trifft nicht Stein oder Holtz an/ das bald wieder zuersetzen ist/ sondern Gottes Ebenbild."

2

Communities face the cold fire

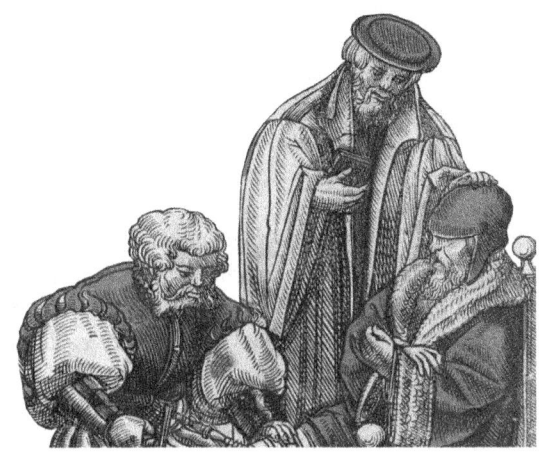

In the summer of 1607, a fifty-year-old man named Stephan Toppinus fell from a wagon. A wheel rolled over his left leg and crushed his calf, baring the shin bone without breaking it. Stephan walked for half an hour on his injury to return home, at which point Fabry von Hilden, a nearby surgeon, was summoned to examine him. Scarcely two days later Fabry noticed that a piece of flesh in the calf was turning blue—a sign of what he called *der heisse Brand*, or "the hot fire." The surgeon immediately cut away the dead flesh in the presence of Stephan's pastor. But this was not enough to prevent the onset of what Fabry termed *der kalte Brand*—"the cold fire." Within two days, a patch of black flesh as wide as a hand appeared on Stephan's calf.

The surgeon resolved to remove the entire lower leg because he expected that the cold fire would spread, a prognosis confirmed when Stephan's foot and more of his calf became black and spongy to the touch. To his lasting regret, Fabry did not have the proper instruments on hand to perform the procedure and left to fetch them. When he returned that afternoon, the cold fire had already climbed too far up the patient's leg to operate. Stephan and his kin and friends demanded that he proceed with the amputation, but Fabry advised them to consult other physicians and surgeons in town to determine the best course of action. By ten o'clock that evening the cold fire had reached the patient's groin, and some five hours later, only the fourth day after his accident, Stephan was dead.[1]

Fabry gave an account of Stephan's troubling case—which he described as "such a raging, cruel [and] terrifying fire, the like of which I had never seen before"—in a letter addressed to Georg Horst, a physician and professor of medicine in Giessen.[2] Had the hot fire and then the cold fire arisen in his patient's leg from a known and external cause alone, or from a hidden and internal cause? In Fabry's opinion, the wound inflicted by the wagon wheel was too minor to account for the ferocity with which the fire had spread. Only the combination of some foul material introduced from outside the body with the contused injury could explain Stephan's rapid decline. He referred Horst to witnesses who could validate this account: the pastor Johannes de Moulin and Master Emanuel Urstisius, a medical student who also boarded with Fabry as his pupil.[3]

The rapidity of the cold fire's spread may have been extraordinary to Fabry, but many aspects of the way the surgeon, the patient, and the patient's friends and neighbors handled the case were quite ordinary. As Fabry was well aware, contusions were more prone to putrefy than other kinds of injuries, and he was vigilant for signs of the hot and cold fires—the dying and final death of Stephan's limb. He combatted the fire as best as he could to save the patient's leg, but once the cold fire set into the bone, his goal shifted from preserving the limb to removing it entirely in order to save the patient. Moreover, the formulation of Fabry's diagnosis and prognosis was not a solitary activity. A number of individuals were not simply present in the room, but were also actively involved. Fabry was accompanied throughout by a medical student who doubled as both assistant and witness. The surgeon performed the excision of dead flesh in the presence of Stephan's pastor, who sought to keep the patient in good spirits. Stephan and his friends were outspoken in their demands for treatment. When Fabry hesitated, he was quick to recommend consulting other practitioners rather than hazard the procedure. Owing largely to the caution he displayed throughout the course of Stephan's illness, the amputation never happened.

The case of Stephan Toppinus draws our attention to medical and social elements that were intertwined in treating a putrefying limb. Fabry's approach in the days following the accident was guided by his medical deductions—as the senior medical expert on site, he connected the changes occurring in the patient's body to early modern concepts of putrefaction. But he did his work in a room full of opinionated people with whom he was in constant dialogue. This chapter explores the medical reasoning and collective discussion that unfolded in cases like this. Scholars have shown that medical practitioners of all stripes worked within wider cultural, political, and social contexts that influenced their practices.[4] We can see the social dimensions of early modern medicine in the intake processes and care of patients at pox houses, the business decisions of apothecaries to extend credit to a customer, and the baptisms that midwives performed in childbirth emergencies.[5] This chapter reveals a particularly powerful manifestation of a larger social community at work in the surgeon's decision-making process surrounding amputation. When treating the hot and cold fires, surgeons relied on firsthand experience and the knowledge accumulated in surgical texts to formulate a diagnosis and prognosis. Once the surgeon detected the cold fire, however, treatment became an increasingly social enterprise as he drew members of the community into conversation about the patient's condition. Their dialogue primarily focused on one simple but weighty question: should the surgeon amputate, or not? Ideally, the decision was communal.

Diagnosing the hot and cold fires

Putrefaction transformed an arm or leg from a living part of the patient into something dead, useless, and dangerous that needed to be excised. A putrefied limb no longer held the vital spirit that animated the body, it could not perform the functions of walking or carrying objects, and—worst of all—its disease inevitably spread if left unchecked. "Because a dead limb is of no more use to the body," Paul Barbette wrote, "then one must remove it so it does not infect the nearby parts."[6] But there were degrees of putrefaction, some of which were reversible. The surgeon had to be careful not to rush precipitously into a procedure before it was absolutely necessary, as Janus Abraham à Gehema warned in his *Wohlversehener Feld-Medicus*. He complained that some field-surgeons resolved too quickly to remove an arm or leg that might still be saved.[7] At the same time, the surgeon could not wait too long.

Timing was crucial when determining the point at which a limb was beyond saving, the point at which the surgeon's task shifted from preservation to removal. This was a challenge. The lines between an injured limb, a dying limb, and a dead one were remarkably blurry in early modern medicine. To decipher signs of decay, the surgeon used the concepts of the hot and cold fires. These were interrelated conditions that could arise independently or could follow from one another, that could exist separately or simultaneously in a limb, and varied tremendously in their severity. Surgical treatises commonly discussed them in conjunction with one another. Laurentius Lose explained that "if you really want to consider this matter, then the hot and cold fire is the dying and death of one or more parts, and as such can be divided into the beginning, progress, and complete end."[8] Together, the hot and cold fires were to some extent a narrative of physical death in an isolated portion of the body.

In the mire of definitions and descriptions surrounding the hot and cold fires, there was one patch of solid ground upon which all surgeons could meet. The hot fire, also known as Gangraena, was the initial decomposing of tissue, and the cold fire, or Sphacelus, was the complete death of a body part, tissue and bone.[9] This distinction, reaching back to antiquity, remained constant throughout the early modern period. The terms were pliable, however, and their usage in treatises could be loose or hyper-specific. They could be conflated with several other conditions, especially St. Anthony's Fire, a disease that could cause flesh to rot and then fall spontaneously from the body.[10] Root causes and recommended cures also varied from author to author. Indeed, for every statement made in a sampling of surgical treatises, we often find two contrary ones.

One of the most popular and influential works on the hot and cold fires was Fabry von Hilden's *Gründlicher Bericht vom heissen und kalten Brand*. First published in 1593, this tract was quickly translated into several languages before it was enlarged and reprinted multiple times within the Holy Roman Empire. Treatises frequently cited it from the turn of the seventeenth century onward. To exercise some discipline over the surgical literature addressing putrefaction, this chapter draws extensively from Fabry's work, which provides a basic framework of definitions and causes recognizable—and often agreeable—to most German-speaking surgeons.[11] Several other treatises, such as Johannes Scultetus's *Wund-Artzneyisches Zeug-Hauß*, Laurentius Lose's *Chirurgisches Hand-Büchlein*, Sebastian Greiff's *Wolbewärte Wundarzney*, Paul Barbette's *Chirurgische und anatomische Schrifften*, and Walther Ryff's *Die groß Chirurgei*, help us elaborate on Fabry's general guidelines.

The hot and cold fires were commonly categorized as kinds of tumors.[12] A tumor was a disease in which a part of the body was improperly enlarged and distended to the point that it could no longer function.[13] As Fabry explained, the classification of Gangraena and Sphacelus as unnatural tumors traced back to Galen's *De tumoribus praeter naturam*.[14] Galen described Gangraena as the initial dying of tissue in a diseased or injured member that gradually spread to nearby parts and led to death. Sphacelus, by contrast, was a condition in which the flesh, muscles, sinews, and bone all putrefied, and in time the putrefaction spread to surrounding parts.[15] Since early moderns often adopted this Galenic classification, surgical treatises frequently included the fires within sections devoted entirely to tumors. In Ryff's *Die groß Chirurgei*, they were listed among such forms of "unnatural tumors" as the Bubo.[16] This organization was also used in the first book of Barbette's *Chirurgische und anatomische Schrifften*, titled "Concerning tumors."[17] Fabry even reported that some scholars considered both Gangraena and Sphacelus as cold tumors because the hot fire commonly developed into the cold fire, which turned the limb "ice-cold and dead."[18]

The term Gangraena, according to early modern authors, originated from the ancient Greeks and meant something that "eats away" or "gnaws."[19] This condition affected the soft parts of the body—including skin, blood vessels, and muscles. It was the beginning or incomplete putrefaction that commonly followed great inflammations.[20] It was usually red and hot to the touch, and the affected flesh became very swollen. As it progressed, the blood-red color faded into white, yellow, or brown, with brown and black stripes running across it. Gangraena was intensely painful and caused horrendous stabbing and throbbing sensations.[21] For all of these reasons—the hot, red, swollen appearance accompanied by tremendous pain—the condition was colloquially called *der heisse Brand*, or the hot fire.

Sphacelus, a term that also originated from the Greeks, attacked both the soft and hard parts of the body, meaning not only the skin and muscles, but also the bone.[22] This was the complete death of a body part, a condition that spread outward over time to destroy neighboring parts of the body.[23] Sphacelus turned a limb gray, blue, and black and was always ice-cold. The texture of flesh and bone turned spongy, the limb emitted a foul odor, and, most important, it lost all sensitivity. Because an affected limb turned cold and because the condition, if left unchecked, would spread, it was called *der kalte Brand*, or the cold fire.[24] A lack of local sensitivity was the most decisive factor in determining if a patient's condition had deteriorated into the cold fire. Although the symptoms of the hot and cold fire could be similar—for instance, an area affected with the hot fire could turn gray—it was the loss of sensitivity that rang the death knell for a putrefying limb.[25]

Distinguishing between the hot and cold fires was a tricky business for surgeons, despite the differences in symptoms. The signs of the hot fire were swelling, heat, burning pain, red coloring, and a superficial putrefaction of tissue. By contrast, the cold fire was characterized by blue and black coloring, ice-coldness, a foul odor, complete lack of sensitivity, and the putrefaction of both tissue and bone.[26] Yet Fabry von Hilden was one of many authors who complained that several practitioners, especially inexperienced barber-surgeons, often confused them. He wrote that "once they call the hot fire cold, another time they call the cold fire hot, and another they call both the hot and cold fire cold or hot without distinction."[27] The profusion of names for each condition reflected this befuddlement. Fabry listed Gangraena, Phagadena, Sphacelos, Cancer, Aschachylos, Estiomenos, Ignis S. Antony, Sideratio, Putrifactio, Corruptio, Mortificatio, and Cancrena as the terms under which the two fires might appear in medical texts.[28] The lack of clarity among practitioners could lead to serious consequences for patients. As Fabry explained, practitioners "thus confuse not only the names, but rather (to the great disadvantage of patients and to their own shame) also the remedies."[29]

One major reason for these terminological mix-ups, according to Fabry, was that the conditions had the same causes, although their course and treatment differed greatly.[30] Both involved the dying away and depredation of natural warmth, and they differed only in that the process began in the hot fire and was completed in the cold fire.[31] "Natural warmth" followed the humoral theory of complexion, which dealt with a balance of elementary qualities of hot, wet, cold, and dry in the body.[32] Laurentius Lose likened bodily warmth to a burning wick in a lamp, which could be suffocated by too much oil, or exhausted when deprived of air.[33]

The number of causes given for this process of dying varied from author to author.[34] Fabry's theoretical orientation was Galenic; like many authors, he framed the issue in terms of the four humors. Treatises influenced by other perspectives could invoke similar causes, but through a different theoretical apparatus. Lose, a Paracelsian, discussed the hot and cold fires with reference to Mercury, Sulphur, and Salt, the three substances Paracelsus taught made up the body.[35] Yet Lose's understanding of the conditions was compatible with Fabry's. After addressing an inflammation of the inner, natural Sulphur in the body in relation to the hot and cold fires, he directed readers to Fabry (*Hildanus*) and repeated Fabry's categories of causes and explanations.[36] Thus the differences seen among treatises do not fall neatly into competing schools of medical thought. Surgeons drew from several sources and, when possible, their own experiences to compile all the ways the hot and cold fires arose in the body. Pinpointing the precise cause of an individual's condition was what mattered. It was the surgeon's first indication of how to treat the patient.[37]

Fabry offered three broad categories of causes. The first was a powerful and sudden change of an open and known quality such as excessive heat, cold, moisture, or dryness. Second was a hidden and unknown quality arising from within or without the body that poisoned the natural warmth and the *spiritus*. The latter referred to a substance made in the heart from inhaled air that moved through the arteries. It served as the vehicle of the vital virtue, which preserved life and could be detected in the rhythm of the heartbeat, pulse, and respiration.[38] Poisoning the *spiritus*, then, meant damaging the conduit of the very thing that maintained life. Fabry's third category was also related to the *spiritus*—specifically the constriction of its movement between the heart and the extremities through the blood vessels.[39]

The first category of causes—a powerful and sudden change of an open and known quality—was chiefly tied to extreme external temperatures that affected the internal elementary balance of the body. Excessive heat could lead to the hot fire because it distorted and dried out the natural warmth, moisture, and blood that nourished and preserved the member. Excessive cold, by contrast, not only pushed the blood back to the heart, but also froze and hardened the limb's sustenance and extinguished the natural warmth, leading to the hot or cold fire.[40] Fabry recounted a case of excessive cold from the winter of 1588, when he was practicing under the physician Jean-Antoine Sarasin and the surgeon Jean Griffon in Geneva. He treated more than fifty German riders and soldiers who suffered from the hot and cold fires after trudging through snow and wading through rivers of freezing water. Several of the patients lost legs, feet, toes, fingers, and the tips of noses and ears.[41]

The application of certain medicines could also cause extreme coldness, particularly in the treatment of gunshot wounds or other contused injuries. Warm and moist medicines promoted suppuration (creation of pus) in a wound, which was essential to healing, whereas "cold medicines" hindered this process and could cause soft tissues to die and blood to congeal, ultimately suffocating the member's natural warmth.[42] Cold medicines included opium, hemlock, nightshade, and wine vinegar.[43] Their misuse often occurred when practitioners, following the Galenic notion of curing through contraries, administered an excessive dose to counter redness, hot skin, and fever in a body exhibiting too much heat. Such an overcorrection impeded the limb's recovery and led to the cold fire. According to Fabry, the practitioner was the primary cause of the cold fire in these cases, as the misuse of medicaments turned an initial—and reversible—putrefaction of a limb into certain death.

The second category of causes came from secret qualities of unknown origins from within or without the body. Following the notion of "bad humors," these could be a kind of poisonous or sharp humor. The four humors—blood, phlegm, yellow bile, and black bile—were fluids that provided nutrition and were vital to the body's operations. They were also the vehicle of complexion, that essential balance of elementary qualities in the body unique to every individual. Bad humors usually indicated a surfeit of one of the four or a harmful secondary humor, which the practitioner needed to expel to preserve the patient's health.[44] When such a humor existed inside the body, it could potentially clump together in the blood and grow foul. This could destroy the *spiritus* and natural warmth of a limb when pushed out to the extremities through the blood vessels. An affected limb soon died. Poisonous humors might also be present in the body at the end of a rapid illness, and if they descended to the feet they could extinguish the natural warmth, destroy the harmony and well-being of a limb, and lead to the hot fire. Fabry also noted that different poxes contained poisonous humors that harmed the extremities and putrefied bones, resulting in open wounds and fistulas.[45] The outbreak of the French pox in the last decade of the fifteenth century led to a slew of specialized treatises which often included instructions for the treatment or removal of putrefied body parts.[46]

Hidden causes that operated from outside the body included the application of certain harmful drugs or venomous bites and stings. As in his discussion of excessively cold medicines, Fabry warned against treating patients with overly strong, caustic, or septic medicaments, such as arsenic, sandarac, aqua fortis, and oil of vitriol. However, the jaws and tails of creatures rather than surgeons' interventions were more commonly to blame for exposure to external toxins. The heat from a starfish's spine, the coldness of a scorpion's sting, and the dangerous complications accompanying the bites of lions, horses, wolves, and rabid dogs were all potential sources of the hot or cold fire.[47] While some surgeons treated every animal bite as poisonous, Fabry distinguished between venomous and non-venomous creatures. Wounds inflicted by a scorpion and an angry bear led to the cold fire for different reasons. A venomous creature's sting contained poison, whereas a large animal's bite crushed flesh and bone together, creating contused injuries that impeded the flow of blood and nutrients.[48]

This touches on the third and last major category of causes: the hindrance of nourishment to a particular part of the body. Contused injuries of any kind fell within this classification. In his observations, the Bamberg practitioner Georg Geelmann (d. 1672) discussed the case of a man who developed the cold fire in his thumb after it was bitten during a scuffle in which he pulled on another man's beard while sticking it in his opponent's mouth.[49] In another case, this one from Ulm in 1642, Johannes Scultetus reported an accident in which a large sack of wheat fell from a house and landed on a woman's leg as she walked by. Her femur snapped in half so that the bone protruded from the skin. She was rushed to the town hospital, where Scultetus treated her for some five months.[50] On the battlefield, gunshot wounds were an increasingly common kind of contused injury, although Fabry's main concern with the hot and cold fires arising from these wounds was the misuse of cold medicines. While some in the early sixteenth century believed that bullets and gunpowder possessed poisonous qualities that caused the cold fire, by the latter half of the seventeenth century many practitioners had rejected this idea.[51] Gehema, for instance, insisted that bullets were not poisonous, and that the hot and cold fires arose from the contusion of blood vessels and tissue alone.[52]

Fabry's third category of causes also included cases arising from shoddy or unskilled medical treatment. Practitioners who prescribed defensive medicines to treat inflammations over an extended period could deprive a limb of nourishment.[53] A more common mistake was binding a patient's limb too tightly when resetting a bone or dressing a wound. Many authors emphasized that bandages wrapped too tightly cut off a limb's nourishment and weakened it.[54] In Sebastian Greiff's *Wolbewärte Wundarzney*, the editor, Johann Mercker, devoted one of his rare annotations to admonishing readers who followed Greiff's directions on dressing wounds to loosen the cords lest they cause the limb to putrefy.[55] To illustrate a similar point, Fabry described a case from 1595 involving a servant in Cologne who fractured his arm between the hand and elbow. The hot and cold fire arose, he recalled, "because the practitioner had initially bound the fracture too tight."[56] Author-practitioners demonstrated a keen awareness of how their own actions could cause a limb to putrefy as surely as frostbite, an animal bite, a gunshot wound, or even the French pox.

The story of dying and death in a limb could have several beginnings, from a falling sack of wheat to a cold winter's night. It could also end differently depending on where a patient's condition fell within a spectrum of decay—that is, whether or not it was reversible. The close relationship between the hot and cold fires made diagnosis a difficult and time-sensitive challenge. In the many—and at times conflicting—instructions found in surgical treatises, a surgeon's experience appeared to be his key advantage. It was the inexperienced barber-surgeon, surgeon, or physician who failed to detect the nuances distinguishing the conditions, or who simply confused the appropriate terminology to describe what was occurring in a patient's body. The unseasoned practitioner could also be the cause of putrefaction through the misuse of medicaments, a botched operation, or the unskilled dressing of injuries. Authors explicitly addressed these individuals with admonitions, tales of malpractice, and detailed lists of definitions to guide a diagnosis.

The surgeon's tools at this stage were a combination of accumulated knowledge about putrefaction, gathered from texts and previous case experience, and a careful sensory analysis of the patient at hand. Through smell, the surgeon judged whether an affected limb emitted an odor and paid attention to see if it worsened over time. He distinguished between differences in the patient's tactile sensations and his own. Was a swollen area merely inflamed, or did it feel squishy? Was the flesh warm or cold against the surgeon's palm? Could the patient feel the surgeon's fingers pressing against the wound? With his eyes, the surgeon studied the patient's limb to find patterns of striated colors, ever vigilant for the appearance of a black spot. Authors offered information with which surgeons could compare and interpret sensory data, both to supplement the inexperience of young barber-surgeons until they built their own repertoire of case experience and to expand and enhance the accumulated knowledge of established practitioners. The importance of recognizing whether a patient suffered from the hot or cold fire and of pinpointing its initial cause could not be overstated. These two factors determined a patient's prognosis.[57]

Fighting fire

Once a patient was diagnosed with the hot or cold fire, the surgeon formulated a prognosis. Drawing on information from the diagnosis as well as the age, gender, and humoral characteristics unique to the patient, the surgeon determined the acuteness of the condition and forecasted how he or she would respond to treatment. Barbette emphasized the weight of this responsibility: "To recognize the outcome of wounds beforehand, especially to know which are mortal or not, is a matter of the highest necessity to the surgeon, because all too often the life of an unfortunate man depends on his judgment."[58] The surgeon tailored the course of treatment to the patient's prognosis, which was a matter of life and death.

A favorable outcome meant the eradication of the hot or cold fire from the body. This was far from a promise of a limb's restoration to its previous, healthy condition. A patient could hope for the preservation of the entire limb—soft tissue and all—if treatment began soon enough. In the later stages of hot fire, treatment involved cutting or burning away the affected flesh, which in some instances could be regrown. For the cold fire, the surgeon removed the dead flesh and shaved off the rotted bone. If it reached the marrow, then the cure required amputation.

Fabry recommended the surgeon factor three points into his prognosis: the nature of the illness, including if it was great or small and its cause; whether the patient was still strong or had already become weakened by sickness, which could be determined by the pulse; and whether the affected site lay near or far from the noble body parts and had a warm and moist, or dry and moderate quality.[59] These were standard considerations when determining a prognosis for any wound or illness. A strong patient with a small affected area located far from the noble members could be cured in a short time and with little risk.[60] The "noble parts," also called the principal parts, consisted of the brain, heart, liver, and sometimes (depending on the author) testicles or ovaries.[61] A weak patient with a large affected area located near one of these noble parts faced a lengthy treatment and risked dangerous complications.[62] As a general rule, then, the closer the hot or cold fire came to the head or torso, the more serious the patient's condition.

Authors drew from their own experiences to offer tips on making an accurate prediction of a condition's progression and the outcome of available treatments. Their recommendations could be general, such as Barbette's note that younger patients were easier to cure than elderly ones.[63] But instructions for prognoses could also be very specific when linked to particular causes. For instance, Fabry reported that a hot fire that developed from dropsy in the leg was difficult and slow to heal, and often turned into the cold fire. A hot fire caused by hidden, poisonous qualities was very dangerous and usually incurable and fatal, foremost when it developed into the cold fire. A hot fire arising from external causes—contusions, fractures, burn wounds, and so forth—was easier to cure than a cold fire, and was also less dangerous than a hot fire from internal causes. If the cold fire appeared in the skull, the patient would likely die in three days, but if the patient lived past the third day then he or she would probably recover. A cold fire that began in the lower leg or foot and climbed above the knee was usually fatal.[64] Medical practitioners could consult these guidelines to formulate and support their own prognoses.

The hot fire was a revocable dying, an incomplete putrefaction in a body part that could be reversed. The key in every case, great or small, was to cure the condition quickly. Barbette warned readers that "when one does not fend off the hot fire in good time, so it changes into the cold."[65] The surgeon's projected countdown to the cold fire's appearance was unique to the individual patient, a clock whose hands moved faster or slower according to the way the patient's elementary balance interacted with the nature (i.e. cause) and symptoms of the hot fire. Treatments provided a holistic therapy characteristic of Galenic medicine, designed to restore balance to the humors, alongside specific activities to combat the hot fire. Techniques were distinguished as universals (*Universalia*) and particulars (*Particularia*).[66]

The universals were the general measures carried out on a regular basis to maintain or improve an individual's overall health. These made up a prescribed diet, a regimen which included not only food and drink, but also sleeping and waking as well as air, work, and rest. Purgation, bloodletting, cupping, and the like were also important components of a diet. The practitioner monitored these aspects of the patient's life by considering humoral makeup, age, gender, and so forth. Practitioners also adjusted the diet to aid recovery when a patient became ill or injured. For instance, Fabry advised that when yellow, choleric humors caused a hot fire, the surgeon should avoid bloodletting altogether. A young patient afflicted with the hot fire arising from an internal hot and dry sickness should consume moist foods.[67] Adjustments made to a patient's diet, then, were intimately linked to the precise cause of the disease, along with the patient's unique characteristics.

Authors disagreed about whether a patient's diet fell under the surgeon's purview when treating putrefaction. This was indicative of the ongoing territorial debates between early modern physicians and surgeons. The extent to which physicians, who ranked above surgeons in the medical hierarchy, were brought into the surgeon's fight against the hot fire in many cases lay with the surgeon. Barbette told surgeons that while air, food, and drink should in general be dry and cool, "as however the causes [of the fire] are different, we leave it to the physician to prescribe an appropriate diet. He also will know well how to distinguish when bloodletting and purgation might be done either [to the patient's] benefit or harm."[68] Gehema also encouraged the surgeon to consult with a physician on choosing the correct medicaments.[69] Others, like Fabry and Joseph Schmid, were more willing to advise surgeons on how to prescribe and regulate a patient's diet. Their own positions in the medical hierarchy may have been a factor in their varying approaches: Barbette and Gehema were physicians, while Fabry and Schmid were surgeons. Note, however, that these matters of authority among practitioners in texts were never clear-cut. Fabry, for instance, also advised the surgeon to consult with physicians in especially difficult cases and criticized inexperienced barber-surgeons who scorned their advice.[70]

While authors may have disagreed over the physician's role in determining the universals, no one suggested that physicians should oversee the particulars of curing the hot fire. Directives to consult with members of other branches of medicine were aimed at the inexperienced practitioner who could not rely on previous observations to guide his work. The particulars included cupping, cutting, the opening of the skin of the affected body part, burning with a cautery iron or sharp and corrosive powders, and administering medicines—especially plasters and ointments—to restore the natural warmth.[71] As with the precision of altering a patient's diet within the universals, therapies to combat the hot fire within the particulars were highly specialized and intended to address not only a patient's individual complexion, but also the specific cause leading to the patient's condition. Authors could provide extensive lists of recipes of topical treatments, each designed to offset a different underlying cause.[72] A hot fire arising from hidden causes, for instance, called for the use of medicaments with hidden properties, such as theriac, a poison antidote. By contrast, in the case of a hot fire arising from a cord or bandage dressed too tightly, the surgeon was instructed to place a poultice of beans, chamomile flowers, egg, and honey over the place the cord had been wrapped, followed by leeches to help draw blood forth again.[73] Knowledge of the fire's underlying cause was critical if the surgeon were to have any hope of countering it.

When the patient's flesh turned black, blue, or greenish, but the putrefaction did not touch the bone, it was a sign that the hot fire was beginning to progress into the cold fire. At this point the goal of treatment shifted from healing an affected area to removing it entirely. The surgeon excised foul material by cutting the flesh away or by using plasters either to chemically burn off the putrefaction or to induce separation. Sebastian Greiff, an advocate of Paracelsian medicine, emphasized treating putrefaction without cutting. Among the numerous recipes his treatise offered, several involved plasters that protected the bone by promoting the division of putrefying and healthy flesh. One such plaster used colophonia (a kind of resin) and liquid myrrh, which was placed on the region where the healthy flesh met the hot fire to cause the diseased flesh to separate from the healthy. After it was removed, the practitioner induced the growth of healthy flesh in its place.[74] Practitioners could also perform treatments to separate healthy and diseased material at the earliest stage of the cold fire, when putrefaction affected only the uppermost layers of bone. The surgeon cut or burned away the rotten flesh and shaved or burned off rotted layers until he reached healthy bone.[75]

The moment a patient lost all sensitivity in the affected part, when the pain of the hot fire vanished and the cold fire reached the marrow of the bone, it was too late to save the limb. As Fabry explained, "since it is impossible to make what is already dead living again and to return it to its earlier condition, one should direct his efforts to this alone: preserving all that is still good and living."[76] In the surgeon's view, this was the pivotal moment when a limb became a zombie-like enemy. The surgeon could not bring the dead back to life, but he could try to prevent the dead from devouring the living.

"The most extreme and single remedy"

The cold fire was the complete and irrevocable death of a limb. "If, however, the cold fire has taken over the entire limb at the foot, the leg or the hand and the arm," Fabry gravely declared, "thus the most extreme and single remedy remains precisely that one cut away not only the flesh, but also the bone, meaning thus the entire limb."[77] The more serious the patient's condition appeared, the more people the surgeon drew into conversation to decide whether or not to take this most extreme measure. The patient, the patient's family and friends, and the surgeon's colleagues all played important roles in establishing the necessity of the procedure and accepting its risks. The decision to amputate was a burden shared by the community.

Surgeons were not of one mind on whether "the most extreme and single remedy" was always the correct course of action. They calculated the likelihood of a patient's survival during and after an amputation by making a second prognosis. The cold fire was fatal unless it was excised; however, depending on its location and extent, such an excision could prove futile in stopping the fire's spread. In addition, the operation could itself be lethal. The risks associated with major amputations of the upper and lower extremities were unparalleled in early modern surgery. Not only were patients in danger of shock and exsanguination during the procedure, but they faced the threat of fever, infection, and burst blood vessels afterward. In its most serious forms, such as the removal of a leg above the knee, amputation required a team of surgeons and assistants, and the results drastically altered the lives of those who survived. All of these factors contributed toward the caution with which surgeons approached the removal of a limb.

Interestingly, the severity of pain an amputation might cause did not appear to be a determining factor. When a patient's life was at stake, the surgeon focused on whether a limb's removal would successfully stop the cold fire's spread, and whether the patient would survive the operation. Pain entered the equation as part of the treatment, including the choice of amputation technique, after a prognosis was made. If the surgeon decided the operation was futile, therapy primarily focused on relieving pain.

Writers worried about whether the surgeon had the right to withhold therapy even from those whose prognosis was certain death. That the patient might die from the procedure weighed heavily in a surgeon's decision not to attempt any kind of intervention. The anatomist Girolamo Fabrizi d'Acquapendente, for instance, told readers that "in such cases I tend to say what I heard from my instructors; that it is better to let the patient die than to kill him."[78] Many authors advised readers to focus on slowing the spread of the cold fire and easing the pain of a doomed patient, advocating for a course of treatment resembling hospice care today. In his treatise, the physician

Jan Muys (1654–1720) described in detail a case in which he decided against amputating the leg of a seventy-year-old man who had contracted a venereal disease in his youth. Throughout his life he experienced cramps in his right leg, and one day they developed into a great pain in his right foot, followed by a rigidity that traveled over his knee in less than two hours. Muys suspected the cold fire and confirmed the diagnosis by scarifying the foot and finding that the patient felt no pain as black and congealed blood oozed from the shallow cuts.[79] "The cold fire had now already come a little above the knee," he recounted, "and meanwhile there was an unbearable pain above the dead parts."[80]

Muys attributed the fire's cause to the bitter fruit of an immoral life: the patient's former indulgence in prostitutes and drinking soured the sanguine humor (blood) and slowed it so that it could not be fully fermented in the heart and then properly circulated to the other parts of the body.[81] Confident in his diagnosis, Muys carefully determined a prognosis. He considered the patient's history, age, and the location of the cold fire above the knee. He judged that the patient's entire *Massa Sanguinea*—the fluid in the veins made up of pure humor blood mixed with the other three humors—was very infected. And he thought of every case of cold fire he had ever known and realized that "no elderly persons whom I knew had been afflicted with this disease had ever escaped death."[82] Muys saw no other choice. "I boldly announced the inevitable death of the invalid to those present and to the kin and friends of the patient," he wrote, "but I promised them to ease the pains as much as possible in the meantime, and if it was possible to prevent it from climbing any higher."[83] As promised, in the patient's last weeks Muys administered decoctions for his pain and applied topical medicines to slow the cold fire's spread. The patient, whom Muys first visited on 26 February, died on 14 March 1681.[84]

To justify his decision to readers, Muys explained the soundness of his judgement. Not only would the patient have been unlikely to survive an amputation, but also the right leg's removal would not have completely excised the cold fire. He reported its appearance in the left foot and both hands in the patient's final days, which he took as proof that all of the blood was infected and would have continued to spread it even if the leg had been amputated.[85] As a Cartesian medical reformer,[86] Muys's concern with the circulation of the blood is apparent throughout his discussion of the case. It plays a pivotal role in his reasoning in the diagnosis, prognosis, and defense of his treatment. Yet even though he was not working strictly within a Galenic framework, his resulting caution toward the risk of a thigh amputation fits comfortably alongside the examples given by practitioners like Fabry von Hilden.

The need Muys felt to reassure the reader that his decision was correct betrays a certain disquiet, an uneasiness that at times led others to give contradictory instructions. The work of Girolamo Fabrizi's own pupil, Johannes Scultetus, provides one such example. In his discussion of amputation in his *Wund-Artzneyisches Zeug-Hauß*, he began by echoing his mentor. If someone was so weak in strength that the surgeon knew "when such an operation would be performed on the patient, he would not only fall into a heart-palsy, but would even die during the cutting: thus then in such a dangerous case and circumstance the removal of the limb should rightly be avoided."[87] Scultetus offered compelling logic for the surgeon to stay his hand in risky cases. It was much better not to lend a hand, or at least to carry out all operations cautiously and thoughtfully, "than when one knowingly kills the patient by means of them."[88] His advice appears simple enough, as does his warning that performing the operation in such dangerous circumstances is akin to intentionally killing a person. Yet, as though unsatisfied, he pressed the matter further by raising a question: "When however there is no hope for the patient to remain alive unless the dead limb is removed by cutting, what then should a respectable and diligent surgeon do in such a case?"[89] Despite his own initial warning to avoid amputation in these circumstances, he ultimately concluded that the surgeon could not abandon a patient to the cold fire's clutches. He implored the reader to prepare the patient with oral and topical medicines to expel harmful vapors and refresh the vital spirit. At that point, it was time to include all those present in the room and face unflinchingly what was to come next:

> When the patient has subsequently improved a little (because to hold off the amputation until he regains his full powers would in truth just be to wait for his certain death), then the surgeon should indicate to those present beforehand what danger the patient is in, [and] thereupon carry out the necessary and required operation with a dauntless mind: because it is certainly better that one ... seize on this doubtful, indeed pitiful, method of cure, than to let the patient die completely helpless.[90]

The instructions Scultetus gave to communicate with "those present" (*denen Umbstehenden*) hint at the first step in a social process leading to an amputation: a series of careful discussions held between the surgeon and the patient, and the surgeon and the patient's family and friends. It was crucial to convey all of the specifics of a patient's condition, including its initial cause. "Such knowledge," Fabry informed readers, "is necessary for the surgeon not only on the ground that he can prevent future incidents as much as possible, but also so that the patient and his kin have all the more hope in, trust in, and dedication to him, because they see that he correctly understands his affairs and art."[91] It was of course necessary to secure the patient's permission to undertake an operation, no matter how dire the situation. Fabry recounted a case in which the failure to gain such consent had fatal consequences. In 1587, a barber-surgeon in Geneva botched the bloodletting of a healthy patient's arm, which soon grew swollen and hot until the cold fire appeared around the incision site. The physicians called to examine him recommended the arm's immediate removal. The patient refused to let them amputate, however, and the cold fire subsequently spread to his shoulder. He died several days later.[92]

The surgeon had to walk a line between addressing the patient honestly and keeping up morale, which was essential for good health. He could speak more bluntly with those close to the patient. Fabry explained that "because however not all illnesses are curable, it is therefore necessary for the surgeon, that he explain himself to the patient's kin, what course the disease will take and what outcome it will have."[93] Treatises warned practitioners against overly optimistic prognoses in order to protect them from accusations of malpractice. Barbette even advised readers to eschew openly declaring a prognosis altogether for certain medical cases—those that were known to display dangerous and unforeseeable turns which could be blamed erroneously on the surgeon instead of on the disease itself.[94]

The patient's family and friends could be the surgeon's greatest allies in moving forward. Those who received the hard news that a limb was irrevocably dead could remain in stubborn and terrified denial until family, friends, and even pastors swayed them not only to acknowledge the reality of their illness, but also to accept the necessity of an operation. The imagination of earlier pain or the fear of amputation could cause the patient to pretend to feel pain in a dead limb.[95] This, coupled with cases in which the patient still had the ability to wiggle fingers and toes, could make winning over the social circle a difficult task.

The surgeon had to convince the patient's family and friends that a limb was completely dead, at times despite what the patient said. Once again it was crucial that the surgeon be able to convey the intricacies of the cold fire, this time to help those present see past the appearance of life in a dead limb. Fingers and toes could retain movement for a long period—some four or five days—after the final death of a hand or a foot.[96] If the surgeon delayed the amputation until movement was lost entirely, the fire would spread in the meantime and destroy even more of the patient's body. Rather than relying on words alone, Fabry recommended that the surgeon perform a demonstration:

> [I]t is very necessary, that the practitioner instruct the friends and relatives about this and make it clear to them. ... Therefore he should prick and cut into the toes or fingers with a knife (without the patient seeing it) and thereby convince the friends that there is no more life present, [and] thus the amputation must necessarily occur.[97]

The surgeon devised a scenario in which members of the patient's social circle could witness for themselves that the patient, despite his or her protests to the contrary, felt no pain in the dead limb. A similar test of sensitivity, performed while the patient could not see the surgeon's hand, could be found in cases of leprosy.⁹⁸ However, there was a fundamental difference in the performance and function of Fabry's demonstration: his was a public display to convince the patient's family and friends, not a diagnostic tool for the practitioner to use in private. This was a shared act of witnessing that was crucial in shifting the surrounding group's perception of the state of the patient's body and how that body should be acted upon.

The exchange between the surgeon and the patient's social circle was the first step toward sanctioning an amputation. The second major step was a consultation with other practitioners to ensure that the procedure was not done precipitously. In his *Feld-Medicus*, Gehema was critical of field-surgeons who acted too hastily. He morbidly observed that there were some so quick with the saw that it was "as though they had a particular pleasure in robbing someone of his limbs."⁹⁹ To prevent such abuses, he warned that amputation was an "extremity" to which "a field-surgeon rightly should not proceed before he has consulted the field-doctor about it, unless the condition of the wound requires a complete and swift extirpation."¹⁰⁰

The small number of physicians typically assigned to an army made Gehema's instructions problematic in practice. High-ranking officers could bring retinues of practitioners with them, but common soldiers had less access to trained care. Gehema complained that one physician was hired to look after an army of twenty thousand to thirty thousand men, while several incompetent field-surgeons—or "barbers" (*Barthscherer*), as he pejoratively called the worst of them—were assigned to individual companies and regiments. He suggested that every army should have at the very least three physicians: one for the cavalry and artillery, and two for the infantry.¹⁰¹ Given that, even then, an army of tens of thousands *might* have three physicians available for consultation, the practicality of demanding that field-surgeons consistently confer with physicians seems questionable. This put surgeons in an awkward predicament. On the one side, they could be found liable for proceeding prematurely because they did not consult a physician. On the other side, they could be reprimanded for waiting too long because they had delayed the procedure until a consultation could take place.

Rules were much stricter in urban environments, since local guilds and municipal authorities passed laws to exert some supervision over amputation. In Munich the town council decreed that barber-surgeons and surgeons were forbidden to remove "an entire limb, neither a hand nor foot, outside of the foreknowledge, advice and counsel of the physicians."¹⁰² Many hospitals, such as those in Augsburg, imposed similar consultation requirements when an amputation was deemed necessary.¹⁰³ Rules for peer-regulation were also common, as with the barber-surgeon guild in Cologne, where a joint examination by no less than four barber-surgeons was required before an amputation could take place.¹⁰⁴

68 *The malleable body*

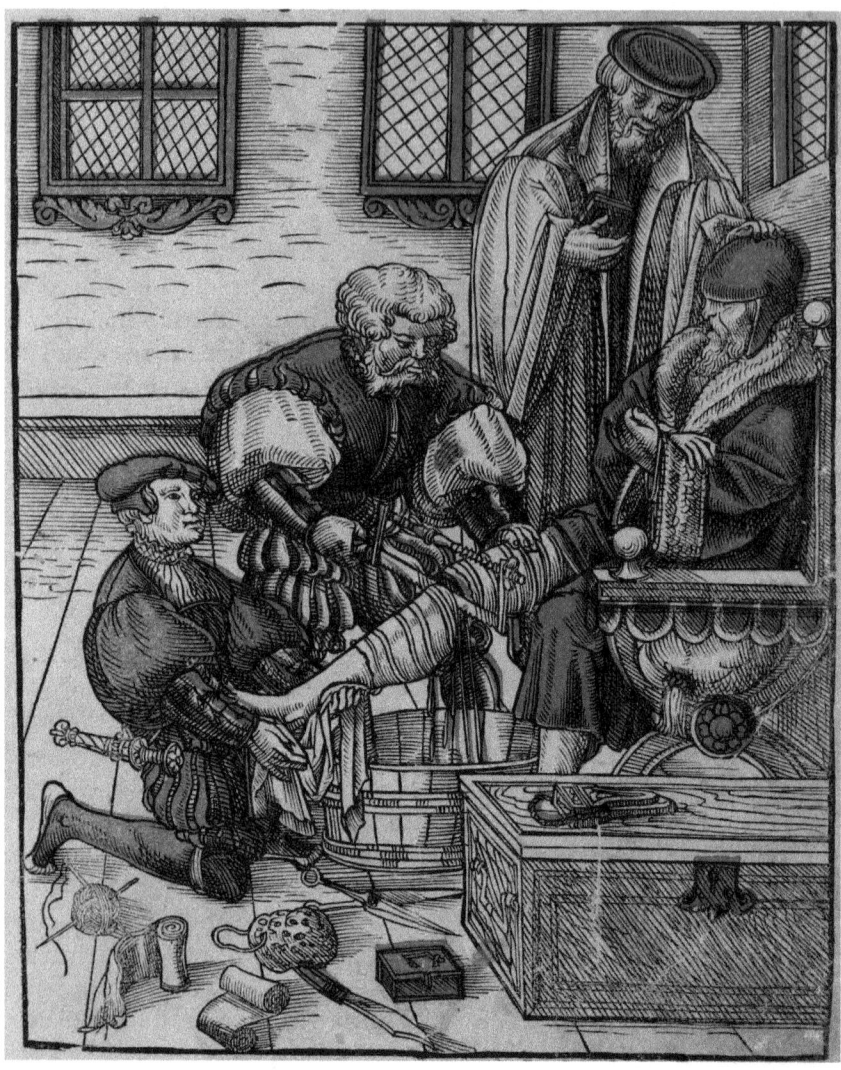

2.1 Leg amputation in Walther Hermann Ryff, *Die groß Chirurgei* (Frankfurt am Main, 1545), title page (detail).

The decision to amputate was ideally one of gathered consensus. A woodcut from Walther Ryff's *Die groß Chirurgei* presents readers with a model of harmony among practitioners when undertaking the procedure (figure 2.1).[105] At the top right, standing above the patient with long robes and a book, is the physician, who rests one hand on the patient's head. To the left of the physician and leaning over the patient's leg is the surgeon, who with a large saw in hand is busy with his task: amputation of the lower leg at the knee. At the patient's foot—and the end of the hierarchical chain linking the performers—is the surgeon's youthful assistant, who obediently holds the lower half of the patient's leg in place while looking uncomfortably off into the distance.

The woodcut conveys a professional hierarchy governing the process of a limb's removal, drawn along a diagonal line that begins with the physician on the upper right and slants downward to the surgeon's assistant on the lower left. The patient strengthens the impression of the diagonal, as his upper body leans back while one leg stretches out at a downward angle. The patient's body connects the three practitioners and reinforces the hierarchical relationship among them as they touch his head, leg, and foot. The patient does not appear particularly uncomfortable: he is not held down or bound to the chair as blood from his leg drips into the wooden tub. With his hat pulled low over his eyes and arms crossed, the patient might even be sleeping. Indeed, there has been speculation that the sponge depicted on the floor is the controversial "sleeping sponge" authors like Heinrich von Pfolspeundt and Hans von Gersdorff described.[106] The tranquil atmosphere of the room contributes to an idealized portrait of agreement and collaboration among surgeons and physicians. The image presents a model operation in which each participant knows his place, and it suggests that the success of the procedure depends upon all involved knowing their roles and cooperating to perform them correctly.

The ordering of the figures not only indicates the authority of the physician over the surgeon, and this procedure, but also presents the roles that distinguish their two branches of medicine in the early modern period. The physician stands holding his book while the surgeon quite literally gets his hands dirty. Viewers are presented with an assortment of surgical equipment: a large chest for instruments with a small carrying case set atop it, scissors, thread and needles, a sponge, rolls of bandages, and a curved knife, not to mention the large bow-saw in the surgeon's hands. Ryff's woodcut is didactic, presenting harmony among medical practitioners as they all work toward a successful operation, illustrating the separate tasks of the physician and the surgeon, and advertising the tools of the surgeon's trade.

The responsibility for amputating a limb was shared among multiple practitioners. Case observations and the instructions of surgical treatises suggest that in severe circumstances, surgeons generally preferred to confer beforehand with peers. Similar to the hot fire, authors also advised consulting physicians when surgeons dealt with the universals of treatment. But the inclusion of the physician in Ryff's woodcut reveals collaboration between physician and surgeon on a matter more urgent than squabbles over the right to prescribe a patient's diet. The single remedy for the cold fire was a rare occasion in which the physician was given ultimate authority over the *particulars* of a surgeon's course of treatment. In theory, the radical nature of an amputation invited the physician into the surgeon's undisputed domain of manual operations. Only after a professional consensus was reached was the surgeon to proceed.

In cases of the cold fire, the surgeon's decision-making shifted from a self-contained process to a collective effort involving several others. This transition underscored the gravity of an amputation. The consequences of prematurely removing a limb, or of doing so incompetently, were dangerous and permanent. Unlike a poorly treated dislocation or a fracture that could be re-set, an amputated leg could not be sewn back on. Besides the danger of blood loss and excruciating pain during the procedure, the potential impact on a patient's quality of life was even more troubling to surgeons. Gehema bemoaned the future of the amputee soldier, for "he [who] loses an arm or leg in his master's service, and is shot lame, so for the most part a pair of crutches and beggary are his consolation and recompense."[107] He warned surgeons of the moral and professional ramifications of a rash procedure. He used strong rhetoric in a pointed effort to arouse and exploit readers' emotions. In a direct appeal, he exhorted them not to "hasten and rush with such a removal of the limb … since otherwise your conscience burdens you, you take on yourself a great responsibility from God and men, and you destroy [your] own honor and reputation."[108] The risks to the patient's life and the surgeon's own career were powerful motivations for practitioners to initiate conversations within the community.

A final step in constructing group consensus was a shared performance of securing spiritual approval and support. Gehema's warnings about the plight of amputee soldiers assumed that patients would survive the procedure. It is likely the vast majority did not.[109] The incredible danger patients faced called for spiritual preparation and divine aid. When describing one case in 1614, for instance, Fabry wrote that "after I called upon God for his aid, in the presence of Master Jacob Goulartius, minister of God, and still many others, I cut off the leg in the femur."[110] References to prayer and the presence of pastors—as seen in the case of Stephan Toppinus in this chapter's introduction—suggest their importance in completing the process of gathering consensus. Prayer before an amputation appears in the earliest printed surgical treatises. In 1517, Gersdorff advised the surgeon to hear Mass beforehand, and to encourage the patient to say confession and receive the Holy Sacrament. Nearly two hundred years and a Reformation and Counter-Reformation later, the Protestant Matthäus Purmann agreed that celebrating the Lord's Supper the evening before an amputation was always beneficial for the patient.[111] Concern for obtaining divine support transcended confessional divides.

The inclusion of prayer within technical instructions was unusual in surgical texts. Introductory chapters on the qualities of a good surgeon, a tradition in medical writing reaching back to antiquity, often elaborated on the surgeon's dependence on God as the Divine Physician and emphasized the piety essential to elicit God's assistance in healing his Christian neighbors.[112] However, in chapters dedicated to manual operations, instructions to assemble the surgeon and his assistants with a pastor, patient, and patient's family for prayer were almost exclusively confined to cases of amputation. Purmann, for example, entwined clinical instruction with consolation and piety in the set of tasks he gave readers to complete before the removal of a leg:

> [L]et the patient—in the presence of the pastor, so that he can comfort him—sit on a comfortable spot, or, what is much better, on a sturdy chair, so that one can walk around him, tie him tight and immobile thereupon, or have your assistants hold him sufficiently, so that he cannot hinder you in the operation; ... As soon as this is done, you and the pastor together with those present can once again through the Lord's Prayer call upon merciful God for [His] assistance and blessing for a desired and favorable operation, so that everything may proceed all the more successfully ... because everyone knows, that without the assistance of the supreme Physician nothing useful and fruitful can be achieved; And thereupon with a necessary prudence and fearlessness accompanied by such assistance, proceed.[113]

Once the patient was firmly tied to a chair or bed, those present came together to pray for the operation's success. The knowledge that God was taking part in the procedure inspired the "fearlessness" Purmann described as necessary for the surgeon to perform it.

Joseph Schmid made prayer the first stage of preparation for the removal of a limb. "Firstly one should have the patient give himself to God, to gain from God the best outcome," he wrote in his *Instrumenta chirurgica*, and "every instrument should also be in readiness beforehand, as namely scissors, knives, saws."[114] Schmid was even more emphatic about the importance of obtaining God's blessing in his *Examen chirurgicum*, intended to train young barber-surgeons and surgeons. The treatise, presented in question-and-answer form, addressed the removal of a limb as follows:

> 270th Question:
>
> However [if] the limb may not be preserved, and by necessity must be cut in half, how would you wish to do it, and to heal the limb?
>
> Answer:
>
> To remove arms and legs is a serious thing, and in need of great consideration. Hence, should I remove a limb, I would want firstly to have the patient furnished with the reverend Sacrament after the Christian custom, in order that God might grant all the more grace to me to perform the work, and to the patient to endure.[115]

Schmid trained apprentices and young surgeons to obtain God's blessing for the procedure before beginning any other preparations, including readying instruments. Nowhere else in his thorough examination treatise, spanning over five hundred pages and addressing every aspect of surgery, did Schmid include instructions of this kind.[116]

By the time an amputation took place, a number of people had already come together to help validate the surgeon's decision. The dialogues intended to affirm the chosen course of action reached their climax with group prayer. The language surgeons often used to refer to those in this moment was *Umbstehende* or *die Umbstehenden*—those standing in a ring.[117] This chain of individuals who stood around the patient was formed link by link as the surgeon drew them into conversation about the cold fire. These were family members and friends (*die Familie, die Angehörigen, die Verwandten, die Freunde*), the pastor (*der Prediger*), the surgeon's assistants (*deine Leute*) or medical student (*der Artzney Candidatus*), in select circumstances the physician (*der Medicus*), and even the surgeon's wife (*seine Hausfrau*). Together, those who made up this ring sought God's support as the Supreme Physician, securing a final group consensus for the operation.

The decision to amputate

Stephan Toppinus never reached the operating bench because his social circle and the medical practitioner treating him never reached a consensus. That the refusal to operate came from the surgeon rather than the patient in this case suggests the caution with which practitioners approached amputation. Indeed, the frequency with which the procedure was carried out in practice is difficult to ascertain. Statistical evidence of such operations and resulting survival rates in Europe do not begin until the eighteenth and nineteenth centuries.[118] However, with the spread of gunpowder warfare, early modern field-surgeons increasingly encountered mangled limbs and contused injuries requiring amputation. These new circumstances at the turn of the sixteenth century were the initial catalyst for experimentation and discussion of limb removal, and the battlefield's importance as a means to gain firsthand experience with invasive surgical procedures only grew over the following two centuries. In civilian practice, the frequency of amputations varied by practitioner and by context. Gersdorff claimed that he had performed between one hundred and two hundred amputations in Strasbourg, particularly in the Antonite hospital dedicated to patients suffering from St. Anthony's Fire.[119] Surgeons treating patients with the French Disease, such as those in specialized pox hospitals, probably also performed amputations at a higher rate than others. Despite complaints of precipitous procedures, surgical literature suggests practitioners generally erred on the side of caution.

A diagnosis of the cold fire launched a series of intense discussions between the surgeon and the patient's circle about how to treat a fatal condition whose only cure was an invasive and risky surgical intervention that, if successful, permanently altered the body. Ryff's woodcut shows order and harmony (figure 2.1), but authors insisted that surgeons had to work to build solidarity through dialogues, demonstrations, and group prayer. Why were surgeons so emphatic about completing this process before proceeding to amputate? Surgeries, and amputations in particular, were messy; they were fraught with mistakes and unforeseen disasters. Fabry recorded one instance of near-disaster in his *Lithotomia Vesicae*, a treatise on bladder stones:

> [A]lthough the patient be tied down sufficiently, at the same time [there] must be arranged several hearty men, who can hold him, so that he not throw himself here and there, and hinder the practitioner in his work. This happened to me once in Payerne, when I was cutting off the leg of a forty-year-old man, and was about to grab the saw and cauteries, then—as the patient began to shout loudly—everyone fled, except my eldest son, who at the time was still a young boy, and [had been] directed to hold the bound lower leg (for the sake of form). If my wife, who at that time was large with child, and was in another room, had not run hither, and gripped and held the patient by the chest, the patient would have fallen into danger, and I with him.[120]

Fabry describes a moment of utter panic in the middle of an amputation.[121] The patient, who has already endured the cutting of flesh on his thigh and waits with a portion of his femur exposed to the open air, begins to scream. The circle of individuals assembled to support the operation disintegrates in terror. We see the tranquil atmosphere of Ryff's woodcut unravel into chaos: people bolt at the sound of the patient's cries, a nervous young boy whose role should have been largely ceremonial is left to hold the lower leg, and a very pregnant woman throws her weight on the chest of a thrashing patient so that her husband can begin to saw. Panic, as Fabry shows, was an ever-present danger lurking at the edges of an operation, threatening to break down order and throw the lives of the participants into peril. This was why the negotiating process surgeons undertook before an amputation was so crucial: it converted *Umbstehende* from bystanders into much-needed assistants. The strength of the circle forged during the dialogues among practitioners, patients, and families made the difference between cooperation and catastrophe.

Reaching a collective decision about amputation operated on several levels. From the surgeon's perspective, it protected him from accusations of carrying out the procedure without sufficient cause or performing it unsatisfactorily. The patient could assess the necessity of the operation in discussions with trusted members of his or her community, hearing from many voices other than the surgeon's. Friends and family, meanwhile, were prepared for the danger and adversity their loved one faced and could use this information in turn to prepare and support the patient before, during, and after the procedure. On an even larger scale, reaching a consensus allayed a general social worry about surgical dismemberment. Authorities in the patient's community—whether a transient military camp or a major urban center—took upon themselves the duty of ensuring that amputation remained a last resort.

Participating in dialogues also created the mindset needed to successfully carry out an amputation. Achieving group consensus banished doubt, bolstered confidence, and checked fear. Scultetus emphasized that the surgeon must proceed "with a dauntless mind," knowing that he was making the best possible decision even when his patient would likely die during the operation.[122] Fabry's insistence that the surgeon explain the cold fire to the patient's kin was intended not only to educate them, but also to inspire hope, trust, and confidence in the procedure and the surgeon's ability to perform it.[123] Sharing the burden of the decision in a series of conversations gradually built a mental state that authors considered necessary for the surgeon and those around him.

The journey to the operating bench reveals broad aspects of early modern medicine as well as features unique to amputation. The principles of diagnosis, the value of previous experience in determining a prognosis, and territorial battles between surgeons and physicians, for example, reflect major points of discussion and practice within surgery more generally. The concepts of the hot and cold fires posed a particularly difficult set of challenges for surgeons because they were often intertwined. Once the cold fire was diagnosed, the surgeon's decision-making process became increasingly collective. Consensus was not always, and certainly not easily, reached. The entry of the surgeon's medical reasoning into social exchange initiated a process of deliberation with unpredictable and at times hostile results. Amputation was a communal event. The burden of its consequences was shared. To some extent, this temporary community was an unusually intense example of the group consultation that occurred in many forms of early modern medical practice, such as childbirth and lying in.

But it also reveals unique concerns. Surgical dismemberment was a desperate and extraordinary measure that resulted in irreversible change. The weight of this transformation pressed early moderns to articulate with fervor and clarity, on multiple levels and from many perspectives, the need for consensus. A patient suffering from the cold fire became the point of intersection in a Venn diagram of overlapping groups: medical, familial, spiritual, and even legal. Amputation took place when the representatives of these different circles reached a collective decision, when they came together to stand in a ring around the patient, prepared to radically and irrevocably alter the shape of the patient's body.

Notes

1 Hildanus, *Wund-Artzney*, 201–202.
2 Ibid., 202: "solcher wüttige/ grausam erschröckliche Brand/ dergleichen ich vor nie gesehen." On Horst: Sachs, *Geschichte*, 4:78.
3 Hildanus, *Wund-Artzney*, 202–203.
4 For a broad treatment: Jütte, *Ärzte, Heiler und Patienten*. For an example of physicians: Schilling and Jankrift, "Medical Practice in Context."
5 Stein, *Negotiating the French Pox*; Strocchia, *Forgotten Healers*, 179–216; Shaw and Welch, *Making and Marketing Medicine*, 81–104; Kosmin, *Authority, Gender, and Midwifery*.
6 Barbette, *Schrifften*, 77: "Dieweil ein erstorbenes Glied dem Leib gantz nichts mehr nutz ist/ als muß man es abnehmen/ damit es andere nahe gelegene Theile nicht anstecke."
7 Gehema, *Feld-Medicus*, 43.
8 Lose and Greiff, *Hand-Büchlein*, 129: "Wann man diesen Sach eigendlich nachdencken wil/ so ist der heisse und kalte Brand eines oder mehrern Theile Absterben und Tod/ und solches kan abgetheilt werden in den Anfang/ Fortgang/ und völligen Ausgang." Lose's discussion is an extended annotation.
9 Barbette, *Schrifften*, 132–133; Herls, *Examen*, 554–555; Purmann, *Chirurgia curiosa*, 637–638.
10 E.g., Paré, *Wund-Artzney* (1635), 415. On St. Anthony's Fire, see Kirkup, *Limb Amputation*, 16–17.
11 I use three German editions: the 1593 (*Gangraena et Sphacelo*), the 1603 (*Gründlicher Bericht*), and the edition published in the 1652 compilation of Fabry's works (*Wund-Artzney*).
12 There were exceptions. See Munnicks, *Praxis Cheirurgica*, 124; Herls, *Examen*, 444.
13 Barbette, *Schrifften*, 87.
14 Fabry is generally accurate about Galen's teaching on this subject. For an introduction to and translation of *De tumoribus praeter naturam*: Lytton and Resuhr, "Galen on Abnormal Swellings," esp. 546.
15 Hildanus, *Gründlicher Bericht*, 30–31.
16 Ryff, *Die groß Chirurgei*, 2r.
17 Barbette, *Schrifften*, 87–155: "Von den Geschwulsten."
18 Hildanus, *Gründlicher Bericht*, 31: "eiskalt und tot."
19 Ibid., 30: "ausfressen," "nagen." See also DeMaitre, *Medieval Medicine*, 99.
20 Hildanus, *Gründlicher Bericht*, 30–31; Ryff, *Die groß Chirurgei*, 2r.
21 Herls, *Examen*, 555. Barbette added that in the last stage, an affected area could turn black: *Schrifften*, 193.
22 Ryff, *Die groß Chirurgei*, 66v. For a detailed etymology: Diab, *Lexicon of Orthopaedic Etymology*, 319.
23 Hildanus, *Gründlicher Bericht*, 31; Ryff, *Die groß Chirurgei*, 2r.
24 Hildanus, *Gründlicher Bericht*, 31–32.

25 Ibid., 32; Herls, *Examen*, 555. Compare to Franz Joël (1508–1579), who used degrees of sensitivity loss to distinguish the cold fire from a dead limb: *Chirurgia oder Wund-Artzney*, 86.
26 Purmann, *Wund-Artzney* (1692), 3:210.
27 Hildanus, *Gründlicher Bericht*, 32: "Sie nennen einmal den heißen Brand kalt, ein anderes Mal den kalten Brand heiß, wieder andere aber sowohl den heißen als auch den kalten Brand ohne Unterschied kalt oder heiß."
28 Hildanus, *De Gangraena et Sphacelo*, 3. Barbette added Necrosis to the list: *Schrifften*, 132.
29 Hildanus, *Gründlicher Bericht*, 32: "verwechseln also nicht nur die Namen, sondern (zum großen Nachteil der Kranken und zu ihrer eigenen Schande) auch die Heilmittel."
30 Ibid.
31 Hildanus, *De Gangraena et Sphacelo*, 7.
32 Siraisi, *Medieval and Early Renaissance Medicine*, 101–102. The natural "warmth" is usually referred to as "heat" in English scholarship, but the early modern German terminology distinguishes between "Hitz," the external element, and "Wärm," the elementary quality within the body.
33 Lose and Greiff, *Hand-Büchlein*, 129–130. A burning flame was a well-established metaphor for the body's innate heat in Western medical literature: Siraisi, *Medieval and Early Renaissance Medicine*, 103.
34 E.g., Barbette, *Schrifften*, 193; Purmann, *Wund-Artzney* (1692), 3:211–217; Fabricius ab Aquapendente, *Wund-Artznei*, 1:128.
35 Lose and Greiff, *Hand-Büchlein*, 127. See also discussion of the cold fire by Johann Agricola (1589–1643), another follower of Paracelsus: *Wund-Artzney*, 507–520.
36 Lose and Greiff, *Hand-Büchlein*, 128.
37 Hildanus, *Gründlicher Bericht*, 78.
38 Siraisi, *Medieval and Early Renaissance Medicine*, 101, 107–108.
39 Hildanus, *Gründlicher Bericht*, 35–36.
40 Hildanus, *De Gangraena et Sphacelo*, 8, 12.
41 Hildanus, *Gründlicher Bericht*, 46–47. See also Hildanus, *Wund-Artzney*, 211.
42 Hildanus, *Gründlicher Bericht*, 41.
43 Hildanus, *De Gangraena et Sphacelo*, 12. See also Barbette on discutient medicines: *Schrifften*, 193.
44 Siraisi, *Medieval and Early Renaissance Medicine*, 104–106.
45 Hildanus, *Wund-Artzney*, 1012.
46 E.g., Renner, *Handtbüchlein* (1559). On the problematic association between the French pox and modern syphilis, see Arrizabalaga et al., *Great Pox*.
47 Hildanus, *Wund-Artzney*, 1012–1013.
48 Ibid.
49 Gelman, *Dreyfache Chyrurgische Blumen*, 458.
50 Scultetus, *Wund-Artzneyisches Zeug-Hauß* (1666), 2:179.
51 DeVries, "Military Surgical Practice," 140–142.
52 Gehema, "Wunden der Soldaten," 744.
53 Hildanus, *Wund-Artzney*, 1014.

54 Scultetus, *Wund-Artzneyisches Zeug-Hauß* (1666), 1:251. For a contrary example: Bontekoe, *Newes Gebäw*, 378.
55 Greiff, *Wolbewärte Wundarzney*, 21.
56 Hildanus, *Gründlicher Bericht*, 67: "Da der Arzt den Bruch anfänglich zu fest verbunden hatte."
57 Ibid., 78.
58 Barbette, *Schrifften*, 157: "Den Außgang der Wunden vorher zu erkennen/ insonderheit wissen/ welche tödtlich seyen/ oder nicht/ ist eine Sache/ die einem Wundärtzt höchst nöthig ist; dann an seinem Urtheil hanget zum öfftern das Leben eines unglücklichen Mannes."
59 Hildanus, *Gründlicher Bericht*, 70.
60 Hildanus, *Wund-Artzney*, 1021.
61 Barbette, *Schrifften*, 220. See also Siraisi, *Medieval and Early Renaissance Medicine*, 107.
62 Hildanus, *Wund-Artzney*, 1021.
63 Barbette, *Schrifften*, 134.
64 Hildanus, *Wund-Artzney*, 1021–1022, and *Gründlicher Bericht*, 72.
65 Barbette, *Schrifften*, 134: "Wann man dem heissen Brand nicht bey Zeiten wehret/ so verendert er sich in den kalten."
66 Hildanus, *Gründlicher Bericht*, 75.
67 Hildanus, *Wund-Artzney*, 1023, and *Gründlicher Bericht*, 76.
68 Barbette, *Schrifften*, 135: "Dieweil aber die Ursachen hier unterschiedlich sind/ als überlassen wir es dem *Medico*, eine dienliche Lebens-Ordnung vorzuschreiben; welcher auch wohl wird zu unterscheiden wissen/ wann das Aderlassen und Purgieren entweder mit Nutzen oder Schaden möchte vorgenommen werden."
69 Gehema, "Wunden der Soldaten," 742–743.
70 Hildanus, *Gründlicher Bericht*, 29.
71 Hildanus, *Wund-Artzney*, 1023.
72 E.g., Barbette, *Schrifften*, 136–140.
73 Hildanus, *Wund-Artzney*, 1041, 1043.
74 Lose and Greiff, *Hand-Büchlein*, 55–58. See also Herls, *Examen*, 561.
75 Hildanus, *Gründlicher Bericht*, 115–116.
76 Ibid., 114: "Da es aber unmöglich ist, das schon Abgestorbene wieder lebendig zu machen und es in seinen früheren Zustand zurückzubringen, soll man seine Bemühungen allein darauf richten, alles das zu erhalten, was noch gut und lebendig ist."
77 Ibid., 117: "Ist aber der kalte Brand am Fuß, am Schenkel oder an der Hand und dem Arm und er hat die ganze Gliedmaße eingenommen, so bleibt als äußerstes und einziges Mittel nichts anderes, als daß man nicht nur das Fleisch, sondern auch den Knochen, das heißt also die ganze Gliedmaße, wegschneidet."
78 Fabricius ab Aquapendente, *Wund-Artznei*, 2:297: "Dann in solchem Fall pflegte ich zu sagen/ was ich von meinen Praeceptorn gehöret; daß es besser sey/ man lasse den Krancken sterben/ als daß man ihn umb bringe."
79 Muys, *Praxis*, 27–28.

80 Ibid., 31: "Der Kaltebrand war nun schon biß übers Knie gekommen/ und indessen war über dem abgestorbenen Theile ein unerträglicher Schmertz."
81 Ibid., 29.
82 Ibid., 31: "keine Alten den Tod entgangen waren/ welche ich wuste/ die jemahls mit dieser Kranckheit befallen waren."
83 Ibid.: "habe ich denen Umstehenden und Freunden des Patienten den unaußbleiblichen Tod des Krancken kühnlich angesaget/ wobey ich ihnen aber versprochen unterdeß die Schmertzen so viel möglich zu lindern/ und wo es seyn könte zu verhindern/ daß es nicht höher hinauff stiege."
84 Ibid., 33.
85 Ibid.
86 See Munt, "Dutch Cartesian Medical Reformers," 88–91.
87 Scultetus, *Wund-Artzneyisches Zeug-Hauß* (1666), 1:206: "wann solche Operation mit dem Patienten vorgenommen würde / er darüber nit allein in eine Hertz-Ohnmacht fallen/ sondern unter wärendem Schnitt gar sterben werde: da solle dann in einem so gefährlichen Fall und Zustand die ablösung deß Gliedes billich vermitten bleiben."
88 Ibid.: "als vermittelst derselben/ den Patienten wissentlich umb das Leben bringet."
89 Ibid.: "Wann aber keine Hoffnung zu haben/ daß der Patient beym Leben bleiben könte/ es seye dann/ daß das erstorbene Glied durch den Schnitt abgelöset werde/ was solle alsdann ein ehrlicher und Gewissenhaffter Chirurgus in solchem Fall thun?"
90 Ibid.: "Wann sich nun der Patient hierauff ein wenig erholet hat/ (dann da man biß zu widererlangung seiner vollkommenen Kräfften mit dem Schnitt inhalten wolte/ wäre in Warheit solches nichts anders/ als auff seinen gewißen Todt warten) da solle der Chirurgus, in was Gefahr der Patient schwebe/ denen Umbstehenden vorher anzeigen/ darauff die nothwendig-erforderte Operation mit unerschrockenem Gemüth vornehmen: dann es ja besser ist/ daß man ... dieses zweiffelhaffte/ ja erbärmliche Hand-Mittel ergreiffe/ als daß man den Patienten gar Hülffloß sterben lasse."
91 Hildanus, *Gründlicher Bericht*, 69: "Solches Wissen ist dem Wundarzt nicht nur aus dem Grunde nötig, damit er künftigen Vorfällen soviel wie möglich vorbeugen kann, sondern auch damit der Kranke und seine Angehörigen desto mehr Hoffnung, Vertrauen und Zuneigung zu ihm haben, weil sie sehen, daß er seine Sachen und die Kunst recht versteht."
92 Ibid., 40.
93 Ibid., 69: "Weil aber nicht alle Krankheiten heilbar sind, ist dem Wundarzt doch nötig, daß er den Angehörigen des Kranken selbst erklärt, welchen Verlauf die Krankheit nehmen und welchen Ausgange sie haben wird."
94 Barbette, *Schrifften*, 221.
95 Hildanus, *Gründlicher Bericht*, 68–69.
96 Ibid., 68.
97 Ibid., 68–69: "ist es sehr nötig, daß der Arzt die Freunde und Verwandten davon unterrichtet und es ihnen klar verständlich macht. ... Deshalb soll er mit einem

Schermesser in die Zehen oder die Finger stechen und schneiden (ohne daß der Kranke es sieht) und damit die Freunde sicher machen, daß kein Leben mehr vorhanden ist, die Abtrennung also notwendigerweise geschehen muß."
98 E.g., Wallis, *Medieval Medicine*, 343.
99 Gehema, *Feld-Medicus*, 43: "als wann sie ein sonderbahres Plaisir darin hätten/ einem seiner Glieder zu berauben."
100 Ibid.: "Zu welcher *Extremität* aber ein Feldscherer billich nicht ehe schreiten solte/ ehe und bevor er darüber den Feld-Medicum consuliret hette/ es sey dann daß die Beschaffenheit der Blessure eine gantz geschwinde *Exstirpation* verheischete."
101 Gehema, *Der krancke Soldat*, sig. A7v–A8r.
102 StdAM, Ratsprotokolle 14, 43r: "ganntze glider alls weder hanndt noch fuess ausserhalb vorwissen, rath unnd guethbedunnckhen der doctoren nit mer abnemmen." Carmel Ferragud explores the involvement of the legal system in amputation in fifteenth-century Valencia: "Wounds, Amputations, and Expert Procedures," 238, 241–247.
103 Stein, *Negotiating the French Pox*, 154–156.
104 Jütte, "Seventeenth-Century German Barber-Surgeon," 186.
105 The woodcut first appeared on the title page of Part I of Ryff's *Die groß Chirurgei*. The image was reused in a chapter on amputation in Ryff's *Letzte Theil der großen Teutschen Chirurgei*.
106 See Königer, *Aus der Geschichte der Heilkunst*, 11. References to soporific sponges in Western medical literature date to the twelfth century at least, but there is little evidence of their use: McVaugh, *Rational Surgery*, 110.
107 Gehema, *Feld-Medicus*, 25: "verlieret er einen Arm oder Schenckel/ in seines Herren Dienste/ und wird lahm geschossen/ so sind meistentheils ein paar Krücken und der Bettlerstandt sein Trost und Belohnung."
108 Gehema, "Wunden der Soldaten," 746: "mit solcher Absetzung der Glieder durchauß nicht praecipitiret und übereilet ... dann sonsten beschwäret ihr euer Gewissen/ ihr ladet eine grosse Verantwortung auff euch für Gott und Menschen/ und ihr bringet euch selbsten umb Ehre und Reputation."
109 Scholars can only speculate about mortality rates among those who underwent amputations in the sixteenth and seventeenth centuries, as the earliest statistical data for such operations in Europe date to the eighteenth and nineteenth centuries. Mary Lindemann suggests the likelihood of survival in the early modern period was as low as 25 percent. Piers Mitchell, speaking of the Middle Ages, points out that while data from nineteenth-century Parisian hospitals shows mortality rates between 39 and 62 percent, depending on the amputation site, whether this bears on patient experiences in earlier centuries is unclear. Archaeological evidence reveals that at least some did survive. Work in human osteoarchaeology has uncovered medieval and early modern cases of healed stumps, and in some instances evidence that the amputee had used a prosthesis over a long period of time. Lindemann, *Medicine and Society*, 266; Mitchell, *Medicine in the Crusades*, 152–153; Wangensteen et al., "Highlights in the History of Amputation," 105–107; Mays, "Healed Limb Amputations"; Baumgartner, "Fußprothese"; Van Cant, "Surviving Amputations."

110 Hildanus, *Wund-Artzney*, 489: "nach dem ich GOtt umb sein hülff angeruffen/ in bey sein Herrn Jacobi Goulartii, Dieners am Wort Gottes/ und noch vieler anderer/ den Schenckel in der dicke abgeschnitten."
111 Gersdorff, *Feldbuch*, 70r; Purmann, *Wund-Artzney* (1692), 3:232. See also Renner, *Artzney-Büchlein*, 223.
112 E.g., Gehema, *Der Qualificirte Leib-Medicus*, sig. A10r.
113 Purmann, *Wund-Artzney* (1692), 3:231–232: "laß den Patienten in Beysein des Predigers/ so ihm Trost zusprechen kan/ auf einen bequemen Ort/ oder/ welches fast besser auf einem festen Stuhl also sitzen/ daß man rund um ihn herum gehen kan/ binde ihm alsdenn feste und unbeweglich an/ oder laß ihm deine Leute genungsam halten/ damit er dich niemals in der Operation verhindern könne; … So bald dieses auch vorbey/ kan der Prediger und Du nebst dem umstehenden nochmals durch ein Vater Unser/ den gnadign GOtt um Beystand und Seegen zu gewünschter und glücklicher Operation anruffen/ damit alles desto glücklicher von statten gehen möge … denn ein jeder weiß/ daß ohne des obersten grossen Artztes Beystand nichts nützliches und fruchtbahres ausgerichtet werden kan; Und alsdenn mit einer nöthigen Vorsichtig-und Hertzhafftigkeit von solchem Beystande begleitet/ procedire."
114 Schmid, *Instrumenta chirurgica*, 169: "Erstlich soll man den Krancken sich lassen GOtt ergeben/ desto mehr von GOtt Glück zu erlangen/ es soll auch zuvor aller Gezeug in Bereitschafft seyn/ als nemlich Scheeren/ Messer/ Sägen."
115 Schmid, *Examen chirurgicum*, 249–250: "270. Frag. So aber das Glied nit mag erhalten werden/ und Noth halben abgeschnitten werden muß/ wie woltestu ihm thun/ unnd dasselbige heylen? Antwort: Arm unnd Schenckel abzunemmen/ ist ein ernstliches ding/ und bedarff gutes auffsehens/ so ich aber ein Glied abnemmen solt/ wolt ich den Patienten zum ersten nach Christlichem brauch mit dem hochwürdigen Sacrament versehen lassen/ damit Gott mir das Werck zu verrichten/ und dem Patienten desto mehr gnad verleihe außzustehn."
116 The treatise includes only two other instances of prayer within manual instructions: Schmid, *Examen chirurgicum*, 126, 230.
117 *Umbstehende* appears analogous to the Latin *adstantes* ("those standing by"), which Winfried Schleiner defines as "the world immediately surrounding" the patient's bed, or "a patient's immediate society." See Schleiner, *Medical Ethics*, 7–8, 32.
118 Mitchell, *Medicine in the Crusades*, 152–153; Wangensteen and Wangensteen, *Rise of Surgery*, 48–51.
119 Gersdorff, *Feldbuch*, unnumbered page between 70v and 71r.
120 Hildanus, *Wund-Artzney*, 952: "ob wol der Krancke gnugsamb angebunden/ müssen gleichwol etliche hertzhaffte Männer/ die ihn also mögen halten/ daß er sich in der *operation* nicht hin und her werffe/ und den Artzt in der Arbeit verhindere/ angeordnet werden. Solches ist mir auff ein Zeit/ als ich zu Peterlingen einem vierzig jährigen Mann hab den Schenckel abschneiden/ und jetzo die Säge und *Cauteria* ergreiffen sollen/ widerfahren/ dann als der Krancke anfahet überlaut zuschreyen/ ist jederman darvon geflohen/ außgenommen mein eltester Sohn/ der dazumahl noch ein junger Knab/ und dem der angebundene Fuß (*pro forma*) zuhalten/ anbefohlen/ und wann meine Haußfraw/ die zur selben Zeit

groß schwanger/ und in einem andern Gemach war/ nicht wär hinzu gelauffen/ und den Krancken bey der Brust ergriffen/ und gehalten hätte/ wär der Krancke/ und ich mit ihm/ übel angelauffen." The anecdote first appeared in Fabry's first edition of *Lithotomia Vesicae* (1626), 167.

121 For the past two decades this anecdote has been frequently misattributed to the Italian anatomist Girolamo Fabrizi d'Acquapendente (Hieronymus Fabricius ab Aquapendente). In his *Greatest Benefit to Mankind*, Roy Porter quotes this passage from the early modern English edition of Fabry von Hilden's *Lithotomia Vesicae* and cites the author as Hieronymus Fabricius ab Aquapendente. Subsequent secondary works use the English quotation through Porter, repeating the misattribution. See Porter, *Greatest Benefit to Mankind*, 187; Dormandy, *Worst of Evils*, 107. The passage Porter quotes appears in Hildanus, *Lithotomia Vesicae* (1640), 93.

122 Scultetus, *Wund-Artzneyisches Zeug-Hauß* (1666), 1:206: "mit unerschrockenem Gemüth."

123 Hildanus, *Gründlicher Bericht*, 69.

3

Visions of the body

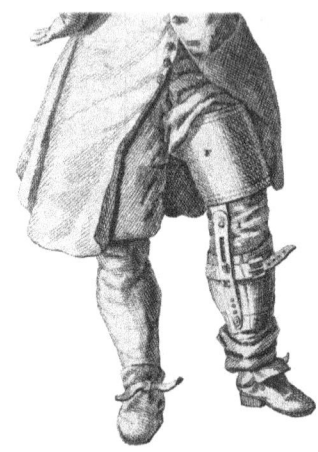

In his *Examen chirurgicum* of 1644, Joseph Schmid uses five hundred and forty-six questions to teach young field-surgeons, barbers, and surgeons about every aspect of the surgical profession. Amputation appears about halfway through the treatise. Schmid first asks how the surgeon should cut off a limb that cannot be saved. This fairly procedural question is followed by one more jarring: "How does it happen, that so many die after one of their limbs is removed?"[1] Any number of horrific answers might spring to the mind of the modern reader. After all, early modern surgeons performed amputations without the aid of antibiotics, transfusions, or standardized sterilization techniques. Schmid's answer targets one issue: the amputation site.

> As I said, it happens because it is a dangerous and worrying thing. When the fire attacks the nerves and muscles, then it runs under the skin in the flesh in such a way that one cannot see or feel it. If the limb is not removed high enough, so that a single nerve is cut off too short, then the fire moves into the nerves and the amputation is useless. Then one must cut the limb again, or [the patient] dies from it.[2]

The fire (*der Brand*) assailing the body is none other than the cold fire, the condition early moderns defined as the complete and concurrent death of tissue and bone. The surgeon had to remove any parts diagnosed with this disease before it infected the rest of the body. In Schmid's response, the fire takes on an insidious character as it spreads unseen beneath the skin. For him, the difficulty of determining where to operate explained the high fatality rate.

Schmid was one of many early modern author-practitioners to instruct on the process of removing a limb. Amputation—and particularly the amputation site—became an increasingly controversial subject in their treatises. Surgeons passionately argued about where and how to cut the body to remove fingers, toes, arms, and legs. These textual debates arose from a changing medical landscape of ever more varied amputation techniques. Hands-on practices both reflected and molded surgeons' attitudes about the body and its malleability— the extent to and manner in which the body could and should be manipulated by the surgeon's scalpel. Like a woodturner fashioning an ornate post, early modern surgeons learned to reshape human limbs with their hands.[3] With saws and knives, needles and thread, they sculpted living, bleeding flesh, and from experience and observation they adjusted their techniques over time. Surgeons expressed their views, experiences, and points of disagreement in their written instructions to others.

Amputation debates in early modern treatises centered on different manual techniques, and the ideas embedded in them. Within the minutiae of surgeons' written instructions are clues to their worldviews, and to how practical and theoretical knowledge informed them. For well over a decade, historians of science have turned to manual practitioners, from engineers to artists, to study the role of craft groups in larger developments associated with the so-called Scientific Revolution.[4] This chapter builds on two distinct, yet interrelated, threads of scholarship connected to this turn. First is recent work examining the nature of early modern artisanal knowledge, which has emboldened scholars to reconstruct and reconsider ways of knowing. Pamela Smith in particular has argued that technical practices reveal how practitioners understood and learned about natural materials and the relationship between their bodies and the world around them.[5] A second crucial area of scholarship from across the social sciences explores knowledge-making practices in early modern Europe, locating sites and actors, many long neglected, that were involved in experimental work in the course of the everyday.[6] This chapter brings surgeons and their operations into these important discussions.

As surgeons operated, knowledge-making practices intersected directly with extreme human experiences and sensations. Like creating a household recipe book or learning metallurgy, invasive surgical procedures were material practices, they were social encounters, they were adjusted by trial and error, and their results were pondered, discussed, and debated, sometimes even in print. Yet they were events not just in the lives of practitioners, but also of *patients*— ones that stirred terror and caused physical pain, had long-lasting repercussions for everyday lives, and could lead to the deaths of the very people surgeons were charged with treating. Their treatises make clear that they viewed their techniques as a unique form of craft knowledge and practice—one in which the living human body was the natural material through which they, as craftsmen, learned, adapted, and experimented. The body, made "in the image of God,"[7] was a natural material with weighty ethical obligations to delineate, and moral consequences to negotiate, at every turn.

Reading surgical instructions requires caution. As we have seen, early moderns considered amputation an extreme measure, but the sources do not allow us to definitively establish the frequency with which it was carried out. In addition, we must remember that the relationship between the textual tradition and actual practice was, as with other crafts, complex. The majority who performed amputations—barber-surgeons, field-surgeons, and surgeons—did not publish treatises. Some authors were not practitioners and compiled knowledge from other works, transmitting a written tradition. Those who practiced presented their experiences within the context of other writers, ancient and contemporary, and could convey techniques of which they did not have firsthand knowledge. Navigating these complexities carefully involves being mindful of them when following, identifying, and analyzing threads of the discourse. Emphasizing the work of those who practiced gives more weight to voices with surgical experience. Focusing on works circulating in the German vernacular allows us to examine a medical dialogue that was accessible to master–apprentice-trained surgeons and barber-surgeons. More important, this was a conversation "vernacular surgeons" contributed to and influenced. These figures were exceptional, but their perspectives were shaped by master–apprentice backgrounds familiar to everyday surgical practitioners in the Holy Roman Empire.

Of fundamental importance is to understand that early modern amputation debates were about practices *and* ideas. It would be naïve to expect a one-to-one relationship between textual claim and daily practice, and impossible to confirm. But that a relationship existed in the early modern period is undeniable. Publishing was, for those with firsthand experience, a way to process, share, and situate one's perspective in a much larger and layered body of written medical knowledge. Lower leg amputation debates in particular suggest that surgical literature trailed broad trends in practice and reflected a multitude of viewpoints influenced by firsthand experience. Early modern surgeons performed amputations more often than their medieval predecessors, and they developed and debated a diversity of techniques unprecedented in European medicine. Their debates reveal a gradual expansion not simply of the variety of methods available, but also of surgeons' expectations of the body's very malleability.

Orders of priorities

Within the fourfold schema defining the manual operations of early modern surgeons, the amputation of a limb was the most extreme form of *Exaeresis*, the removal of what was superfluous to the body.[8] Mangled or putrefying limbs belonged to the same category as external objects that penetrated the body—bullets, splinters, shards of glass—and as excess materials the body generated—cancerous lumps, bladder stones, or a dead fetus. In the most technical sense, a dead limb was not just useless and dangerous to the patient's body, but was alien to it—a separate and foreign body unto itself. Surgeons referred to the procedure to remove it as *abschneiden*, to cut away or cut off; *die Abnehmung*, taking off or removal; *abnehmen*, to take off or remove; *hinweg schneiden*, to cut away; *Ablösung*, removal; and occasionally even *amputieren*, to amputate.[9]

Early moderns did not invent surgical dismemberment, nor were their instructions the first to appear in Western medical literature. Ancient Hippocratic writings and the Galenic corpus advised treating putrefaction with cautery in nearly all circumstances. Amputation, reserved for the most dire situations, was to be carried out in dead flesh, to preserve the healthy and avoid hemorrhaging, or at the nearest joint, for a speedy operation.[10] But these texts did not explain *how* to perform the procedures.[11] From antiquity, Aulus Cornelius Celsus (c. 25 BCE–c. 50 CE) and others remained cautious, warning readers of the risks.[12] Celsus, who briefly discussed his technique, suggested cutting between living and dead tissue, removing some healthy flesh in the process rather than risk leaving any diseased behind.[13] Later, Islamic writers like Albucasis (936–1013) elaborated on their techniques in works well known in Europe.[14]

By contrast, many European surgical works of the late medieval period devoted very little space to amputation.[15] Several influential authors, including Lanfranc of Milan (c. 1240–c. 1306), did not address it at all. For those who did, non-invasive treatments were preferred, and often a scant few lines instructed readers on what to do when these were not possible. Authors might vaguely suggest that the surgeon should remove all putrid flesh and cut away some healthy with it, as Celsus had advised.[16] Guy de Chauliac (c. 1300–1368) told readers to disarticulate at the joint when possible, or in dying flesh if the putrefaction was far from the joint, but clarified that he avoided amputations and instead tightly wrapped a dead limb until it detached of its own accord.[17] Henri de Mondeville (c. 1260–1320) engaged with the problem of amputation at greater length than most of his contemporaries, pondering the advice of Avicenna and Razes on operating at the joint in every case to best ensure the complete removal of putrefaction. In a description closely matching that of Albucasis, he explained how to perform the procedure, including the use of two bands placed above and below the incision site.[18] Exceptions aside, discussions of amputation in late medieval European surgical treatises shared a centuries-long tradition of caution, brevity, and consideration of the amputation site.

Medieval surgeons treated penetrating wounds from arrows and crossbow bolts, and sharp or blunt-force trauma from other weapons, including swords, axes, and spears.[19] While many of these remained in use in some form, injuries from gunpowder weapons presented new challenges from the fifteenth century onward.[20] Artillery and handguns could tear apart bodies in ways that required immediate amputation, but even more dangerous was the susceptibility of even minor gunpowder injuries to infection and putrefaction. The impact of bullets and flying debris created contused wounds that crushed blood vessels, shattered bones, and introduced foreign matter.[21] Most, if not all, of the first generation of early modern surgeons to publish treatises, including Hieronymus Brunschwig (c. 1450–c. 1512), Hans von Gersdorff (1455–1529), Francisco de Arce (1493–c. 1573), and Ambroise Paré (c. 1510–1590), had experience in military campaigns.[22] In time they applied this experience to civilian practice. These new injuries, along with other developments related to the rising social status of surgeons, contributed to a newly intensified focus on amputation procedures in surgical literature. Eventually numerous amputation methods appeared in print, and a need and willingness to perform them spread among practitioners.

Over the course of the sixteenth and seventeenth centuries, author-practitioners developed passionate schools of thought about where and how to remove a limb. The most influential German authors on the subject included Hans von Gersdorff, Fabry von Hilden, Johannes Scultetus, and Matthäus Purmann. There was also a healthy German market for works composed in France, Italy, and the newly born Dutch Republic, among other places. At times these authors' instructions evoked a world in which practitioners could choose whichever techniques they desired. But that world existed only in theory. In practice, surgeons were often limited in time and resources, particularly on a naval vessel under fire, in a hospital tent crowded with desperately wounded soldiers, or on a house call in a remote location. But in the world of surgical treatises, when bloody scenes were muted into tranquil black type, surgeons could lay out all of the factors affecting an operation and instruct on the proper way to attend to them.

Amputation methods reflected different ways of prioritizing variables, such as the amount of time to operate, the risk of hemorrhaging, the pain a technique inflicted, and the condition of the stump afterwards. The location and extent of an injury or the cold fire were especially important. Each method consisted of a linked series of practices which together dealt with all of these variables in a strategic order that inevitably emphasized certain concerns over others. The development and dissemination of diverse techniques made it possible for surgeons to specialize in one set of practices or to reorder their priorities on a case-by-case basis. While some rejected particular methods in acrid language, many treatises surveyed the available options and acknowledged the advantages specific to each.

One central concern faced every surgeon: how to balance the harm and pain of surgery against the requirements for recovery. Choosing an amputation technique which placed a patient in greater peril to avoid complications during recovery, and vice versa, was essentially a decision about priorities: whether the surgeon should prioritize immediate or future risk. A struggle between the two appears most evident in debates over rapid amputation techniques and strategies to prevent exsanguination. A method that rendered the procedure itself faster and less painful could result in a painful stump that required a longer recovery period, whereas a method that took longer and caused intense pain could lead to a stump that healed relatively swiftly.

Fabry von Hilden and Johannes Scultetus fiercely debated rapid amputation techniques, using arguments typical of the larger discussion. Fabry opposed these procedures. The mallet-and-wedge procedure, for example, prioritized speed and minimal pain during the procedure over potential complications from the resulting stump. This method involved laying a patient's finger, hand, toe, or foot on a table or bench, setting a wedge on the digit or limb, and then striking the wedge with a heavy mallet to simultaneously separate soft tissue and bone. Fabry warned of its indelicacy and danger, both of which stemmed from the inexperience and ignorance of those who used it. "It is not fitting," he scolded, "for a respectable and diligent practitioner to perform such a crude and unseemly work and to treat his wounded [patients] like an executioner."[23] At times, executioners did use wedges and mallets to carry out sentences involving the removal of hands or fingers. Although the judicial practice of chopping off hands was rare in the Holy Roman Empire by 1600, the amputation of fingers remained common.[24] The punitive use of the technique made it violent, clumsy, and even disreputable. Rapid amputation was incongruous with the professional behavior Fabry expected of the experienced medical practitioner, who should never swing instruments and wildly chop at patients in the brutal manner of a hangman.

The second ground for Fabry's opposition was closely linked to the first: not only was the practice "crude" and "unseemly," but it was also very dangerous. The sophisticated practitioner should know *why* this was so. Fabry explained in detail that rapid amputation crushed and tore the flesh and nerves, and often caused the bones to splinter up to the next joint. Treating the resulting damage required an enormous amount of effort to avert the life-threatening complications of inflammation, spasms, and intense pain. Even if the operation went well, it could take a year to remove all of the splintered bone fragments.[25] Fabry illustrated this with an anecdote involving an inexperienced barber-surgeon in Cologne who struck off a hand with a chisel. The patient suffered chronic pain, and it took more than a year and a half for the bone fragments to come out.[26] Even if the wedge-and-mallet technique were not crude, Fabry argued that the lengthy recovery it required far outweighed its expediency.

He repeated these objections in a critique of practices in which surgeons used forceps to pinch off fingers and toes. His argument addressed the surgeon's unique role in medicine as one who inflicted a new injury in order to treat an existing one. When surgeons amputated by crushing the member between a pair of sharp tongs or beneath a wedge, they caused a contused injury. By contrast, they caused incised and lacerated injuries when they used a knife and saw. Healing these, Fabry explained, was simpler. Pinching off a digit, although speedily accomplished, could not be performed without violence, contusion of the tissues, bones, and vessels, and danger for the patient.[27] The stakes were high. The damage caused by the use of pincers on the big toe of Jaques Bolon, a poor charcoal-burner, forced him to use crutches for years.[28] Fabry advocated a lengthier, complex, and more painful amputation for fingers, hands, toes, and feet because it minimized the risk of long-term complications. Ensuring the patient's swift and sure recovery was more important than the speed and pain of the procedure itself.

Other surgeons valued the minimization of immediate rather than future risk. Scultetus instructed on performing rapid amputations matter-of-factly in his *Wund-Artzneyisches Zeug-Hauß*. In the first half of the treatise, chapters center on various surgical instruments and procedures appearing in numerous detailed illustrations. The numbered figures in Plate 53, which move the viewer's eyes counterclockwise through the engraving, display three operations to save putrefying forearms, a tray of tools to amputate below the wrist, and procedures for amputating a hand or finger and dressing the stump (figure 3.1). Scultetus explained that the sixth figure, which appears on the lower left, "shows how a hand, which has been entirely overtaken by the cold fire, is set out on a high and round tree-stump or block, in order to chop it off near the heads of the great and small forearm bones, which are still healthy (*against the opinion of Hildanus and indeed with successful progress*) by means of a mallet made of the hardest wood and an iron chisel."[29] Scultetus's glib aside to Hildanus, the Latinized version of Fabry's name, assured readers he was aware of Fabry's critique and vaunted his own authority by dismissing it.

In contrast to Fabry, who cautioned readers about the long-term complications involved, Scultetus focused on the procedure and the early stages of closing and bandaging the stump. He did so for both the mallet-and-wedge technique and the use of pincers. In another plate, which displayed the instruments most necessary for amputation procedures, Scultetus presented "a great pair of tongs with which a dead or cancerous hand, finger, foot and toes is frequently pinched off without the use of a knife."[30] He showed the pincers in action in Plate 53, where disembodied hands on the lower right use them to remove a thumb (figure 3.1). This image also illustrated a case history appearing in the *observationes* of the second half of the treatise, where he suggested that he learned the technique from his mentors at Padua, Girolamo Fabrizi d'Acquapendente and Adriaan van den Spiegel. He cross-referenced

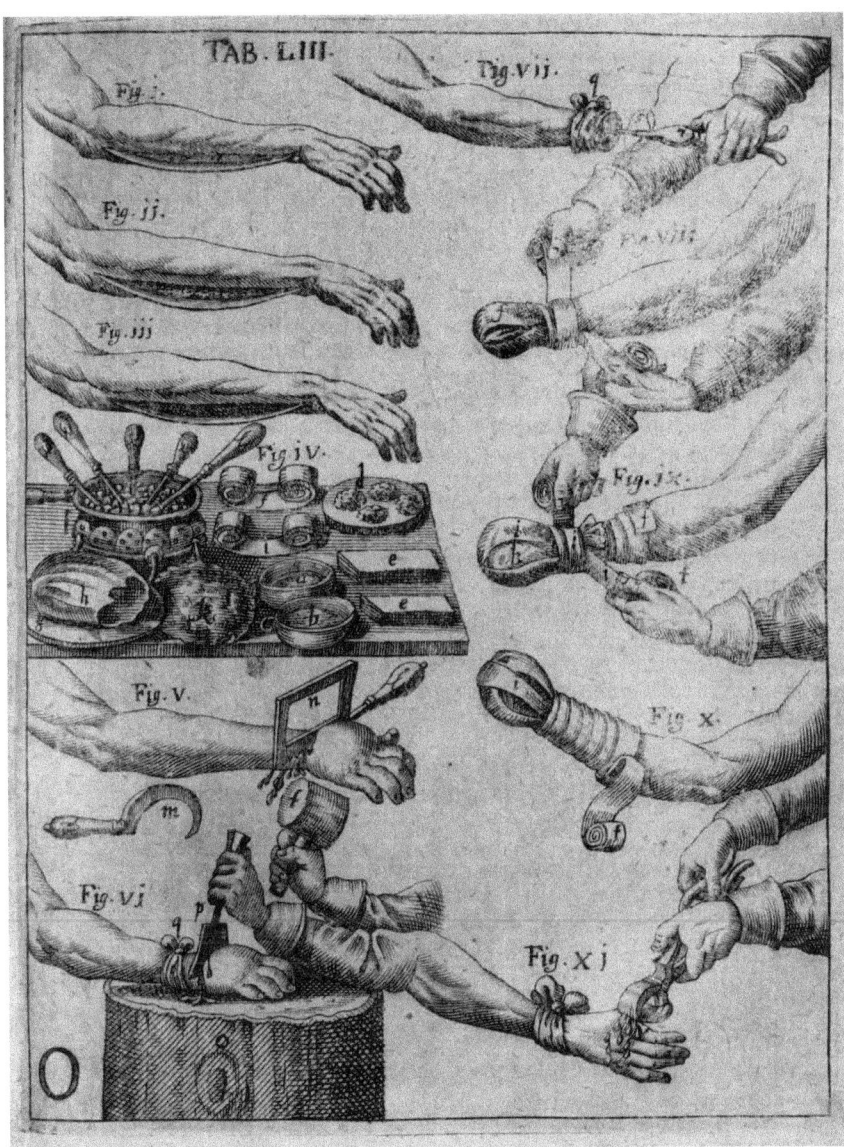

3.1 Hand amputations in Johannes Scultetus, *Wund-Artzneyisches Zeug-Hauß* (Frankfurt am Main, 1666), Tab. LIII.

the figure in his description of a case in which Spiegel used a pair of forceps to pinch off a monk's left thumb.[31] Scultetus linked these techniques not to the brutal, unsophisticated work of the executioner, but to the prestige and fame of learned anatomists. References to his university mentors bolstered the apparent wisdom of rapid amputation methods by reminding readers that he was a doctor of both medicine and surgery, and that renowned physicians in Padua practiced and taught the techniques he recommended.

Methods of staunching blood loss, or hemostatic methods, provoked similar debates. Preventing exsanguination was the greatest challenge the surgeon faced when closing and dressing a newly formed stump. The major methods of closing blood vessels were cautery, corrosive or caustic medicines, and ligature. Iron cautery, distinguished from corrosive medicines as *cauterium actuale* (actual cautery), was the use of red-hot iron instruments of various shapes and sizes to burn off tissue or to close blood vessels.[32] Although some authors referred to unskilled practitioners who used a broad piece of iron to cauterize an entire stump at once, the common and much more accepted practice utilized small instruments intended to precisely target individual blood vessels.[33] Iron cautery was the fastest and most immediately effective method, but a cauterized stump healed more slowly than one whose bleeding was staunched in other ways.

Later in his career, Fabry promoted the use of a red-hot knife to amputate and cauterize simultaneously, a controversial technique for which he became famous in German-speaking literature.[34] In the large collection of observations published in his *Wund-Artzney* of 1652, he recounted the case of a youth who developed the cold fire in his leg. The patient's condition called for the removal of the limb above the knee, the riskiest amputation site on the body due to the presence of major arteries and the size of the femur. Once the patient and his leg were tied to a bench, Fabry paused. That hemorrhaging would be fatal for this particular patient seemed clear. When he could delay no longer, he took action:

> I straight away gripped the leg with my left hand, and laid bare the flesh up to the bone with my right, but not with the shearing blade ... but rather with a cautery iron, which had the form of a knife. ... Through the help of this iron, I removed the flesh, and at the same time stilled the blood; When now the flesh was cut off up to the bone, I took the saw in my right hand, and cut off the bone successfully with it, and although this operation was difficult, God be praised, nothing adverse befell me.[35]

He described his use of the curved cautery knife, displayed in an accompanying illustration, as a creative response to the needs of his young and sickly patient. Surgeons often shuffled their priorities as circumstances required. The order of priorities embedded in Fabry's use of the cautery knife contradicted the emphasis that he—in most other contexts—placed on the creation of a healthy stump.

Fabry insisted that there were no adverse effects from cutting soft tissue with a red-hot knife, but others were less convinced. Cornelis Solingen argued that though "Hildanus greatly praises his *Cauterium cultellare*, or cautery iron shaped as a knife ... the skin and muscles, etc., are shriveled together" by the instrument, causing the same damage as a wide cautery iron.[36] The author used Fabry's own words to further condemn the practice, explaining that "as he himself admits," the blood vessels could reopen, forcing the surgeon to apply a small cautery iron to close them one by one. "Thus," he concluded, "I hold that the use of this instrument cannot be good and beneficial."[37] Solingen's critique, which goes on at length, refers to the unreliability of the cautery knife and condemns the shriveled, scarred surface it created. The complaint, similar to Fabry's own objection to the damage caused by rapid amputation, underlines the potential cost of placing the immediate risk of hemorrhaging above the creation of a healthy stump.

Cauterium potentiale (potential cautery) applied corrosive or caustic medicines, such as quicklime mixed with soap, that caused tissues to burn.[38] These were particularly useful to surgeons treating reluctant patients who lived in terror of the cautery iron. According to Paul Barbette, cautery by iron was "far surer than one done with caustic medicines, yet because of the patient's fear one is commonly forced to take the latter in hand."[39] Fear of iron cautery was so widespread that Solingen suggested the surgeon should "set the brazier filled with glowing coals and cautery irons to the side of the patient, so that he does not see them."[40] By contrast, corrosive medicines were less terrifying and reportedly caused minimal pain.[41]

But some practitioners vehemently objected to the use of corrosive medicines, citing it as a dangerous and unreliable technique. Jan Muys observed its deleterious results during the French occupation of the Dutch city of Arnhem from 1672 to 1674. In his *Neue Vernünfftige Praxis der Wund-Artzney*, he claimed that six thousand Frenchmen were buried within two years because the practitioners treating patients in the town's main hospital used powder of vitriol of Cyprus. "They lie in a garden," he continued ominously, "where every year after their deaths the insignia of their kingdom, that is, lilies, still grow from the remains of their bodies."[42] Muys not only rejected the "French use" of corrosive medicines, but also advised surgeons to apply the iron cautery sparingly.[43] Instead, he lauded the skillful employment of ligation.

The ligation of blood vessels was the most time-consuming and difficult method to perform during an amputation, but if successful the stump healed much faster and with less pain and complications than one burned by iron or corrosive powders. Ligation involved the use of forceps to draw out the blood vessels individually. Then, keeping the vessels shut with a clamp, the surgeon would tie them closed with thread.[44] Scultetus illustrated the procedure in Plate 53 of his *Wund-Artzneyisches Zeug-Hauß*, where a disembodied hand in the top right grasps a pair of forceps (figure 3.1). This method traces back to Celsus, but surgical treatises of the medieval and early modern period rarely mentioned it until Ambroise Paré included it in his widely influential works of the mid-sixteenth century.[45] Because this technique took longer to perform, surgeons recommended its use only on strong patients who stood a good chance of surviving a lengthy operation.[46] Despite its benefits, the pain and length of the procedure made this method, according to Solingen, "cruel and unmerciful."[47]

At times, the surgeon's approach was guided solely by expediency. Solingen, for instance, argued that ligation was virtually impossible to perform during combat on a naval vessel where there were limited instruments, too many patients, and little time. "In sea battles one uses cautery the most," he explained, "because it is the easiest, most convenient and readiest means for the surgeon." The author clarified this was not an idle preference, but a necessity dictated by circumstance. "One cannot aid all patients at once, so that while you help one, the other lies and bleeds," he reasoned. He assured the reader he had seen and experienced it enough to know that ligation simply took too long.[48] A former naval surgeon, Solingen used his firsthand knowledge to situate the reader in a particular context in which the surgeon must prioritize speed, taking into account the survival not just of the *individual* patient undergoing surgery, but also the *many* patients waiting for aid.

However, when surgeons had the time and means to choose, their treatises suggest it was a matter of preference. Those in favor of iron cautery emphasized its speed and reliability. It ensured a patient would not die of hemorrhaging before the surgeon finished dressing the stump and that the blood vessels would remain closed afterwards. Practitioners who advocated corrosive medicines claimed that they were less painful and aroused less fear than the red-hot iron. The patient-friendly advantages of corrosive medicines outweighed their unreliability. In contrast to both iron and chemical cautery, ligation staunched blood loss without inflicting burn wounds. Those who favored it prioritized a relatively swift and easy recovery over the risk of a prolonged operation. Ligation was the boldest of these hemostatic methods in its readiness to hazard a patient's life in the short term to minimize complications. Its failure to become part of common surgical practice suggests that early modern practitioners were largely unwilling to prioritize future over immediate risk when exsanguination was at stake.

Understanding the priorities embedded in different surgical techniques enables us to locate flashpoints in amputation debates. Consider disagreements over rapid amputation methods and hemostatic techniques. Should the surgeon minimize the immediate risk to the patient's life during a procedure, or work to head off potential complications during recovery? Surgeons' responses were always guided to some extent by real-world issues—time, tools, the severity of the patient's condition, and so on. On a deeper level, these conflicting priorities also reveal attempts to define what was best for patients and to articulate the surgeon's role in their recovery. Surgeons were concerned about their patients' survival, but they were also concerned about the changes their instruments made to their bodies. After all, those most concerned with the dangers of a complicated recovery often implicitly discussed the construction of a "healthy" stump. In an amputation, surgeons did not simply *remove* something. Through the act of removal, they *created* something, too. Surgeons' instructions are as much about how and what to *create* as they are about how and what to *remove*.

Lower leg amputation

The lower leg was the most controversial area for amputation in the early modern period. Surgical treatises devoted far more attention to it than to any other kind of limb removal precisely because there were so many ways to do it. Patients' experiences could vary radically, and the operations could result in radically different stumps. Depending on the surgeon, a patient with a putrefying toe or two could lose part of the foot, the whole foot at the ankle, or the entire lower leg at or a little below the knee. A surgeon's choice of amputation site reflected his views on both the patient's body and his own role in preserving the patient's health.

The removal of other body parts was relatively uncontentious. Surgeons generally agreed that in an upper limb amputation, whether a finger, hand, or arm, the operation should target only dead flesh. This basic principle ensured a shorter and less dangerous procedure, preserved as much of the patient's healthy body as possible, and created a stump suitable for an artificial hand.[49] There was no such consensus in the removal of a lower extremity. A leg amputation was simply more dangerous and difficult to perform. It took longer, required larger instruments, involved greater risk of hemorrhaging, and called for more assistants. Ideally, the network of kin, community members, and medical practitioners brought together during the decision-making process leading to an amputation remained in place during the operation. The tremendous physical and emotional effort called for a minimum of three or four assistants to pass instruments, adjust ligatures, apply bandages, provide moral support, and, crucially, to hold the patient still.[50] Another important distinction involved what came *after* the procedure. Unlike the stump of an arm, a leg stump had to be capable of bearing a great deal of weight if the patient acquired an artificial limb.

One influential approach was what we might call the "hand's-width method," which took place three to five fingers below the knee, or roughly a hand's width (*eine Handbreit*).[51] Surgeons who performed this technique used a knife and a saw. The knife, which was often curved, cut through soft tissue—skin, flesh, muscle, sinew, blood vessels, and so forth. Once he reached the bone, the surgeon carefully scraped off the thin layer of connective tissue protecting its surface (the periosteum) before turning to his bow-frame saw.[52] A woodcut from Gersdorff's *Feldbuch*, labeled "Sawing" (*Serratura*), illustrates the point in a procedure when the surgeon has finished cutting the soft tissue with a knife and has changed instruments in order to saw the bone (figure 3.2).[53]

Visual depictions in treatises like Gersdorff's were not intended to be faithful representations of the stress, messiness, and pain of an amputation. However, some elements of Gersdorff's woodcut correspond to the textual instructions of surgeons. The illustration shows two ligatures—which one surgeon described as strong, thin cords similar to the kind women use for their hair—positioned on either side of the amputation site.[54] This technique, also found in late medieval surgical literature, kept the skin taut for a more precise incision between the cords. The ligature would have been incredibly tight to dull local sensitivity and to prevent hemorrhaging. In the woodcut, the surgeon's assistant supports the lower leg while the surgeon saws, using one hand to steady the knee. Authors often advised the surgeon either to appoint an assistant to draw the flesh upward to bare the bone, or to use a leather sleeve fitted to the patient's thigh for the same purpose. The flesh was drawn upward not only to give better access to the bone, but also to ensure that there would be healthy flesh to fold back over the severed bone to create a generous cushion for the stump.[55]

The hand's-width method represents a particular and significant historical perspective. It was introduced into the medical discourse by vernacular surgeons in the latter half of the sixteenth century and very likely originated in the practices of surgeons trained by apprenticeship. The most influential authors who first instructed on it at length in print, Ambroise Paré and Fabry von Hilden, did not suggest it was novel. They identified aspects of the procedure, such as concerns for removing all diseased flesh or the use of two ligatures around the amputation site, within ancient and medieval sources.[56] What made this method distinct, from the perspective of the textual tradition, was that it located the amputation site a little below the knee regardless of how much or how little of the lower leg was diseased. This approach maintained a strong presence in surgical literature through the following century, gaining advocates from guild-trained and university-educated writers. By that time, some authors referred to it as "the instruction of the ancients," as though it had been practiced since time immemorial.[57] The appearance of the method in surgical literature and contemporary perceptions of it over time suggest it was an ongoing craft practice that was codified in print as vernacular surgeons published treatises. The technique and the underlying principles its advocates described blended lessons familiar from late medieval teachings and a sensibility both more practical and mechanical than the inherited textual corpus. Its longevity demonstrates the powerful appeal of its guiding rationale, its compatibility with and roots in the Galenic tradition, and, most important, its apparent utility.

To those unfamiliar with the history of amputation, the possibility that a patient could lose his or her entire lower leg when only the foot was gangrenous

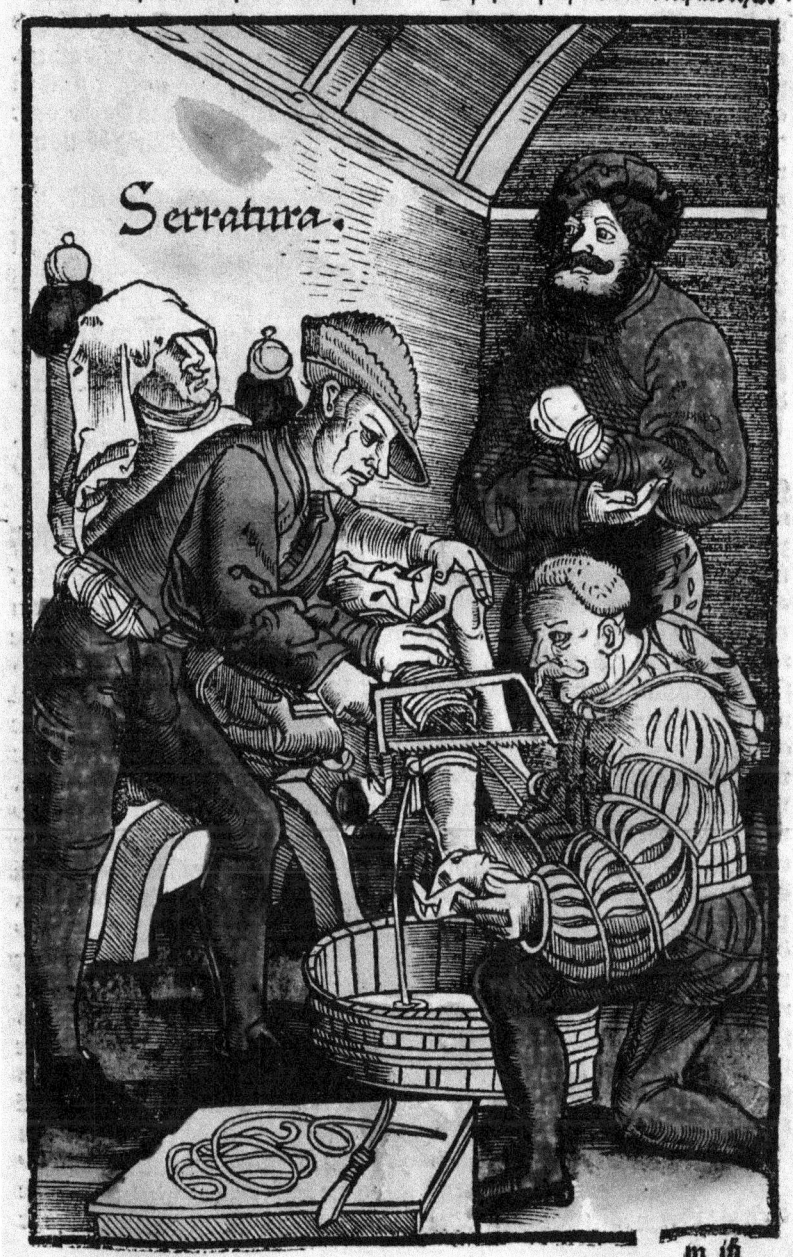

3.2 "Serratura" in Hans von Gersdorff, *Feldbuch der Wundarznei* (Strasbourg, 1517).

may sound illogical and even tragic—like a grisly Monty Python parody of premodern medicine. But, as several early modern surgeons argued, the hand's-width method had a practical foundation intended to serve the patient's best interests. Advocates explained that lower leg amputation should always be performed a hand's width below the knee—or, as one put it, "where the garters [*Hosenbänder*] are worn"—because it provided the ideal placement for a prosthesis.[58] By amputating below the knee, the surgeon saved the patient's joint. Since antiquity, many had considered the joint to be the easiest amputation site, but operating there rendered it useless to the patient. It was ultimately better, as one physician explained, to take the more difficult path and operate at least two finger widths from the nearest joint whenever possible.[59] Prioritizing the patient's future convenience above the surgeon's present was a major concern. Matthäus Purmann, who agreed that amputating at a joint was easiest, strongly opposed it: "I say to all these [who amputate at the joint], one must look herein not to [the surgeon's] convenience, but rather to the benefit and service of the limb and of the body."[60]

The hand's-width method created a short stump below the joint, which several authors considered crucial to the patient's future mobility. They argued not only that it was harder to fit and use prostheses on longer stumps, but also that patients experienced greater trouble with them in general. Fabry warned such stumps became so cumbersome that some were driven to face the danger of a second amputation to cut them closer to the knee.[61] Paré pointed to the example of a captain whose foot was shot away by an iron ball in a naval battle: the wound healed, but the long stump was "more troublesome and debilitating." Time passed, and the captain made a difficult decision. "Since the leg was more functional higher up," Paré recounted, he had it removed "about five fingers under the knee." The operation was a success, as the captain "could afterwards use it much better and move it more swiftly than before."[62] He explained that a long stump required the patient to rely on a crutch in addition to whatever form of prosthesis (if any) was fitted to the leg. The surgeon who left a long lower leg stump therefore forced the patient to walk with greater difficulty on three feet instead of two.[63]

The kind of three-legged amputee Paré described can be seen in many early modern images depicting the poor, sick, and lame. One noteworthy example is a woodcut from Gersdorff's *Feldbuch* that accompanies an explanation of St. Anthony's Fire, a disease which could cause rotting flesh that at times separated spontaneously from the healthy (figure 3.3). In the image, an afflicted man supplicates St. Anthony, patron saint of the ailment. The fire on the supplicant's outstretched hand indicates the disease that has taken his right foot and left a long lower leg stump. The leg is bent at the knee with the length of the stump resting *parallel* to the ground on a wooden prosthesis with a wide and narrow socket that cradles the entire lower leg. The figure uses a

Visions of the body

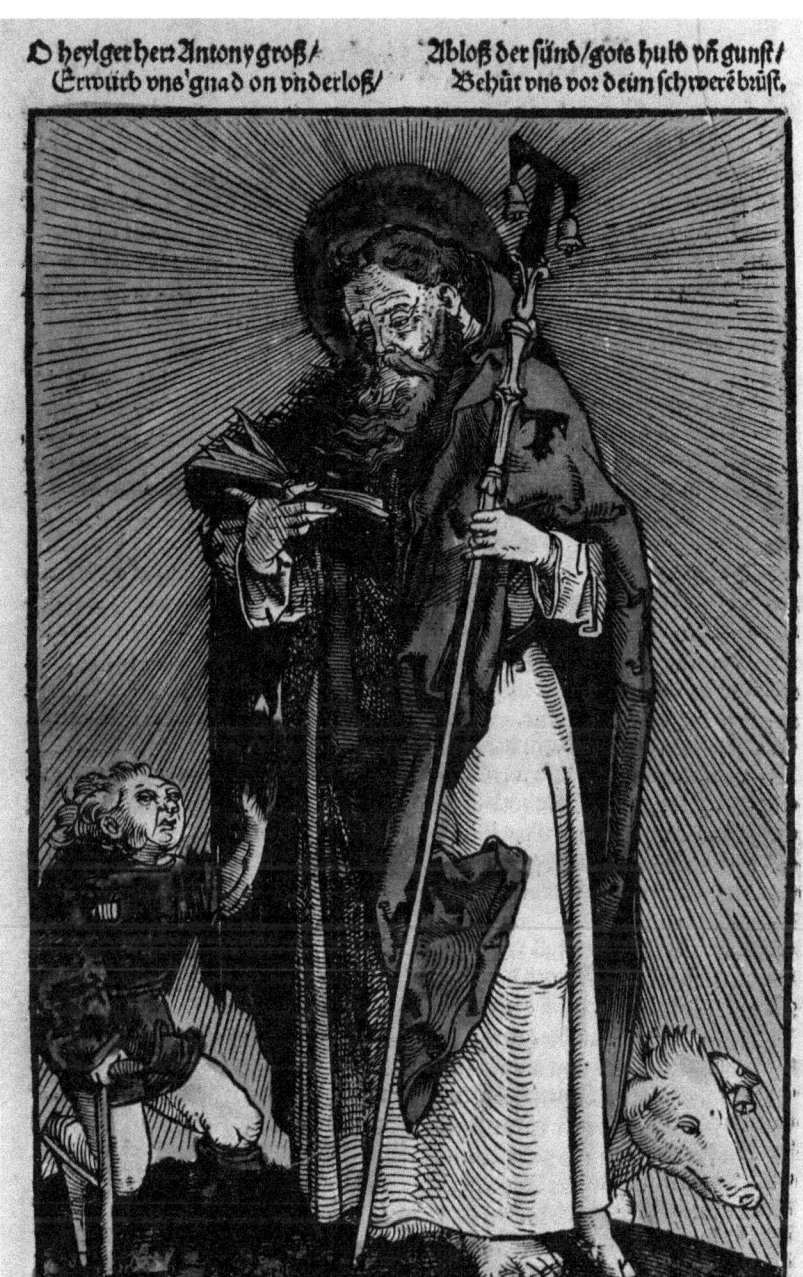

3.3 St. Anthony's Fire in Hans von Gersdorff, *Feldbuch der Wundarznei* (Strasbourg, 1517), 65v.

crutch on his right side, presumably to stabilize the awkward weight distribution with an additional vertical support. This image employs the combination of objects as a device to suggest suffering and one in need of aid. It also suggests a hindered state of mobility that advocates of the hand's-width method sought to avoid.

By taking away flesh that could be saved, the method reshaped the patient's leg so that it could perform its natural functions of standing, bending, and walking. This set of priorities did not go unchallenged, and the defensive arguments made on its behalf suggest that it was not the prospect of an easier procedure that caused practitioners to reject it. Rather, efforts to defend the hand's-width method suggest that surgeons felt uneasy when they removed the healthy along with the unhealthy. To remove more than was necessary was contrary to the approach they took to protect the body in other procedures.

Fabry acknowledged this tension, which preyed on the minds of surgeons when they determined amputation sites: "although the surgeon should spare the human body as much as possible, nevertheless it is certain that such a remaining stump of the leg, which he could yet preserve to some extent, causes the patient great inconvenience after the cure."[64] His contemporary, Paré, said the same. As a general rule, surgeons should spare the healthy body from the iron and always cut as little as they could from it. "Yet," he continued, "because of the action and ornament of the remaining healthy part of the limb, one cannot always obey and follow this advice."[65] Those who advocated amputating just below the knee were reasoning not only with young practitioners and stubborn colleagues, but also to some extent with their own consciences. Their guiding justification emphasized practicality on behalf of the patient.

Paracelsian treatises in the mid-sixteenth century, Paduan texts after them, and Dutch works in the seventeenth century all challenged the hand's-width method. Advocates for alternative approaches came from inside and outside the Holy Roman Empire and belonged to dynamic networks of education and exchange. Although the resulting limbs could differ, all of these alternative methods preserved longer stumps. It is impossible to estimate the proportions of amputees with long or short lower leg stumps in early modern Germany, and examples of both appear in visual sources and the archaeological record.[66] Depictions of amputees with long stumps in paintings, medical and religious woodcuts, and popular broadsheets from the Thirty Years' War suggest they were not an uncommon sight in illustrations.[67] The priorities underlying the techniques that created them were varied. Chief among them were maintaining the material integrity of the body, safeguarding the patient's survival during the procedure, and a compromise between preserving the healthy body and providing for future mobility.

Certainly, not every alternative technique was concerned first and foremost with preserving the healthy body or its future mobility. Some aimed at accelerating the process of amputation, like the mallet-and-wedge method. Indeed, the "Botallo manner," named for the surgeon Leonardo Botallo, was the same method applied on a grander scale: an arm or leg was placed between two blades, which were then rapidly pressed together by the drop of a great weight.[68] Like the mallet-and-wedge technique, the Botallo manner had its share of critics. Purmann witnessed a case in which a dropped blade failed to sever a bone on the first try, as well as another botched procedure in which the knives turned inward and cut a limb unevenly.[69] He ultimately dismissed the technique as unreliable since "it can happen faster and quicker [than amputation by saw], whenever it goes well; but who can promise us that it will work properly five times in ten?"[70]

The Botallo manner was rare and risky. For the most part, those who criticized alternative amputation techniques did not accuse their proponents of opting for what was easier or faster. In fact, Purmann criticized other alternative procedures for being *too* lengthy. When selecting an amputation site, he advised surgeons not to leave patients with long stumps because "the patient must wear a wooden leg." A great amount of flesh under the knee not only hindered walking, but also "an artificial lower leg" would not attach as well as it would higher up. At this point his explanation turns to problems with the procedure itself: "Not to speak of the bones, which are far apart in the middle of the lower leg and make for a long operation, which is not the case closer to the knee, and [the operation] goes faster and better."[71] The rapid Botallo manner was dangerous and unreliable, but the knife-and-saw technique used far below the knee was difficult, lengthy, and inconvenient for a prosthesis. Purmann therefore favored neither.

Practitioners who used a knife and saw to amputate a leg mid-shin followed yet another set of priorities. They were not convinced it was in the best interests of patients to lose more of their bodies than was absolutely necessary for their survival and were unwilling to reshape a limb to the surgeon's own design. Some of them were Paracelsians. The surgical writings of the controversial Paracelsus promoted non-invasive techniques to treat injuries and open wounds. He instructed surgeons to allow the body's natural healing power to work and base their therapies on an artful manipulation of sympathies and correspondences found throughout nature. The Paracelsian weapon-salve, for instance, was a technique rooted in sympathetic medicine in which the practitioner applied ointment to the weapon that caused a patient's injury rather than the injury itself.[72] Paracelsians were averse to amputation, instead favoring treatments intended to induce separation of corrupt and sound flesh without the use of a knife.[73]

When there was no hope of inducing separation, Paracelsians used the knife sparingly.[74] Sebastian Greiff instructed surgeons to cut off dead and insensitive flesh entirely, but in such a way "that you touch nothing living."[75] After giving a series of recipes to apply to the surface of dead matter, he informed readers that they now had also "a short account, help and advice for cutting away bone, [such] that you can completely abstain from the cut of the knife."[76] This approach, which made no distinction between an upper and lower extremity, or between a digit and a limb, preserved as much of the healthy material of the body as possible. There was certainly precedent for sparing all living flesh in the learned textual tradition, but the emphasis on inducing separation through chemical treatments, with recipes for plasters with nitre and alum, added a Paracelsian flair. Greiff's vague and uncategorical advice indicates how little he expected the surgeon to intervene in the body's form, instead allowing the body's powers of healing to determine its contours. This perspective on amputation, which persisted into the latter half of the seventeenth century, was primarily concerned with keeping healthy material intact rather than providing for future mobility.

Paracelsians like Greiff offered no hint of the role of the patient's immediate safety when targeting only dead flesh. By contrast, the patient's safety was the ultimate priority undergirding the "manner of Aquapendente," an amputation technique that came into vogue at the turn of the seventeenth century.[77] This newly popularized method involved cutting into the dead part of a limb a short distance from the healthy flesh and sawing through the rotted bone. Once the bone was removed, the surgeon applied a wide cautery—a red-hot iron instrument as wide as the raw stump—to burn off the remaining dead matter until the patient could sense heat and pain. Whatever remained of the dead flesh would separate itself from the living within three to four days.[78] This method ensured that the putrefied parts—and *only* the putrefied parts—were removed.

The question of whether to cut into dead, as opposed to living, flesh was not new.[79] Neither was the method of cauterizing foul material remaining on the stump until the patient sensed pain.[80] What was new was the network of highly educated practitioners connected to the University of Padua and its renowned medical faculty who promoted the widespread use of this technique and argued that it was as good—or better—than that of Celsus, Galen, and the ancients. Many surgical treatises identified this method with the influential physician and anatomist Girolamo Fabrizi d'Acquapendente.[81] Fabrizi succeeded the famous anatomist Gabrielle Fallopio (1523–1562) as professor of anatomy and surgery in Padua. He popularized the amputation technique which became synonymous with his Latinized name in his role as instructor at the university, in his widely disseminated publications, and, particularly in the German context, through the writings of his German pupil, Johannes Scultetus.[82]

It is difficult to judge how prevalent the practice of the Aquapendente method was in Germany outside of Scultetus's town of Ulm. Two prominent examination treatises aimed at young surgeons did not even include the option of cutting into dead flesh as an appropriate answer to the question of where and how to perform an amputation.⁸³ Whether or not it entered general practice, the Paduan-promoted technique was regularly discussed in surgical literature of the seventeenth century and would have been known at least in theory to most practitioners capable of reading in the vernacular.⁸⁴

Followers of Girolamo Fabrizi saw many advantages to his technique. Amputating in the insensitive, dead region of a limb rendered the cutting and sawing painless. Burning off the remaining putrefied matter removed flesh and cauterized blood vessels simultaneously: when the heat reached close enough to the healthy flesh for the patient to feel it, the ends of healthy blood vessels were already sealed. Consequently, its advocates argued, performing an amputation in dead flesh caused very little pain, could be executed quickly, and minimized hemorrhaging.⁸⁵ This technique prioritized the immediate safety and comfort of the patient. Like the Paracelsian approach, it used the location of the cold fire to determine the length of the stump so that any healthy flesh was spared. Furthermore, the natural separation of healthy and dead flesh in the three days following the procedure cast the body in a self-regulating role.

The greatest appeal of the Aquapendente method was that it practically removed the risk of exsanguination. When operating in healthy flesh, the battle to prevent massive hemorrhaging began the moment the curved knife penetrated soft tissue. Even with a tight ligature in place, the surgeon had to work as swiftly as possible to remove the limb and close the ends of the open blood vessels. Once the initial incision was made, any delay could be lethal. In his *Examen chirurgicum*, Joseph Schmid advised readers to have two identical sets of instruments on hand for sawing. The surgeon should do this, he explained, "so that when one [saw] breaks, he immediately would have another, otherwise the patient would bleed to death while one had to fetch another."⁸⁶ The Aquapendente method largely eliminated the battle against hemorrhaging by cutting into flesh with fouled vessels that only oozed stinking, dark liquid. If the bow-frame saw snapped in half, if a ligature slipped unexpectedly, or if anything else went wrong, the patient would not be in any additional danger.

Critics of amputation in dead flesh pressed the issue of the patient's troubled medical future following the procedure. They argued that even if it successfully excised the cold fire, the use of cautery irons to burn the surface of the entire stump could lead to several complications.⁸⁷ Fabry von Hilden, who included a detailed rebuttal to the technique in his *Gründlicher Bericht*, warned that cauterizing in this way created a hard scar of melted skin, flesh, and muscle that caused inflammation and inflicted unbearable pain. Even worse, the resulting stump would include a bone that ended without the protection and padding of extra flesh sewn over it. When the surgeon cut into dead flesh, the entire limb—flesh and bone—was severed in a straight line, and the remaining two or three finger widths of putrefied material were burned off simultaneously.

If the blisters caused by the iron cautery did not heal, the end of the bone was in danger of protruding through the open ulcers of the stump. As Fabry concluded, "the scar [on the stump] remains fragile and is harmed by the wooden leg time and again."[88] At the heart of these critiques of the Aquapendente method was a condemnation of its perceived disregard for the patient's future comfort and mobility. It created a stump that could not bear an artificial limb without constant injury.

Johannes Scultetus was eager to refute Fabry's scathing assessment of a surgical practice that he championed as a signature teaching of his university mentor, and he devoted a section of his *Wund-Artzneyisches Zeug-Hauß* to the matter.[89] Rather than defend the Aquapendente method on each point, he instead attacked the technique of cutting into living flesh, which he argued could not be performed without great violence and danger to the patient and the healthy flesh. The ligatures tied tightly on either side of the amputation site, intended to dull sensitivity and prevent hemorrhaging, could deprive a healthy section of a patient's limb of nourishment and cause it to putrefy. Moreover, Scultetus pressed, often when the surgeon believed he was cutting into healthy flesh, the first incision revealed foul tissue hidden beneath the surface. When this happened, he had to make further cuts up the leg until he found the flesh entirely healthy, a process that could turn into a lengthy and incredibly painful prelude to the amputation. If the surgeon decided against making a second or third cut to find healthy flesh, then the foul tissue would have to be burned away with a cautery iron.

Scultetus was concerned not only with the amount of time Fabry's method took, but also with the danger of blood loss it entailed: "more time is required to draw forth the blood vessels with forceps and to tie and stitch them with thread (moreover, when one also loosens and removes the ligature, sometimes so much hemorrhaging follows that if one does not evenly touch the remaining blood vessels with a cautery iron, it can never be stilled)."[90] In other words, the effort to create a healthy stump able to bear a prosthesis was not worth the risk of exsanguination.

The exchange between Fabry and Scultetus expressed contrasting views of the surgeon's duty to the patient. Fabry's objection to the Aquapendente method rested on the likelihood that cautery would leave the patient unable to adopt a wooden leg. Scultetus's critique of the "ancient method" rested on the immediate danger it caused, and his response to Fabry suggests that he was more concerned with the patient surviving the procedure than with anything else. Scultetus concluded that "the manner of the Paduan surgeons and of Hieronymus Fabricius" was far better than that "of the ancient surgeons."[91]

Changing attitudes toward technology among practitioners in the latter half of the seventeenth century made possible a compromise between competing orders of priorities in lower leg amputations. Surgeons who wrote of artificial legs that functioned better when positioned as close to the ankle as possible presented a new perspective. According to these authors, based largely in the Dutch Republic, long stumps were no longer debilitating. With the aid of new technology, they could be more convenient for the patient than short ones. With the right prosthesis, that is, the surgeon could preserve the patient's healthy body in a way that also provided for future mobility. Solingen explained that

> when a cold fire is in the foot or toe, and a tumor arises above the ankle or joint ... then one must not wait long with removing the leg, lest the entire leg be infected, for if anything one can still spare the length of the leg or arm (albeit such is entirely averse to the instruction of the ancients, who wanted one always to amputate the leg four or five finger-widths below the knee). For one can yet fasten instruments, like a foot, to the amputated leg, with which the patient can walk comfortably. This happens much more easily when the shin bone or lower leg is still long, since indeed the longer it is the better, because thereby the patient can better move the attached foot.[92]

His description depicts the hand's-width method as an old and inflexible technique whose guiding rationale no longer reflected the prostheses then available. Of course, the inherited textual tradition of ancient and medieval writers did not insist on or discuss placing the amputation site a hand's-width below the knee. But by the late seventeenth century, surgical literature treated the hand's-width approach as conventional.

Growing confidence in new instruments and artificial limbs altered views about the superiority of what had come before. Jan Muys reported that "before this one always amputated the leg a little below the knee, even when the cold fire had not yet infected a third of the leg, but now one preserves the length of the leg as much as possible, because today instruments have been devised that can conveniently be applied far below the knee of an amputated leg."[93] Authors like Muys referred to "new" prostheses to defend the preservation of the lower leg, just as early advocates of the hand's-width method had used wooden prostheses to insist on short stumps.

Details of the design and manufacture of instruments which purportedly made a long stump ideal are noticeably absent from surgical literature until the last decade of the seventeenth century. Solingen, one of the greatest supporters of saving the length of the leg on account of these devices, mentioned them only in passing. For instance, he explained that when an amputation "occurs in the lower leg under the knee, one can do a better job of putting a wooden or copper foot on it."[94] This passing remark about a copper foot may be a hint that, as with the artificial hands we will discuss in Chapter 5, technologies and techniques were often in use long before evidence of them appeared in print. Previous references to prostheses for lower extremities in surgical treatises were confined to wooden supplements of varying lengths. One notable exception is the "rich man's leg" included in Paré's sixteenth-century book on artificial body parts, which displayed an articulated but impractical above-the-knee prosthesis made of iron.[95]

Perhaps the earliest detailed description of a prosthetic device used to defend longer stumps was the artificial foot illustrated in the influential treatise of Pieter Verduyn (1625–c. 1700), a Dutch surgeon who first published his *Dissertatio epistolaris de nova artuum decurtandorum ratione* in 1696. A year later, it appeared in German translation as *Neue Methode, die Glieder abzunehmen*. Verduyn's "new method" was flap amputation, which expanded on the traditional practice of preserving an excess amount of healthy flesh during an amputation in order to protect and cushion the end of a severed bone.[96] Rather than use a curved knife to cut the soft tissue around the bone in a straight line, Verduyn instructed the surgeon to spare a flap of flesh down the calf. An assistant pulled away the extra flesh while the surgeon sawed the bone. Once the limb was severed and the wound washed in warm water, the flap was drawn back down and folded over the end of the bone.[97]

Verduyn's "new method" largely followed the same principles of the hand's-width method. Not only did he provide a cushion for the stump, but he also used ligatures above the amputation site and operated only in healthy flesh. Verduyn's treatise promoted the use of what he referred to as a "French tourniquet," a thick band on the upper leg that was tightened by twisting a stick.[98] The tourniquet, still a familiar device today, was intended to apply enough pressure to temporarily close blood vessels and prevent hemorrhaging. A surgeon who followed the Aquapendente method would have objected to this kind of ligature, which was placed high on the upper leg, because it temporarily cut off nourishment to the healthy flesh below it.

Verduyn advised that "one must take care to remove no leg that is already completely corrupted by the cold fire or other sicknesses, since all work and effort is here in vain."[99] Instead, surgeons should always perform amputations in warm, healthy flesh. Verduyn shared the fears of earlier critics that cutting in dead flesh might not excise all of the cold fire, and that even if it did, the resulting stump would be a misery for the patient. Flap amputation was a way of manipulating healthy flesh to fashion a stump according to the surgeon's design. Verduyn and those who adopted his method chose to alter the shape of a patient's body beyond the necessary removal of putrefied tissue. This was an approach that those who favored the hand's-width method shared. But Verduyn's choice of amputation site on the lower leg asked the surgeon to do exactly what advocates of the hand's-width method rejected: amputate as far as possible from the knee. He claimed that the longer the stump, the easier it was to fit and use an artificial leg. "[O]ne can very conveniently attach an artificial foot with a stocking to the remaining stump and furnish a shoe so artful that it appears to be quite a natural foot," Verduyn explained, "whereon he [the patient] can walk as well as his other leg."[100] His assertion about the prosthesis is not just that it is a feasible substitute, but that it appears "natural" and allows for an easy gait. To create a short stump that prevented a patient from using such a device would impede his or her future mobility. "Here it should be remembered," Verduyn advised, "that one leaves the stump as long as possible, so that the artificial foot can be fastened the more firmly."[101]

The treatise illustrates the ease and natural appearance of such a device in a detailed engraving of a gentleman standing serenely with the aid of an artificial leg (figure 3.4). His trouser is pulled up and his leather stocking pulled down to suggest how conveniently patients could conceal the upper leg harness, the buckles of the lower leg, and the metal brace which connected the artificial foot to the thigh. The gentleman gestures to a diagram of the device to better exhibit its components. These are labeled with letters corresponding to explanations in the text. According to Verduyn, the prosthesis comprises a wooden foot attached to a curved copper plate. Iron rods on either side of the leg connect the plate to a harness tied to the patient's thigh, and a non-locking joint enables the patient to bend his knee uninhibited.[102]

The illustration envisions the patient post-amputation as rehabilitated, relaxed, and provided with both the bodily form and artificial instruments to appear and move as if the procedure never happened. Verduyn was vocal about his concern for the patient's future mobility. He established this at the very outset of his treatise, which began with a list of equipment required to perform an amputation. A preliminary checklist to prepare for an operation was common in surgical literature, but Verduyn's inclusion of "an artificial foot made of wood or other materials that is not too heavy" was unique.[103] He incorporated the fabrication and application of an artificial limb into the amputation procedure itself. His goal was to fashion a stump that could accommodate a prosthesis designed to give the patient the look, feel, and gait of a natural leg.

It is tempting to see in Verduyn's engraving a satisfying culmination of two centuries of surgical experimentation. But such a conclusion would be far too clean for a problem as messy as surgical dismemberment. In the same decade in which his copper-footed gentleman made his first appearance, Purmann's *Chirurgischer Lorbeer-Krantz oder Wund-Artzney*, which criticized long stumps, entered its second edition. Barbette's *Chirurgische und anatomische Schrifften*, which described "the manner of Aquapendente" at length, also began circulating in its fourth German edition that same decade. Only a few years before, new editions of the works of both Scultetus and Fabry had appeared in German and Latin.[104] A patient suffering from the cold fire in a lower extremity faced a wider spectrum of surgical possibilities at the close of the seventeenth century than at the beginning of the sixteenth. Far from reaching a consensus about a

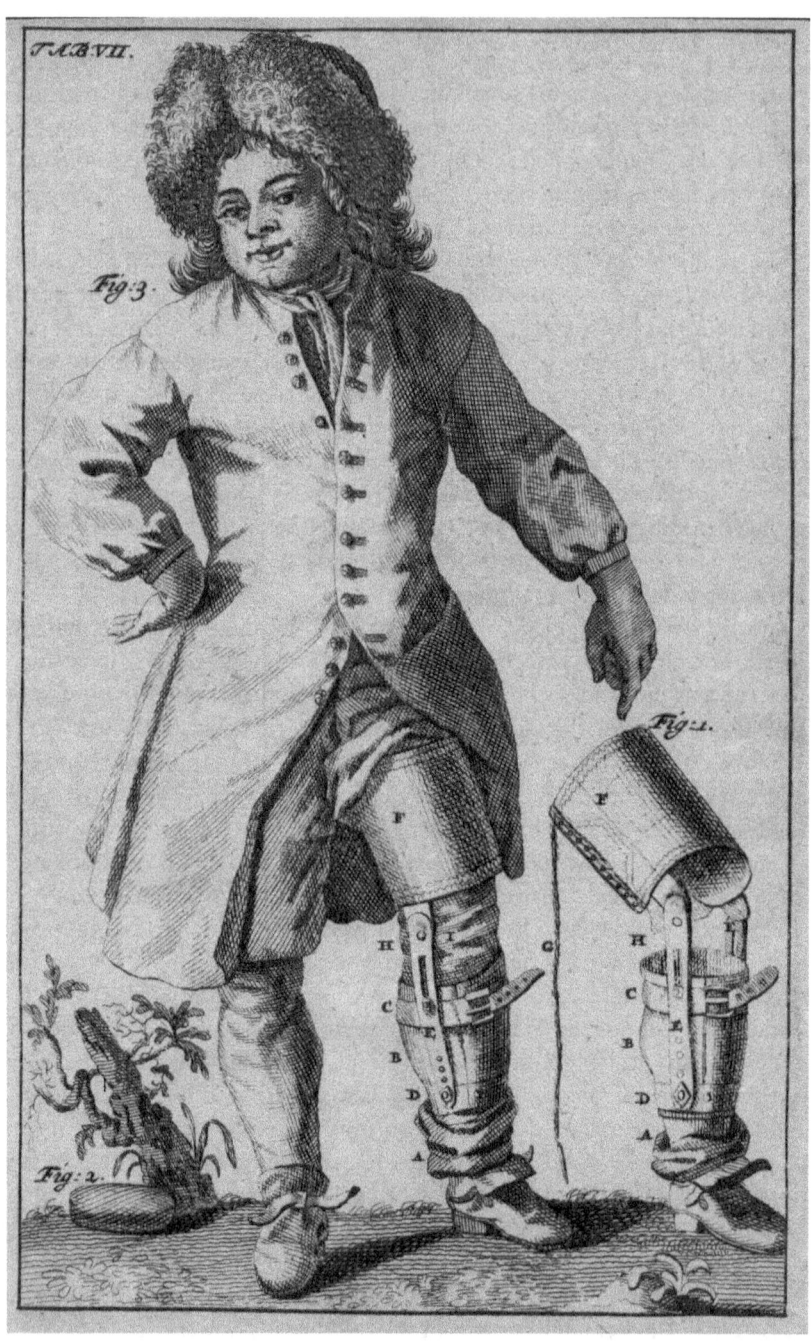

3.4 Patient with prosthetic leg in Pieter Adriaanszoon Verduyn, *Neue Methode, die Glieder abzunehmen* (Amsterdam, 1697), Tab. VII.

uniform approach, the surgical literature increasingly made space for a body that could be altered in drastically different ways.

The meanings of debate

Early modern surgeons worked by trial and error to learn and modify approaches to amputation that were tailored to the unique challenges the removal of an extremity posed. They did not base their decisions to cut, saw, sew, and burn solely on the exigencies of the moment. They also took inspiration from multiple sources—their teachers, their experiences in practice, and their reading. Guided by a calculated list of priorities, a chosen method reflected what was *more* important in their eyes. This could change on a case-by-case basis. Practitioners, particularly field-surgeons, were creative by necessity, and the spectrum of amputation techniques circulated in the vernacular offered them the flexibility to adapt to the individual circumstances and needs of each patient. Their treatises reveal the slow formation of a code of professional ethics, a series of proposals for how the surgeon should respond to a putrefying body in every conceivable context. These printed assertions were built from and part of the greater knowledge-making practices surgeons carried out with every operation.

The epistemological value of surgeons' amputation techniques lay in the connection, created and present as they operated on individual patients, between developing an embodied knowledge of how physical, bodily matter worked and an intimate questioning of what it meant to be human more broadly. As they cut apart bodies and sewed or cauterized tissue back together, and as they observed and theorized over the results, they implicitly and explicitly considered what features were elemental to human life and living in human society. Through their amputation techniques, they explored different ways in which the physical body belonged to or supported those features. And in every procedure they undertook, they continued to work through the challenge of determining the surgeon's role in these matters. The crossing of these two kinds of problems, of physical matter and the human, constantly being worked out and reconsidered during surgical procedures, was at the center of the surgeon's way of making knowledge and developing meaning.

Amputation debates do not offer one linear story, but rather a series of overlapping stories. Three are of especial importance. The first is methodological. Surgical instructions shed light on how early modern surgeons thought, and how their thoughts differed from one another. Amputation methods reflected different visions of surgical practices and priorities: the surgeon who viewed the body as almost endlessly malleable and the surgeon who took it as a constraining system to be interfered with as little as possible; the surgeon who designed a complex and multi-staged operation and the surgeon who preferred a simple and radical procedure. Each vision defined the best interests of the patient in a specific way that adjusted the nature and scope of the surgeon's task. This could encompass the patient's present and future safety, physical and emotional comfort, material integrity, and ability to perform everyday activities. Surgeons did not articulate the sum of these interests—what we might call "well-being." Rather, we find it implicitly, in their arguments about the advantages and especially the disadvantages of various techniques.

Disagreements about methods for removing the lower leg show us that an amputation was about much more than simply excising the cold fire. The controversy surrounding the choice of amputation site in lower leg procedures practically vanished when discussing the upper extremities because sparing as much of the arm as possible preserved healthy flesh, was safest for the patient, and provided the best placement for an artificial hand all in one. As Purmann explained:

> At the arm however the flesh must on the contrary be spared, so that one can so much more conveniently put on an iron hand, and also the damage is not so very noticeable, moreover it [the amputation] is also not so dangerous lower [on the arm] as above, on account of the heavy bleeding.[105]

The advantages he cited in preserving the length of an upper extremity directly conflicted with one another in the lower leg. The hand's-width method selected a site that was higher on the limb than necessary in order to craft a stump capable of bearing a prosthesis. This site posed a greater risk of hemorrhaging and required the removal of healthy flesh. Alternative methods of amputation that arose in the early modern period resisted this order of priorities in different ways. They reasserted the surgeon's mission to protect the healthy body, a feature championed in the textual tradition since the Hippocratic corpus. Some of their methods, like that of Aquapendente, also insisted on the unrivaled importance of the patient's immediate safety. Still others advanced new attitudes toward available prosthetic technology.

The vision embedded in the hand's-width method was of the body as a vehicle of motion. The leg was defined by its function as an instrument of mobility rather than as a material entity vital to the patient's person. If a small fraction of the lower leg could serve the patient's needs better than a larger one, then there was no reason to preserve as much of the lower leg as possible. The surgeon trespassed on medicine's aim to safeguard the healthy body in order to provide for the patient's future well-being, which in this context was nearly synonymous with mobility. Practitioners aggressively intervened in the body's form to ensure the patient could maneuver the limb long after the operation was over.

Alternative approaches to lower leg amputations presented a different relationship of the surgeon to the patient, the body, and nature. Some techniques limited the surgeon's power to intervene and narrowed the temporal scope of his concerns to focus primarily on the patient's immediate needs.

These insisted that nature should determine the amputation site, at times even placing the body in a self-regulating role. The view of the leg as an instrument of motion, and the imperative to provide for future mobility, were absent from the instructions of those who preserved as much of the patient's healthy leg as possible. An important exception appeared in the latter half of the seventeenth century, when the views of Dutch practitioners advocating for the conservation of long stumps because of their utility to the patient began to circulate in the Holy Roman Empire. Attitudes toward new technology made possible a compromise between the priorities of the hand's-width and alternative methods of lower leg amputation.

In other words, surgical instructions give insight into surgeons' views of the body and help us map their ideas over time. They also reveal a different form of early modern medical theory than scholars usually discuss. Rather than a corpus of formal thought, codified in authoritative texts, surgical instructions reveal implicit approaches to the body developed through practices. These were operational theories about what the parts of the body were for and how far they could be changed. Though not explicitly codified in learned or craft literature, these theories actually guided surgeons' hands and instruments.

The second story amputation debates tell is of a shift in the available technology, and in attitudes toward it. Advocates of the hand's-width method and later champions of alternative methods from the Dutch Republic were concerned about the stumps surgeons created. They gave increasing attention to how altered body parts interacted with artificial materials, and they shared the priority of reshaping the patient's body to bear a prosthesis. But their attitudes toward prosthetic limb technology formed a fault line between them. Dutch surgeons like Muys, Solingen, and Verduyn emphasized the importance of technological progress in prosthetic devices to explain why early moderns could and should break with the past and spare the length of the lower leg. Surgical treatises offer few details about the "new" prostheses used to defend the preservation of the lower leg. But their impact on advocates for longer stumps is clear.

The chronology of shifting centers of medical influence outlined in this chapter coincides to a remarkable extent with scholarship on technological leadership, a long-established concept in economic history that social historians of early modern Europe have found useful. Among social historians, the theory refers to a discrete geographic region that initiates the development of new technologies in a wide range of areas. Scholars have argued that technological leadership moved in succession from northern Italy to Germany, to the Dutch Republic, and then to Britain between the late Middle Ages and the mid-eighteenth century.[106] The correlation between this timeline and that of surgical debates may offer a way to connect medical literature and experience to larger historical narratives of change.[107] At the very least, it identifies new territory for further exploration.

Finally, amputation debates tell a story about the rising challenge to Galenic medicine. Ancient and medieval surgical treatises were of course by no means monolithic in their discussions of amputation. Nevertheless, the growing number of techniques examined at increasing length in early modern treatises was linked to broader intellectual and methodological conflicts within medicine that created a less coherent approach to surgical thinking. Some author-practitioners incorporated elements deemed useful from different approaches without adopting any one of them wholesale. Others adhered more strictly to a specific viewpoint, which then guided their instructions. Drawing from multiple approaches, they brought a rich panoply of voices into conversation about the challenge of limb loss.

Renaissance anatomy at Padua, for example, taught Galenic writings even as its proponents challenged Galen's infallible authority. Girolamo Fabrizi d'Acquapendente, whose name became synonymous with an amputation method, belonged to a network of anatomists who uncovered structures of the human body that Galen had not seen or recorded. His career, as Cynthia Klestinec shows, particularly highlighted the environment of intense competition in the late sixteenth and early seventeenth centuries as anatomists vied with one another over approaches to anatomical demonstration.[108] Johannes Scultetus, the staunch German defender of the Aquapendente method, came out of this complex institutional and intellectual context. This informed his learned approach to surgery, which worked within the Galenic tradition while arguing that his mentors' techniques surpassed the ancients.

Rival theoretical models to Galenic humoralism, namely forms of iatrochemicalism and iatrophysics, surfaced in debates over the lower leg. The Paracelsian perspective, which sought to preserve all healthy flesh, sprang from an attack on the learned Galenic tradition. Paracelsus spurned ancient texts and insisted medical practitioners look to nature and experience to learn the art of healing. In his teachings a chemical natural philosophy, an early pillar of the iatrochemical school of thought, supplanted humoral theory. The vast majority of his works did not appear until after his death, but his surgical writings were widely circulated. Three editions of his *Große Wundartznei* appeared during his lifetime; thirty-one in total appeared between 1536 and 1656. Surgery, then, was a major way by which Paracelsian ideas entered German culture.[109]

The competing methodology of iatrophysicists, who drew on the laws of mechanics to understand the body, also appears within amputation debates.[110] Jan Muys, who praised new prosthetic technology and advocated for long lower leg stumps because of their utility, was a widely influential Cartesian medical reformer.[111] He not only defended Descartes at length in his prefaces, but also integrated him into the main body of his surgical text, placing the philosopher alongside practicing surgeons. In a case history concerning a gunshot wound, Muys manages to reference Descartes's *Principia philosophiae* on gunpowder and then advise readers to consult Fabry von Hilden and Johannes Scultetus about instruments to extract bullets.[112] Muys's German translator, Christoph Horch (1667–1754), declared in his preface that physicians and surgeons had been freed from the erroneous foundations of the four humors and were now supported by and grounded in the solid foundations of the true philosophy.[113]

Amputation debates draw out another critical perspective to the inherited textual tradition: vernacular surgeons from master–apprentice backgrounds. The hand's-width method shows the new influence they wielded in the wider textual discourse. Their voice, though difficult to hear and by no means representative of a uniform school of thought, is crucial to any discussion about the gradual dismantling of Galenism. In theory, removing some healthy flesh during an amputation was not incompatible with the received Galenic tradition. Since antiquity, even as authors instructed on sparing as much healthy flesh as possible, they also discussed disarticulating at the nearest joint, thereby removing some healthy flesh, to ensure the complete removal of disease or a swifter procedure. But, as Nancy Siraisi suggests, "in reality, amputation of limbs through living tissue was probably rare before the sixteenth century."[114] The boldness of the hand's-width technique was entirely in the amputation site, chosen not for speed or safety, nor because of the extent of the cold fire, but to create a useful stump that could bear a prosthesis. This principle, expressed at length in surgical treatises in the latter half of the sixteenth century, did not come from the inherited textual tradition, and its goal was antithetical to previous discussions of disarticulating at the joint. Its guiding rationale was markedly more mechanical and practical than earlier teachings: its advocates espoused a vision of the body as a vehicle of motion.

That the technique gained support over time among authors from both master–apprentice and university-educated backgrounds reflects the compatibility of this perspective with Galenic medicine *and* new strains of natural philosophy arising in the sixteenth and seventeenth centuries. Barbette, for example, received his doctorate from the University of Leiden and was a close friend of Francois de le Boë Sylvius, a leader in the iatrochemical school of thought whose work attempted to create a chemical foundation for Galenic humoralism and whose ideas also drew from Cartesian matter theory.[115] Barbette's description of the body as a clock is one sign of this influence.[116] Purmann, by contrast, trained by apprenticeship and served as a field-surgeon for several years. Christoph Horch, who as we have seen was a passionate follower of medical Cartesianism and translated Muys's work, spent time as a student in Breslau to learn from Purmann.[117] The orders of priorities in the hand's-width method and in the approach in seventeenth-century Dutch treatises like Muys's, after all, aligned. Even though one advocated for a short stump and the other for a long, they shared the goal of shaping a limb capable of movement. This suggests that the sensibilities advanced by vernacular surgeons who treated the leg as a vehicle of motion were compatible with the mechanistic view of Cartesian medicine and predated it by half a century in print.

Taken together, these overlapping stories of visions of the body, attitudes toward technology, and competing approaches in medicine point to a greater meaning in amputation debates. They signify a gradual and far from inevitable process in which the human body became more flexible in form, its limbs more adaptable to artificial supplements, its texture more pliant to the surgeon's instruments. Authors of early modern surgical treatises were not unified in their views about the extent to which and the manner in which one should manipulate the body in an amputation. The more surgeons experimented, learned, discussed, and disagreed about techniques, the more different ideas about the body circulated and came to be considered side by side. The multiplicity of methods recorded in any single treatise reflected surgeons' abilities to ponder modifying the body in many different ways at once. The result was an expansion of surgical possibilities for amputation between the sixteenth century and the close of the seventeenth.

Without a doubt, hands-on practice was essential to the substance and the ebb and flow of textual debates. Yet whether treatises mapped accurately onto widespread surgical practice may be impossible to discover. A competitive medical marketplace could have encouraged different authorial strategies, such as situating oneself within a distinguished, learned tradition or presenting oneself as an innovator. What these debates can tell us for certain is that the contours of the amputee body underwent significant alterations in the early modern period. Surgeons learned from and experimented with the natural material of their patients' bodies. More remarkable still, with their tools and treatises, they actually created a new kind of body. A malleable body.

Notes

1 Schmid, *Examen chirurgicum*, 252: "Wie kompts/ daß deren viel sterben/ nach dem das Glied abgenommen ist?"
2 Ibid.: "Darumb wie ich gesagt hab/ ist solches ein gefährlich unnd sorglich ding/ dann so jetzt der Brand die Nerven und Maußfleisch angriffen/ laufft etwan der Brand under der Haut im Fleisch ubersich/ daß man es aussen nicht sicht/ noch spüren mag/ So man dann das Glied nit hoch genug abnimbt/ also daß ein eintziger Nerven zu kurz abgeschnitten wird/ laufft der Brand in dem Nerven hindersich/ daß also der Schnitt vergebens ist/ daß man das Glied noch ein mal abschneiden muß/ oder darvon stirbt."

3 Sachs, *Sixteenth-Century Book of Trades*, 182–183.
4 E.g., Roberts et al., *Mindful Hand*; Long, *Artisan/Practitioners*. On connections among surgeons and artisans in this period: Stolz, *Die Handwerke des Körpers*; Cavallo, *Artisans of the Body*; Kinzelbach, "Erudite and Honoured Artisans?"
5 Smith, *Body of the Artisan*.
6 E.g., Leong, *Recipes and Everyday Knowledge*; Rankin, *Panaceia's Daughters*.
7 Hildanus, *Wund-Artzney*, 937: "das Ebenbild GOTTES."
8 Barbette, *Schrifften*, 1. See chap. 1 for Barbette's fourfold schema.
9 Hildanus, *Gründlicher Bericht*, 117, 163; Paré, *Wund-Artzney* (1635), 421; Purmann, *Wund-Artzney* (1692), 3:229.
10 Galen, *Opera omnia*, 718; Ferragud, "Wounds, Amputations, and Expert Procedures," 247–248; Krajbich et al., *Atlas of Amputations*, 1:3; Wangensteen and Wangensteen, *Rise of Surgery*, 16–18.
11 Gurlt, *Geschichte*, 3:794.
12 Ferragud, "Wounds, Amputations, and Expert Procedures," 248.
13 Celsus, *De Medicina*, 3:469–471; Gurlt, *Geschichte*, 3:794.
14 Mitchell, *Medicine in the Crusades*, 153; Ferragud, "Wounds, Amputations, and Expert Procedures," 248.
15 Ferragud, "Wounds, Amputations, and Expert Procedures," 248–249.
16 E.g., Borgognoni, *Surgery of Theodoric*, 2:37.
17 Chauliac, *Cyrurgie*, 412–413.
18 Mondeville, *Chirurgie*, 564–568; Albucasis, *On Surgery and Instruments*, 562–566; Gurlt, *Geschichte*, 3:795.
19 DeVries and Smith, *Medieval Military Technology*, 5–41; Woosnam-Savage and DeVries, "Battle Trauma."
20 DeVries and Smith, *Medieval Military Technology*, 137–163; Lindemann, *Medicine and Society*, 131.
21 Kirkup, *Limb Amputation*, 105.
22 See Bynum and Porter, *Companion Encyclopedia of the History of Medicine*, 2:970–971.
23 Hildanus, *Gründlicher Bericht*, 118: "daß einem ehrbaren und fleißigen Arzt nicht geziemt, solch ein grobes und unschickliches Werk zu verrichten und seine Verwundeten wie ein Scharfrichter zu behandeln." Joseph Schmid also complained of inexperienced practitioners using mallets in the manner of hangmen: *Instrumenta chirurgica*, 180.
24 Harrington, *Faithful Executioner*, 64.
25 Hildanus, *Gründlicher Bericht*, 118.
26 Ibid.
27 Ibid., 118–119.
28 Hildanus, *Wund-Artzney*, 701.
29 Scultetus, *Wund-Artzneyisches Zeug-Hauß* (1666), 1:202–203, Tab. LIII, Fig. 6: "Die VI. Figur weiset/ wie die von dem kalten Brand gantz eingenommene Hand/ auff einem hohen und runden Stotzen oder Block (o.) dargeleget wird/ umb solche/ nächst an denen noch gesunden Häuptern/ der grossen und kleinen Elenbogen Röhren (wider deß Hildani Meynung/ und zwar mit glücklichem

Fortgang) vermittelst eines auß dem härtesten Holtz gemachten Schlegels (t.) und eines Stemm Eisens (p.) abzuhauen" (emphasis mine).

30 Ibid., 1:39, Tab. XX: "ein gar grosse Pfetz-Zang/ mit welcher ein abgestorbene/ oder mit einem Krebsschaden behaffte Hand/ Finger/ Fürfuß und Zähen/ ohne Gebrauch eines einigen Messers zum öfftern abgezwickt wird."

31 Ibid., 2:212.

32 Joseph Schmid reported that in cases of the highest necessity, all surgeons used actual cautery as a fail-proof method to stop massive hemorrhaging: *Examen chirurgicum*, 135.

33 For an illustration: Scultetus, *Wund-Artzneyisches Zeug-Hauß* (1666), 1:Tab. XIX.

34 Pierre Franco and Giovanni Andrea Della Croce also discussed amputating with a heated sickle knife in the latter half of the sixteenth century: e.g., Della Croce, *Wund-Artzney*, 106.

35 Hildanus, *Wund-Artzney*, 489: "so hab ich alsbald mit der lincken Hand/ den Schenckel ergriffen/ und mit der rechten das Fleisch biß auff das Bein ledig gemacht/ aber nicht mit dem Schermesser ... sondern mit einem brennenden Eysen/ welches die Form eines Messers gehabt. ... Durch hülff dieses Brenneysens/ hab ich das Fleisch abgeledigt/ und zu mahl das Blut gestellt; Alß nun das Fleisch biß auf das Bein abgeschnitten/ hab ich hernach die Seg in die rechte Hand gefast/ und das Bein glücklich damit abgeschnitten/ und ob zwar solche verrichtung schwer war/ so ist mir doch/ Gott sey Lob/ nichts widriges darbey begegnet."

36 Solingen, *Hand-Griffe*, 394: "Hildanus lobet sein Cauterium cultellare, oder Brenn-Eisen welches als ein Messer gestalt ist/ sehr/... die Haut und musculi &c. zusammen geschrumpelt werden."

37 Ibid.: "wie er selbsten gestehet," "so halte ich davor/ daß der Gebrauch von diesem Instrumente nicht gut und dienlich kan seyn."

38 Barbette, *Schrifften*, 38, 45.

39 Ibid., 69: "weit sicherer als das jenige/ so mit etzenden Artzneyen (*potentiale*) geschicht/ doch wird man gemeiniglich wegen der Furcht des Krancken gezwungen/ dieses letztere vor die Hand zu nehmen."

40 Solingen, *Hand-Griffe*, 376: "Auch muß man die Feuerpfanne mit glüenden Kohlen und Cauterien/ oder Brenn-Eisen darein/ zur Seiten des Patienten setzen/ damit derselbige sie nicht sehe."

41 Barbette, *Schrifften*, 45.

42 Muys, *Praxis*, 319: "sie liegen in einem Garten/ in welchen auch noch nach ihre Todte alle Jahr aus der substantz ihrer Cörper die insignia ihres Reichs/ das seynd Lilien/ hervor wachsen."

43 Cornelis Solingen also characterized the use of vitriol of Cyprus as a French practice: *Hand-Griffe*, 397.

44 Scultetus, *Wund-Artzneyisches Zeug-Hauß* (1666), 1:203.

45 E.g., Celsus, *De Medicina*, 3:417–419.

46 Solingen, *Hand-Griffe*, 394.

47 Ibid., 396: "grausam and unbarmhertzig." By contrast, Solingen's contemporary Jan Muys suggested that cautery irons were seldom used and reported that he

had seen the ligation of blood vessels performed safely and successfully: Muys, *Praxis*, 319.
48 Solingen, *Hand-Griffe*, 392: "In Seeschlachten gebrauchet man zum meisten das Brennen/ weilen solches das leichteste/ gemächlichste und fertigste Mittel vor dem Chirurgo ist," "man alle Patienten nicht zugleich helffen kan/ dann indem man einen hilffet/ so lieget der andere und blutet."
49 Jessen, *Wund-Artznei*, 182; Hildanus, *Gründlicher Bericht*, 118.
50 Solingen, *Hand-Griffe*, 372–388; Schmid, *Instrumenta chirurgica*, 174; Hildanus, *Gründlicher Bericht*, 128.
51 Hildanus, *Gründlicher Bericht*, 117; Paré, *Wund-Artzney* (1635), 420–421; Barbette, *Schrifften*, 77; Herls, *Examen*, 563.
52 Schmid, *Instrumenta chirurgica*, 176. See also Sachs, *Geschichte*, 2:185–201.
53 On the treatise and the circulation of its images: Panse, *Feldbuch der Wundarznei*.
54 Herls, *Examen*, 564; Schmid, *Instrumenta chirurgica*, 170; Hildanus, *Gründlicher Bericht*, 127; Renner, *Artzney-Büchlein*, 223.
55 Hildanus, *Gründlicher Bericht*, 128; Schmid, *Examen chirurgicum*, 251.
56 E.g. Hildanus, *Gründlicher Bericht*, 127; Paré, *Wundt-Artzney* (1601), 531.
57 Solingen, *Hand-Griffe*, 384–385.
58 Hildanus, *Gründlicher Bericht*, 117.
59 Barbette, *Schrifften*, 77.
60 Purmann, *Wund-Artzney* (1692), 3:229: "Ich sage zu diesen allen/ man muß hierinnen auf keine Bequemligkeit/ sondern auf den Nutz und Dienst des Gliedes und Leibes sehen."
61 Hildanus, *Gründlicher Bericht*, 117.
62 Paré, *Wund-Artzney* (1635), 421: "mehr beschwerlich unnd verhinderlich," "denn dienstlich war/ besser hinauffwertz," "ohngefähr fünff Finger unter dem Knie," "er nemlich denselbigen nachmals viel besser brauchen unnd hurtiger bewegen können/ denn zuvor."
63 Ibid.
64 Hildanus, *Wund-Artzney*, 1046: "Dann ob wol der Wundartzt deß Menschen Leib/ so viel müglich ist/ verschonen soll/ so ist dennoch gewiß/ daß solcher übriger Stumpff deß Schenkels/ den er etwan noch würde erhalten können/ dem Krancken nach der Heylung grosse Ungelegenheit zufüget." Compare to Purmann, *Chirurgia curiosa*, 655.
65 Paré, *Wund-Artzney* (1601), 531: "Jedoch kann man diesem Rath von wegen der Wirckung und Zierthe/ deß ubrigen und gesundten Theils deß Gliedts nit allwegen nachkommen und folgen."
66 Archaeological evidence in medieval and early modern Europe shows a variety of lower leg amputation sites. One example from Denmark (c. 1500) occurred ten centimeters above the ankle; another from Germany (eighth century) at the knee joint; and two examples from Switzerland (11th–15th centuries) at the ankle. See, respectively, Ladegaard Jakobsen, "Cripple from the Late Middle Ages," 21; Keil, "Eine Prothese"; Ulrich-Bochsler and Baumgartner, "Über drei Funde von Amputationen." For a later example from Canada that addresses the effect of prosthesis use on a lower leg stump 78 mm below the knee (approximately a

hand's width): Lazenby and Pfeiffer, "Effects of a Nineteenth Century Below-Knee Amputation."
67 E.g., Bruegel the Elder, *The Beggars*, 1568, oil on wood; Issickemer, *Buchlein*, title page; Harms et al., *Deutsche Illustrierte Flugblätter*, 2:418–419, 492–493.
68 Botallo, *Zwey Chirurgische Bücher*, 2:297.
69 Purmann, *Chirurgia curiosa*, 655–656.
70 Purmann, *Wund-Artzney* (1692), 3:235: "es geschwinder und hurtiger geschehen kan/ wenn es wol angehet: Aber wer kan uns versichern/ daß unter 10. malen es 5. mal recht angehet."
71 Ibid., 3:230: "der Patient eine Steltzen tragen muß," "ein gemachter Fuß," "Geschweige der Röhren/ die unterwerts im mitlern Theile weit voneinander stehen und eine langsame operation machen/ welches näher dem Kniehe nicht ist/ und hurtiger und besser ... gehet."
72 Pagel, *Paracelsus*, 148; Vekerdy, "Paracelsus's *Great Wound Surgery*."
73 E.g., Lose and Greiff, *Hand-Büchlein*, 55–58; Agricola, *Wund-Artzney*, 519.
74 E.g., Agricola, *Wund-Artzney*, 223–224.
75 Greiff, *Wolbewärte Wundarzney*, 27: "daß du kein lebendigs berürest."
76 Ibid., 29: "hastu nun auch kürtzlichen Bericht/ hülffe und Rath zum Beinabschneiden/ daß du der scherffe des Schermessers gar wol entrathen kanst."
77 Surgical treatises referred to this technique as "the manner of Aquapendente." Keeping to this spirit, I refer to it as the "Aquapendente method."
78 Barbette, *Schrifften*, 78–79.
79 Wangensteen and Wangensteen, *Rise of Surgery*, 18.
80 Girolamo Fabrizi d'Acquapendente and Cornelis Solingen both credited the papal surgeon Giovanni da Vigo (c. 1450–1525) as the first to give a detailed method of amputating in dead flesh and using cautery to burn off the remaining putrefaction: Fabricius ab Aquapendente, *Wund-Artznei*, 2:299; Solingen, *Hand-Griffe*, 406. For Giovanni da Vigo's original discussion: *Practica in chirurgia*, fol. 125r.
81 Barbette, *Schrifften*, 78.
82 In Fabrizi's surgical works (published under his Latinized name Hieronymus Fabricius ab Aquapendente), he showed remarkable reserve toward invasive procedures long established in medical literature, although he otherwise drew heavily from ancient authorities, particularly Celsus and Paulus of Aegina. His publications demonstrate awareness of the technique of ligating blood vessels, but it was not discussed in his work on amputation, nor did he cite the contemporary authority Ambroise Paré. See Gurlt, *Geschichte*, 2:447–448.
83 Herls, *Examen*, 563; Schmid, *Examen chirurgicum*, 249–250.
84 For example, Paul Barbette advocated amputation in healthy flesh at least two fingers below the knee, but for certain cases he also explained and advised the use of the Aquapendente method: *Schrifften*, 77–79.
85 Ibid., 78–79.
86 Schmid, *Examen chirurgicum*, 253: "so dann eine verbrech/ er alsbald ein andere hätte/ sonsten würde sich der Patient zu todt bluten/ biß man ein andere holen müste."

87 Fabry von Hilden argued that the procedure risked failing to excise all of the cold fire since the corruption spread faster deep along the bone, where it was not visible externally: Hildanus, *Gründlicher Bericht*, 119–126.

88 Hildanus, *Gründlicher Bericht*, 124: "Deshalb bleibt die Narbe schwach und wird immer wieder durch die Stelze beschädigt."

89 Scultetus, *Wund-Artzneyisches Zeug-Hauß* (1666), 1:204–205.

90 Ibid., 1:205: "längere Weil oder mehrere Zeit erfordert wird/ die Puls-Adern mit dem Zänglein herfür zu ziehen/ und mit dem Faden umzubinden und zu verknüpffen/ (über das/ wann man auch die Binde aufflöset und abnimmet/ so erfolget bißweilen ein solches verbluten darauff/ daß/ wann man die übrige Gefässe der Adern nicht ebenmässig mit glüenden Eisern dupffet/ solches nimmermehr kan noch mag gestellet werden)."

91 Ibid.: "der Padoanischen Wund-Ärzten/ und deß Hieron. Fabricij Manier," "der alten Chirurgorum."

92 Solingen, *Hand-Griffe*, 384–385: "wann ein Kalterbrand in den Fuß oder Zehen ist/ und sich eine Geschwulst über die Enckel oder Knöchel zeiget/ ... man alsdann nicht lange mit dem Abnehmen des Beines warten muß/ dann sonsten der gantze Fuß angestochen wird/ da im Gegentheil/ man noch die Länge des Fusses oder Armes sparen kan/ (ob gleich solches der Alten Befehl gantz zuwider ist/ als welche wollen/ daß man das Bein allezeit solle vier oder fünff Fingerbreit unter dem Knie abnehmen) dann man kan noch Instrumenten als ein Fuß/ an das abgenommene Bein feste an machen/ mit welchen der Patient gemächlich gehen kan/ welches viel gemächlicher geschiehet/ wann das Schienbein oder Unterbein noch lang ist/ dann je länger es ist/ je besser ist es auch/ dann der Patient damit desto besser den angesetzten Fuß fortschieben kan."

93 Muys, *Praxis*, 320: "Vor diesen hat man allezeit den Schenckel ein wenig unterm Knie abgenommen/ wenn gleich der kalte Brandt noch nicht das dritte Theil desselben inficirt gehabt/ aber jetziger Zeit erhält man so viel müglich die Länge des Schenckels/ weil man heutiges Tages instrumenta erdacht hat/ welche dem weit unters Knie abgenommenen Schenckel füglich können appliciret werden."

94 Solingen, *Hand-Griffe*, 413–414: "wann solches an den Fuß unter den Knie geschiehet/ so kan man besser einen höltzernen oder kupffernen Fuß dran machen."

95 Paré, *Wund-Artzney* (1635), 750.

96 The concept of flap amputation had been published nearly two decades earlier by the English surgeon James Yonge (1647–1721) in his *Currus triumphalis*. Yonge's treatises do not appear to have been translated, printed, or circulated within the Holy Roman Empire in the seventeenth century, and Verduyn's treatise does not indicate any familiarity with Yonge or his work.

97 Verduyn, *Neue Methode*, 17–18.

98 Ibid., 16–17.

99 Ibid., 15: "Dan man muß sich wohl vorsehen/ daß man keinen Fuß absetze/ der durch Kalten-brand oder andere Kranckheiten schon gantzlich verdorben ist; dan alle Arbeit und Muhe ist hier umbsonst."

100 Ibid., 24–25: "man an den übergebliebenen Stumpf gar bequem ansetzen kan einen gemachten Fuß mit einem Strumpf und Schuh versehen/ welcher so künstlich/ daß er scheinet ein rechter natürlicher Fuß zu seyn/ worauff er so wohl als auf sein ander Bein gehen kan."
101 Ibid., 25: "Derohalben ist hier zu erinnern/ daß man den Stumpf so lang lässet als möglich/ damit der gemachte Fuß desto fester könne angebunden werden."
102 Ibid., 31.
103 Ibid., 14.
104 Purmann, *Wund-Artzney* (1692), 3:230; Barbette, *Schrifften*, 78–79; Hildanus, *Opera observationum et curationum*; Scultetus, *Wund-Artzneyisches Zeug-Hauß* (1679); Scultetus, *Armamentarium Chirurgicum* (1693).
105 Purmann, *Wund-Artzney* (1692), 3:230: "Am Arme aber muß das Fleisch im Gegentheil geschonet werden/ damit man desto füglicher eine eyserne Hand anmachen könne/ und auch der Schaden nicht gar zusehr gemercket werde/ zudem ist es auch unten so gefahrlich nicht/ als oben/ wegen des starcken Blutens."
106 Davids, "Shifts of Technological Leadership"; Ames and Rosenberg, "Changing Technological Leadership."
107 For example, in the latter half of the seventeenth century, the Dutch Republic was a site of medical innovation on multiple fronts: Ragland, "Experimental Clinical Medicine."
108 Klestinec, *Theaters of Anatomy*, 56–57, 143–144, 160. Klestinec has also examined the private anatomies of Giulio Casseri to explore meanings of embodied knowledge and experience in anatomy and surgery: "Practical Experience in Anatomy."
109 Gunnoe Jr., "Paracelsus's Biography"; Vekerdy, "Paracelsus's *Great Wound Surgery*," 78; Pagel, *Paracelsus*, 126–152.
110 De Moulin, *History of Surgery*, 100.
111 Muys, *Praxis*, 3–4, 140, 187; Munt, "Dutch Cartesian Medical Reformers," 33, 88–91. For Cartesian medicine in the broader Dutch context: Schmaltz, *Early Modern Cartesianisms*, 228–283.
112 Muys, *Praxis*, 156.
113 Ibid., unpaginated.
114 Siraisi, *Medieval and Early Renaissance Medicine*, 157.
115 De Moulin, "Paul Barbette," 507, and *History of Surgery*, 99; Ragland, "Chymistry and Taste."
116 Barbette, *Schrifften*, 221.
117 Horch takes pains to identify this connection at the close of his dedication: Muys, *Praxis*, sig.)(5v.

4

After the operation

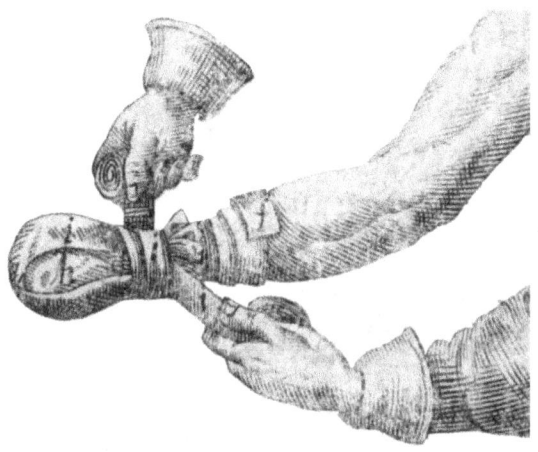

The prolific artist Jost Amman attempted to capture the whole of surgery in his title page illustration for Paracelsus's *Opus Chyrurgicum* of 1565 (figure 4.1).[1] The image, which has little to do with Paracelsian subjects, presents a series of self-contained scenes taking place in a hospital sickroom. Medical practitioners dominate the foreground. From left to right, a surgeon amputates the leg of an open-mouthed patient, two physicians and an apothecary are engrossed in discussion, and another surgeon treats a head wound. Each conveys bustling activity, from the motion of the saw to the physician's wide gesticulation with a uroscopy flask. The background features another kind of medical drama. Two of the four beds lining the walls are occupied. The patient on the left is the picture of unrest. He lies with one hand on his head, an arm crossed over his body, and his knees bent. A woman, perhaps a member of the hospital staff, approaches him through the open door. On the right is another patient who lies still, hands folded in prayer and head turned slightly to look at the figure at the bedside. Christ, crowned with heavenly rays, stands with both palms turned in a sign of blessing, healing, or both. His presence not only reminds the viewer of God's role as the divine physician, but also suggests that a patient's fate was ultimately unknowable to mortal practitioners, a point surgeons often made.

Surgical treatises offer the historian a perspective on early modern amputees not unlike the view from Amman's woodcut. The largest figures drawn

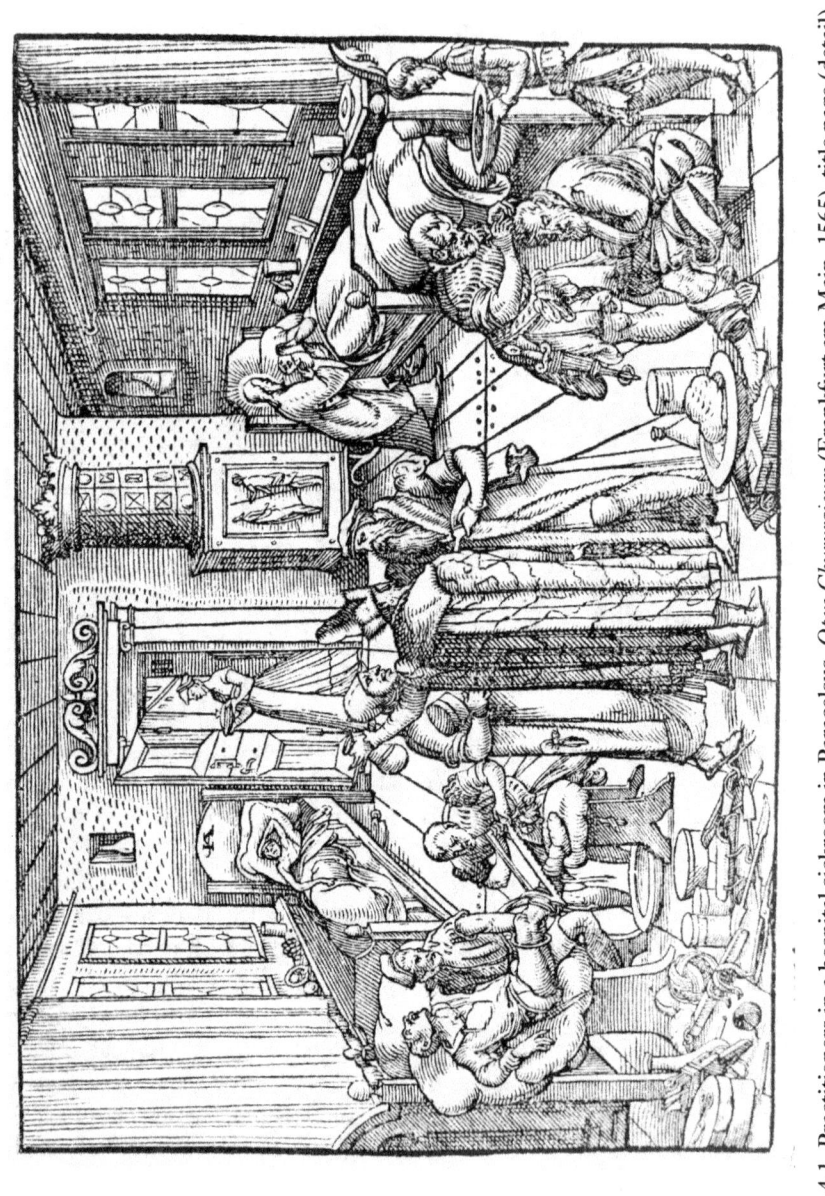

4.1 Practitioners in a hospital sickroom in Paracelsus, *Opus Chyrurgicum* (Frankfurt am Main, 1565), title page (detail).

in the greatest detail are practitioners operating on patients. The more time that passes after a procedure, the smaller and less clear the figures become. Convalescing patients appear at a distance. Those who recover are somewhere beyond, through the door and out in the world. For all of its limitations, this vantage point reveals much about how surgeons conceptualized the body during recovery from an amputation and thereafter.

Recovery, for surgeons, meant a healed stump. Their treatises provided detailed instructions on how to care for the stump and attend to the various complications patients experienced following the procedure. What came after the stump healed was typically addressed indirectly, if at all. Here, Amman's room with an open door is a useful analogy. Inside the room, the surgeon has firsthand encounters treating patients and draws on these experiences to learn about the body. Looking out the door, he can spot passersby at a distance and reflect on what he sees or hears secondhand. Moreover, the door remains open. A patient whose stump heals might leave a surgeon's care only to return later to address an injury to the stump or an entirely unrelated ailment.

This chapter explores how surgeons went about asking and answering questions concerning amputees' bodies in surgical literature. I examine two issues. The first involves the puzzling experience of sensations in amputated limbs. This appears within discussions of convalescence, as surgeons sought to combat a myriad of symptoms threatening recovery. In our analogy of Amman's woodcut, the surgeon is busy at work inside the room, analyzing firsthand experiences. By contrast, the second issue turns on surgeons' abstract ideas about the future of amputees whose stumps had healed, and thus were no longer convalescing patients. Here the surgeon looks out the door, drawing on his accumulated knowledge of surgery and the body to interpret and reflect on activities outside of his everyday practice. At the heart of both issues was the recognition that a limb amputation removed something surgeons could not replace. They grappled with the implications of irrevocable bodily alteration in ways that were pragmatic, intellectual, and cultural. Their experiences informed their understanding of how the body could respond to a major surgical intervention, but equally important was an existing corpus of medical knowledge. Articulating their understandings of the body after an amputation held significance for surgeons' broader conceptions of it as a site of change.

What follows, then, examines the construction of medical views about the body after an amputation and surgeons' attitudes toward amputees. The orientation of our approach, which emphasizes *construction*, draws inspiration from disability history to distinguish surgeons' ideas and discussions, on the one side, from the lived experiences of amputees, on the other.[2] It is an emphasis that leads to a deep engagement with surgeons' intellectual worlds, which emerged at the intersection of the grisly realities of practice and formal speculation. As historians of medicine have shown for early modern physicians, surgeons could use writing as a form of epistemic practice.[3] Through their writing, they brought their experiences into conversation with a corpus of textual knowledge, leading them to consider their hands-on activities in light of a surprising number of broader discourses, including theories of embodied cognition and the boundaries of art and nature. Two important aspects surface from their conceptions of the body after an amputation: the adaptability of the body to change, and the body as a composite of natural and artificial parts, potentially capable of constant change.

Early modern "phantom limbs"

Surgeons treated patients for many types of complications in the hours, days, weeks, and months following an amputation. During post-operative convalescence, the period when the stump healed, patients often required constant attention. This dangerous and uncertain time began when assistants helped place the patient in bed or, for field-surgeons, perhaps a pallet on the ground. In an ideal setting, surgeons might drape black cloth over windows to dim the room, and sprinkle water and herbs to keep it cool.[4] Actual conditions could be deplorable, as Janus Abraham à Gehema's field book suggests in its insistence that surgeons protect convalescing patients from vermin.[5] The most immediate threat all practitioners guarded against was the reopening of major blood vessels.[6] This was why the practitioner, as one author instructed, always needed to have someone with the patient to ensure "he does not move, cough, sneeze, shout loudly, laugh, talk too much, consume hot food and drink or let his body be covered too heavily, especially with warm cloths, but rather that he keeps well still."[7] An assistant might also apply uninterrupted pressure to the bandages for the first twenty-four hours.[8]

And that was only the beginning. Bone splinters did not emerge until thirty to forty days after the procedure.[9] Along the way, various symptoms might arise, including fever, inflammation, and even putrefaction of the stump. Some of these were serious but rather straightforward to treat. The surgeon applied a cautery iron to close reopened blood vessels, used a scalpel to cut away putrefying flesh, or took up forceps to remove bone splinters. But for one complication in particular, the surgeon's chest of instruments offered no obvious solution. What did one do when a patient complained of pain in a limb that had already been amputated? What if that patient insisted that the amputation never occurred? And *why* did such things happen? These were questions that Fabry von Hilden and the physician Michael Döring (d. 1644) addressed in an exchange of letters Fabry later published in a collection of surgical observations.

Although only a handful of authors tackled it at length in print, the issue was far from obscure in early modern Europe. René Descartes, who held a keen interest in medicine, occasionally drew on it to bolster his arguments about mind–body dualism.[10] Others approached such sensations by focusing on the power of the imagination, the finer anatomical points of sensory perception, or theories of human cognition. Medical practitioners' concerns on the subject, however, often came from a distinctly practical context. Their discussions were rooted in confronting and explaining how the body adapted to change, and how to treat patients who were adapting to changed bodies.

These authors did not have a single term to refer to these bewildering sensations. Historical and medical scholarship has traditionally considered any pre-modern mention of the subject within the modern category of phantom limb phenomenon (PLP). Phantom limbs, as Cassandra Crawford writes, are "those ghostly appendages that can persist sometimes with uncanny realness long after fleshy limbs have been traumatically, surgically, congenitally, or electively amputated."[11] They allude to experiences that amputees have described in turns as frightening, painful, annoying, and even comforting. Scholars often cite the sixteenth-century work of Ambroise Paré as the first "clinical" description of PLP in Western medicine. Although Paré's report of phantom sensations has often been treated as an isolated example in medical literature until the nineteenth century, recent scholarship suggests that the early modern context was more complex.[12] Figures like Fabry and Döring prove this irrefutably.

The phrase "phantom limb" is as slippery as is it is compelling. Since the American Civil War surgeon Silas Weir Mitchell coined it in the late nineteenth century, both the medical reasoning offered to explain it and the ways amputees have described their experiences of it have frequently changed.[13] Indeed, studies of amputees in the twentieth century show these experiences could differ greatly from decade to decade.[14] In other words, even today, the term designates a nonuniform experience deeply tied to culture, society, and historical moment. It is in this colloquial and culturally contingent sense, rather than in the mode of retrospective diagnosis, that the notion of phantom limbs is useful for historical analysis. Our exploration of early modern phantom limbs approaches experiences and meanings surrounding perceived sensations of removed body parts from the perspective of early modern surgeons. Fabry and Döring enrich our nascent understanding of this subject and illustrate that in the German-speaking lands, Paré belonged to a wider surgical conversation in which other writers held equal authority.

Döring gave a vivid description of one amputee's experience in his correspondence with Fabry. They knew each other well: Döring boarded with Fabry in 1608 and considered himself a pupil of the renowned surgeon.[15] In March and August of 1610, he sent two letters about the case of a seventy-year-old pastor. While he discusses events leading to the removal of the patient's left lower leg, the bulk of his text addresses what followed. The affair unfolds in a village a few miles outside Giessen, a town in central Germany, where Döring served as a professor of anatomy and botany. On his counsel two surgeons performed the amputation. The pastor's subsequent convalescence was riddled with pain and various complications. Making matters worse, these setbacks occurred against a backdrop of constant infighting among practitioners. When the stump became infected, the pastor asked for Döring's advice. He dutifully recommended "what is read in the book [of Fabry von Hilden] about the hot and cold fire."[16] Then his tone turned withering: "But what do the surgeons do? First they disdain my advice."[17] We might note that this tug-of-war offers a glimpse into how vernacular texts could (or could not) influence practice. Döring based his advice on Fabry's treatise, but the surgeons resisted it until the pastor and his family insisted. The account of the patient's recovery is filtered through Döring's annoyance with the other practitioners involved.

The pastor himself was preoccupied with a different matter. Painful and bizarre sensations began almost immediately after the amputation. After surgeons bandaged the stump and laid the patient in a bed, Döring recounted, he "complains about nothing more than that his big toe—and his big toe alone—hurts him."[18] What was bewildering was that it was the *left* big toe, belonging to the amputated leg. The pastor then "felt with his fingers in the place of the bed where his foot had always rested, as he wished thereby to persuade those present to believe all the sooner."[19] The scene recalls the way in which surgeons would prick a dead limb with a needle or scalpel to show observers no sensitivity remained before an amputation procedure. In a tragic inversion of this, here the pastor reaches for an empty spot on the bed to prove to the room that his pain existed, even if its perceived source no longer did.

The sensations multiplied. According to Döring, the symptom spread from the toe, "long since cut off," to the entire leg.[20] Though his comment may appear offhand, he was carefully recording a sequence of events. Before amputating the leg, the surgeons first tried to excise the cold fire by removing the pastor's toes alone.[21] Döring clarified that the phantom sensation began in the body part that had been separated from the pastor the longest, yet it did not occur until just after the entire lower leg was removed. The patient remained adamant about his experience as the sensations grew to envelope the rest of the missing appendage, and Döring eventually intervened:

> Because I heard that the patient wanted to argue so persistently, by good chance a story occurred to me, which you, my good Sir, if I am not mistaken, told me yourself. ... That is, the leg of one like him had been removed, [and he] believed nothing other than that he had not yet lost it, and therefore wanted to rise from the bed. But when he fell to the floor, he learned from his injury and not without danger that he had the leg no more. So as I told this to the patient he immediately started to burst out: he feared very much that the same might befall him.[22]

Döring's approach to the situation was to normalize the experience for his patient by assuring him that others had felt these sensations and developed the same mistaken notions. This immediately suggests two crucial points about early modern phantom limbs. The first is that the subject was not unfamiliar to practitioners: Döring had a story of another patient to draw on when treating the pastor. He even suggests it came from a prior conversation with Fabry. The second is that, at least in this case, the practitioner's response was not to deny the amputee's sensations, but to prevent dangerous misadventures by persuading him not to act on them.

The episode sparked excited curiosity in the physician, who was eager to share what he witnessed. He wrote to Fabry only ten days later, devoting his entire first letter about the patient to "what namely a marvelous power is in the imagination [*Einbildung*] and the common sense."[23] By the latter, Döring meant the internal sense that integrated the five external senses into a general sensation.[24] He was discussing sensitivity and imagination together. These could exist in body parts long since removed, and they presented a range of experiences. They could be "troublesome," or one might grow "used to them, as if [the absent parts] were still present." One could "either hate or love" them.[25] Fabry published the letter in a collection of observations in a chapter titled "Of false imaginations encountered in the nursing of those who had a limb removed." Fabry's response appears in the subsequent chapter under a similar title.[26] This suggests they were sharing, discussing, and puzzling over specific phenomena they had encountered in amputees during convalescence.

Imagination, *die Einbildung*, was a word laden with meaning in early modern intellectual and medical discourse. Unpacking its significance sheds light on the specific actions Döring took in response to the elderly pastor as well as Döring and Fabry's general discussion. The two practitioners consistently referred to the imagination in the context of phantom limbs, rather than terms indicating madness, insanity, or delirium found readily enough in other examples of their correspondence.[27] *Die Einbildung* could be used in different ways, some more precise than others. It could, for example, more generally mean a fantasy. Döring used it this way to snipe at the surgeons treating the pastor as foolish men who fancied they possessed great knowledge.[28] A "false imagination" (*ein falsche Einbildung*), as Fabry labeled sensations in amputated parts, indicated a delusion in which one's perception of something was not true. But the language of imagination to describe this delusion attaches an entire apparatus of assumptions about the body and human cognition that provides important nuance for how the authors understood it. Imagination was an internal sense of the mind whose purpose was to perceive what was not present.[29] One could see a tree in a nearby field using sight, an external sense. But one could close one's eyes and still see a likeness of that same tree through the imagination. One could even change its colors from green to blue. It worked by receiving information about objects in the physical world and producing non-material forms of them—called phantasmata—that could be manipulated and stored in the memory.[30]

Scholars debated the hierarchy and functions of mental powers through the sixteenth and seventeenth centuries, giving increasing emphasis to the imagination. It could serve as one of several internal senses, including common sense and memory, or it could encompass the entire role of the internal sense, connecting the body to an immortal rational soul.[31]

The medical implications of the imagination's power led authors to examine seriously its ability to induce illness, maintain health, support recovery, and even alter a fetus in the womb.[32] In this context, the imagination and emotions often could not be disentangled. They were understood to work closely together. Emotions were "cognitive-physiological events, located in the mind and the body simultaneously."[33] Fundamental to Galenic medicine was that different temperaments, created by an individual's unique humoral makeup, were associated with various mental and physical dispositions. Thus Cornelis Herls wrote that those with a melancholic temperament (a predominance of black bile) were "sad, gloomy, sullen [and] fearful."[34] Changes in the balance of humors or their qualities altered one's health and mood. However, the humors and one's temperament alone did not determine one's emotions, which required the practitioner's constant consideration. As one of the six nonnaturals of Galenic medicine, they were as essential to one's health as moderating sleep or exercise.[35] The predominant Aristotelian view defined them as perturbed movements of the body's various spirits, material substances whose powers or functions included motion, cognition, warmth, and nourishment.[36] Joy, anger, fear, and sadness, created by the spirits moving about in an intense or disorderedly way, could potentially harm one's health, causing fever, palsy, various pains, and other conditions. Paul Barbette, for example, warned in a discussion of plague that one must moderate sadness, fear, and anger because they could violently transform the blood, a mixture of the four humors, and render one susceptible to the disease.[37] While early moderns advanced several theories about the precise process, they generally agreed that both the internal senses—which determined if an object was good or bad—and physical changes in the body were at work.[38] How the spirits moved depended on the assessment made by the imagination and other internal senses. Paré drew on the example of joyous laughter. Joy came from the heart as it dilated, he explained, sending heat and spirits through the blood to the body. But what caused the heart to dilate in the first place? The internal senses interpreted something a person had seen or remembered as an object of happiness and amusement and conveyed this to the heart.[39] Intense emotion that altered the substance of the spirits could impact good cognitive function, as this relied on the animal spirits seated in the mind.[40] The relationship between the mental powers, emotions, and the health of the body was a never-ending cycle of complex and mutual influence.

Concern for the emotional state of patients in surgical treatises reflected a robust engagement with this psychosomatic strain of early modern medicine.

If the imagination could stir the emotions, it could also calm them. If patients could be convinced they would survive a procedure, it might materially help their bodies endure. The way surgeons discussed caring for patients during and after an amputation exemplifies this. The desire to distance the patient from what was happening to his or her body sat uneasily beside the need to keep the patient alert during the operation. While early printed treatises by Hieronymus Brunschwig and Hans von Gersdorff advocated for a kind of anesthesia through the inhalation of an infusion of opium, mandrake root, henbane, lettuce, and hemlock from a "sleeping sponge," many later authors either discouraged the use of narcotics or advised on how to administer only enough to ease pain and prevent hemorrhaging.[41] Patients needed to have as much strength as possible to survive the shock of the procedure. Surgeons kept them awake to keep strong their heartbeat and pulse, the indicators of the vital spirit. If they fainted, surgeons tried to revive them, even resorting to pulling on their hair at the temples and calling them by name.[42] To mitigate their terror, authors instructed surgeons to hide cautery irons from them, and to blindfold them before making the first incision.[43] Some recommended including "a brave and eloquent man" in the procedure solely to encourage the patient.[44] As the relationship between the mental powers and the emotions was mutual and could create all manner of bodily symptoms, the power of positive thinking was no empty adage. It could save a life.

Positive encouragement also played a vital role in the patient's recovery. Apart from the reopening of blood vessels, restlessness and unnatural wakefulness posed the greatest threats to the healing process.[45] Sedatives eased physical discomfort and promoted sleep, but emotional distress also required diligent attention. Comforting words consoled patients consumed by sadness. "If the patient is sad, full of grave thoughts and he has dark moods, which is almost constantly the case with amputation," Fabry wrote, "one should attempt every method to cheer him up and please him with entertaining conversations and respectable company."[46] The picture Fabry paints matches the autobiographical account of the knight Götz von Berlichingen, who lost his right hand in 1504.[47] In deep despair during his convalescence, Götz prayed for God to let him die. Friends visited him at his bedside to share news and to praise him for the exploits that led to his injury.[48] "Many more comrades came to me," he recounted, "so that for two or three days I had little rest—it was like a pilgrimage to me. And many good people came, who knew me and saw how I fared."[49] Though Götz's hyperbolic style emphasizes his social importance rather than his injury, he nonetheless conveys a concerted effort among friends and acquaintances to offer emotional support. From the surgeon's perspective, their visits had salutary effects on his health.

Döring's approach to the elderly pastor fits well within this psychosomatic context. To Döring, both the patient's sensations and the appropriate therapeutic response to them were rooted in an understanding in which the imagination, emotions, and health were intertwined. Thus, by working to normalize his phantom sensations, the physician kept his patient calm and provided a compelling story to educate him about the dangers of the delusion. It is significant that Döring described the pastor's fearful response. This was not a sudden fright or all-consuming terror, which could cause grave harm. Instead, the physician's story focused the patient's anxiety on what could happen if he acted on the sensations by attempting to walk. The anecdote encouraged the pastor to put himself in the place of the unfortunate man who unwittingly injured himself. Should he wake up alone and unsure of whether the amputation had taken place, the apprehension Döring's story instilled could have worked as a powerful deterrent against experimenting to find out.

Another patient faced this very struggle in a case Fabry described in response in April 1610. Jacob Denisio, a patient from Payerne, had his right leg removed up to the knee. Afterwards, he "imagined he suffered all over from great pains on the instep, heel and toes."[50] Fabry continued:

> But, what is astonishing, near the end of his treatment, when he awoke from a period of sleep and wanted to go to the bathroom, he began to doubt himself and to deliberate (for there was no one around him) whether he could rise from bed alone, or if he still had both his feet or not. Finally, as he concluded to himself that he still had both feet and lacked nothing, he tried to rise from bed. But he found himself hideously deceived: he immediately fell under the bed and severely wounded the stump.[51]

Jacob's injury underscores our authors' persistent warnings that surgeons appoint assistants or family members to watch over patients night and day. It also points to Fabry and Döring's shared concern for the danger of patients acting on phantom sensations.

Some practitioners handled the delicate psychological state of patients during convalescence with great care. Others did not. In his *Wund-Artzneyisches Zeug-Hauß*, Johannes Scultetus referred to a case he witnessed during his student days. He wrote that a local count broke both bones of his right shin and developed the cold fire.[52] Pietro de Marchetti (1593–1673), an anatomist at the University of Padua, performed an amputation "while the patient did not perceive it, indeed knew nothing of it."[53] (The patient may have agreed the procedure could happen when the surgeon deemed him fit.) Marchetti followed the method of Aquapendente, cutting into the dead flesh and burning away what remained of it with cautery irons. Scultetus's emphasis on the patient's obliviousness during the procedure could have been, at least in part, a strategy to highlight the advantages of this technique for minimizing pain. No one informed the count of his condition until he started to complain of pain in his amputated foot:

The third day after the leg was removed, the patient complained of what great pains he suffered in the big toe of his right foot. The surgeon, smiling, answered that he was not a little astonished at how he, the patient, could complain about his big toe, which had already been buried for three days. As the patient heard this, he was so terrified by it that he immediately fell into a severe swoon.[54]

The shock and terror the amused Marchetti induced in his patient contrasts starkly with the gentle dialogue between Döring and the elderly pastor. Whereas Döring normalized the experience of phantom sensations and sought to reassure and inform, Marchetti mocked the count's experience and surprised him with the news of his procedure. The result was a sudden and extreme emotional disturbance with severe bodily symptoms, showcasing the dramatic and dire impact the emotions could have on a patient's health. Scultetus offered no further comment on the count's delusion.

Döring and Fabry showed more interest in the phenomenon. Using the language of imagination, they engaged with a deeper intellectual discussion about phantom sensations to try to explain them. In his response to Döring, Fabry drew on a treatise on arquebus wounds by the French physician Laurent Joubert (1529–1583). This work did not circulate in the German vernacular, and Fabry probably read it in French. Joubert explored a series of questions about pain in an amputated part that culminated in a striking metaphor of a mirror. In a mirror one sees oneself where one is not. In a similar way, animal spirits gathering sensations through the nerves can reflect pain from one part of the body so that it appears to be in a different place than it truly is.[55] Fabry simplified and summarized Joubert's position:

> The animal spirit which flows through the nerves represents, as it were, the sensitivity of the amputated limb into which it should flow; however, because it can come no further, it goes back again to the common sense, causing a false imagination.[56]

In other words, an amputation disrupts the route the animal spirits expected to take when moving through the nerves, leading to miscommunication. The animal spirit assigned to travel to an amputated limb returns to the common sense, located in the mind, reporting sensory data for pain in the stump as though it came from the amputated part the spirit could not reach.

Drawing on his own practice, Fabry linked the phenomenon to a transitional period during the body's recovery from the procedure. "It is not astonishing that those who have a large limb—like an arm or leg—removed [and] still suffer pain, inflammation or other symptoms in the stump imagine the finger or toe hurts them," he wrote to Döring, because "this occurs to almost everyone whose limb is cut off."[57] "However when the cure is over," Fabry explained, "similar imaginations rarely occur."[58] The implication is not only that the healing of the stump and severed nerve endings results in fewer distressing symptoms for the common sense to sort, but also that the process for collecting and interpreting sensory data adapts. Perhaps the animal spirits cease attempting to reach a portion of the nerves that has been cut away, the common sense learns to read the representations of the animal spirits more accurately, or some combination of the two.

The true wonder, according to Fabry, was when a patient's body did *not* adapt. He cited the case of Jacob Denisio particularly because the phantom sensations persisted long after his stump had healed. "Two years after his complete cure," Fabry wrote, "he avowed and testified before Herr Merula, servant of the Word of God, and before others ... [that] he often believes he still has pains in his foot, instep, and shin."[59] Even Denisio's harmful fall from bed appeared remarkable because it happened toward the end of his treatment when, Fabry noted, the patient "felt well and had neither fever nor any pains."[60] Significantly, he did not assume the symptom's cause changed simply because of when it was experienced. He echoes Joubert in his clarification that Denisio's false imagination "did not come from a madness or loss of reason."[61] Implicit here is the expectation that when the stump was nearly healed, and certainly years after it finished healing, the initial confusion an amputation created for embodied processes of sensation and cognition dissipated. Denisio's experiences during and after convalescence were extraordinary to Fabry because they presented a body that seemed to heal without fully adjusting to the impact of a major surgical intervention. It suggests he understood the human body as something generally inclined to be adaptable—as disposed to, capable of, and even expected to change. This is consistent with his preference for the hand's-width method of amputation, which reshaped lower legs to facilitate patient utility rather than to preserve the healthy body. He expected the body—in most cases—to adapt.

No single explanation could fully account for the bewildering sensations of early modern phantom limbs. Fabry drew from Joubert's work when corresponding with a physician, but elsewhere he referred to multiple possible causes. Paré, who wrote about the subject twice in Book 11 of the German edition of his collected works, was particularly influential because of the therapeutic he advised. In a chapter on the signs of the complete death of a limb, he described "false sensitivity" after amputation as astounding. Patients, he wrote, "complain after several days—indeed several months—about the amputated limb, as though it still was present and hurt them, which is a wondrous and almost unbelievable thing, had I not myself seen [it] with my own eyes and heard from patients."[62] He returned to the subject again in a chapter on the treatment of a stump after amputation, directing readers on how to bandage it and what topical medicines to apply. For patients who imagined long after a limb was removed that it was still attached to their bodies and complained about pain, the surgeon should smear the entire spine and the limb with an ointment.[63] Pain in amputated limbs appears here as one of many possible complications that could arise. Thus, rather than an illustrative case history, he instead provided a detailed recipe for his ointment and instructions on its use, noting that it also treated convulsion, paralysis, rigor, and other ailments of the "nervous members."[64]

Couched as a parenthetical aside is Paré's explanation for this symptom's cause. "In my opinion," he asserted, it "originates from nowhere else than because the severed nerves contract toward their source and thus cause a pain like the spasm."[65] This reasoning fits within his broader understanding of the way muscles and nerves contracted back toward their "source" (i.e. the brain or the spine) when damaged.[66] In his discussion of wounds of the nerves and nervous parts, for example, he explained that if a nerve was cut only halfway, then the part still attached to the body would contract this way, causing great pain because of the sympathy between the brain and the nerves.[67] A spasm or convulsion (*ein Krampff*) caused by pain likewise displays an intricate connection between injury, pain, nerves, and the brain. It occurred when damaged nerves, either punctured by a sharp object or exposed to extreme cold, experienced so much pain that they contracted toward "their source, the brain, and desire from it help and support as if from their parent."[68] Paré interpreted phantom limbs within this context of damaged nerves physically moving and changing in response to injury. His explanation was distinctly different from, though not incompatible with, Joubert's discussion of the movement of animal spirits through the nerves. Other areas of Paré's treatise demonstrate his familiarity with the role of the animal spirits in conveying sensory data, but his analysis of phantom pain focuses on the nerves rather than the substances that moved through them.[69] His approach was pragmatic: he concentrated on material damage to the structuring parts of the body that the surgeon could treat.

Therapeutics also assumed prominence in Fabry's *Gründlicher Bericht*. He discussed spasms without explicitly referring to phantom limbs. The key to discerning the wider dialogue with which he was engaged rests in the connection between the two. He devoted one of a series of chapters on complications arising after an amputation to spasms. One form occurred when damaged nerves caused one or more body parts to feel by sympathy the pain in another injured part.[70] The passage lists three explanations for the appearance of this particular kind of convulsion. It could arise from pain, swelling, and inflammation of the stump. It might also occur because the severed nerves contract. Finally, such spasms happened "because the spirits of the brain (called the animal spirits), when they move down to the stump and there go no further, retreat back unruly and contrary," affecting the activity of the nerves.[71] Fabry offered multiple explanations without contradiction, at some points echoing Paré and at others Joubert. Yet his ultimate goal was therapy. No matter the cause, Fabry advised, the surgeon should refer to his previous chapters for methods to mitigate pain, dispel swelling, and check inflammation.[72] In addition, he provided the recipes for two ointments which together make up more than half of the passage. One he presented as his own, and the other, transcribed in full, is from Paré's discussion of phantom limbs.[73]

Delusions were dangerous. Surgeons had to treat the symptom of phantom pain before it could cause harm. In his letter to Döring, Fabry recounted the tragic case of a sixty-year-old man he treated in a district of Payerne. He removed the patient's left arm up to the elbow. "In the third day," Fabry wrote, "in my absence he stretched the arm (because he imagined that he still had it and nothing was cut off), and wanted to extend and grip, not knowing about the [amputated] hand."[74] The blood vessels reopened, causing heavy hemorrhaging, and he died a few days after. Cases like this are why Fabry consistently emphasized practical instruction, from his *Gründlicher Bericht* to his correspondence with Döring more than ten years later. A shift in audience altered his rhetorical strategy, but not his overarching message. When writing for practicing surgeons and barber-surgeons, he gave more attention to Paré; when composing a letter to a learned physician, he referenced Joubert. In both cases, he stressed the importance of treatment and focused the bulk of his attention on it. "It is enough for me," he declared to Döring, "when future surgeons remember to be diligent and watchful that their patients do not move the stump because of such a false imagination and thereby cause hemorrhaging and very great pains."[75] His instructions focus on guiding practitioners' *responses* to false imaginations.

The rationale surgeons developed to understand these symptoms shaped their approach to treating those who experienced them. False imaginations were somatic events invisible to the naked eye, yet comprehensible to the surgeon. Discussions of early modern phantom limbs highlight the body as an active site of change, responding and adapting to surgical alteration rather than a passive object worked upon by the surgeon. They also suggest the active role of patients in keeping their bodies at rest during a tremendously difficult time. Surgeons could apply ointments, alleviate pain, and promote the healing of the stump, but they could not keep a patient from acting on phantom sensations. Fabry and Döring's correspondence suggests the most powerful tool for the diligent surgeon was an honest conversation with the patient.

With early modern phantom limbs, two very different kinds of dialogue intersected: complex theories about embodied cognition among intellectuals, and therapeutic recommendations among practitioners. Vernacular surgeons contributed to both. Consider two vastly different publications from the late seventeenth century. Cornelis Solingen (1641–1687) wrote in his general surgery that after a limb amputation, "it is often very necessary, that a barber-surgeon's assistant keeps vigil over the patient, because the patient gets from time to time false imaginations in sleep, whereby the stump of the leg is moved, and from it follows a new hemorrhaging."[76] He refers readers to Fabry together with Joubert, a university physician, for more information. Meanwhile, in 1693, a student at the university of Tübingen composed a master's thesis entitled *Paradoxa Sensatio* on "the pain of an amputated limb."[77] The work, written in academic Latin, cites as authorities Fabry and Paré alongside Descartes and Johann Bohn (1640–1718), professor of anatomy at Leipzig.[78]

For practicing surgeons, treating symptoms of phantom sensations was part of a larger battle of the senses, emotions, and health waged during an amputation and through convalescence. Blindfold patients from frightening instruments, fill their ears with comforting words, drug them to help them sleep. This struggle could be seen as the surgeon's attempt to control the patient's body by mastering and manipulating the senses. But that was only half of the story. Discussions of phantom limbs reveal practitioners learning about a body adapting to change—a process that surgeons could not control at all, but only attempt to understand as they treated patients' symptoms.

Patient to amputee

Yet the ways surgeons grappled with the body as a site of change was not simply reactive, responding to complications that arose during convalescence. It was also speculative. Surgeons pondered the future responses patients might make after their stumps had healed. In the sixteenth and seventeenth centuries, this was largely a theoretical exercise unconnected to the activities of medical practitioners. To return to our analogy of Amman's woodcut, they were looking out the door at passersby rather than describing their own firsthand experiences. Indeed, authors of surgical treatises who devoted detailed attention to post-operative convalescence said little of patient interactions afterwards. They do not provide instructions or offer case histories about working with amputees to regain mobility or learn new ways to perform everyday tasks.[79] Evidence that surgeons were involved in the process of acquiring artificial limbs is likewise vanishingly small. Medicalized rehabilitation of amputees, in which practitioners oversee physical therapy, occupational therapy, and adoption of prostheses, is a modern concept.[80] Early modern surgeons' discussions of transitions out of post-operative convalescence do not necessarily reveal much about the experiences and perspectives of amputees. But they do shed light on medical thinking. Even more significant, they suggest that surgical discourse about amputees held broader implications for how practitioners conceived of the body, and of interventions that could be made to it outside of surgery. They discussed the body as a site of possibilities even as they defined the limits of surgery. These two seemingly divergent lines of thought intersected sharply because of the ways surgeons addressed a deceptively simple question that permeated the entire period of convalescence: What comes next?

Surgeons ensconced the issue within their conceptual world of operative techniques and treatments. An entire category of operations in early modern surgery dealt with putting the dismembered or mutilated body back together. Authors defined *Anaplerosis* as the reconstitution of that which is lacking by birth or accident.[81] This medical construction identified certain human bodies in opposition to a perceived norm and gave solutions for bringing them closer to that norm. Placing amputees within it reveals how the authors of surgical treatises approached those who survived an amputation: something was now lacking and should be restored. Thus, in the frontispiece of the 1693 edition of Johannes Scultetus's *Armamentarium Chirurgicum, Anaplerosis* is represented by a young man who raises his left arm to model an artificial hand fastened to his forearm by a number of straps. But prostheses were only one way to restore body parts. In fact, they received far less attention in surgical writing than reconstructive surgeries on the nose, ear, eyelid, or lip. Authors repeatedly distinguished between these two kinds of restoration—reconstructive surgeries and prostheses. One was real and true (*recht*), the other artificial and false (*falsch*).

In essence, the distinction referred to the material used. Reconstructive surgeries used human flesh to reshape portions of the face. These could serve primarily aesthetic or physiological purposes. Operations to repair cleft lips, which affected the ability to speak, eat, and drink, involved both.[82] The nose's function and the morality of restoring a maimed nose were matters of debate among humanist physicians, but these intellectual niceties did not preoccupy surgeons who discussed rhinoplasty in the German vernacular, beginning with Heinrich von Pfalzpaint's manuscript of 1460.[83] His treatise described a form of skin-grafting traditionally credited to a family of practitioners in Sicily. Gaspare Tagliacozzi (1545–1599), a professor of surgery and anatomy at the University of Bologna, famously laid out the technique in his *De Curtorum Chirurgia per Insitionem* (1597).[84] Many subsequent authors either referred readers to Tagliacozzi or described his method at length. The grueling procedure, which took place over three or four months, involved taking an attached flap graft from the patient's forearm and sewing the free end of it around the nasal cavity. The flap, which remained connected to the forearm to continue providing nourishment to its partially severed end, was kept in place by binding the patient's arm over his or her head until the surrounding blood vessels took root in the extended skin. The surgeon then reshaped the skin and eventually severed the connective flap completely. Authors suggested that in extraordinary cases, the same technique could be used for ears and lips.[85] Though well known in treatises, "true" restorations were not common in practice, for they were intensely painful, time-consuming, and fraught with uncertainty.

The notion of replacing like with like led some to elaborate on the nature of the human body. In his treatise of surgical observations, Janus Abraham à

Gehema asked whether one could refill a deep wound with the flesh of another person or animal.[86] The question follows the logic of true restoration: if a surgeon uses human flesh to replace human flesh, does it really matter *whose* flesh is used? He answered with a case history:

> The nose of a Polish nobleman was cut off by another nobleman with a sword. He persuaded one of his subjects with promises of a none too displeasing reward [that] he should allow a chunk of flesh be cut from his arm. The poor subject resolved to do it: the arm of the peasant was bound to the face of the nobleman, and from it a nose so artfully cut, as if it had been formed by a sculptor. However, this curious invention would not go right, but rather the affixed nose soon putrefied again, and the unhappy nobleman had to manage with only a wooden nose, which was given a natural color by a painter.[87]

The description of the procedure indicates it may have been an attached flap graft with the peasant's arm bound to the nobleman's face. Clearly, this attempt to use one person's flesh in place of another's failed.

In Gehema's analysis, the logic of true restoration appears sound in theory but difficult in practice. The only obstacle to using another person's flesh was the fragility of human blood vessels. One could cut a claw from a capon's foot and graft it onto the creature's head without difficulty; likewise, one could graft a branch from one tree onto another and it would bloom. These feats were possible because one could make incisions into a capon or a tree without damaging the vessels through which nourishment flowed. "In the human body, however," he expounded, "such vessels are so delicate and subtle that they can be completely disarranged and displaced by the least injury, whereby then the *circulation* of the blood and humors is hindered, and no growth can occur."[88] Gehema was not alone in contemplating why the human body's materials could not easily be exchanged with that of others: similar discussions appear in the treatises of Matthäus Purmann and Jan Muys.[89]

An attached flap graft using the patient's own flesh to reshape a nose was difficult. Using another person's flesh in a graft was fine in theory but unlikely to succeed. But performing a true restoration of an amputated limb was incomprehensible. In Galenic medicine, the hard and structuring parts of the body (considered spermatic) could not regenerate, while flesh and fat (considered sanguinary) could. The former came from a combination of female and male sperm in the early stage of an embryo, while the latter developed from a form of nurturing blood that existed through all stages of life. Spermatic parts included bones, cartilage, veins and arteries, organs, and more.[90] Surgeons took note of these distinctions.[91] Paré, observing that spermatic matter could not regenerate, advised readers not to cut away lightly parts which came from sperm because they could not be restored.[92] Nature could sometimes *repair* spermatic parts by substituting other material. When a broken bone healed it was not because the spermatic substance regenerated, but rather because nature employed matter, made from a humor thicker than the material which produces bone, to form "a hard and thick callus" that restored the continuity of the part.[93] In other words, bone did not regrow even a little. While some authors disputed whether a nose could be reconstructed because of its spermatic parts,[94] there seemed little room for doubt that a limb amputation removed something that could not be regenerated or grafted back on. Surgical treatises did not even broach the subject when discussing true restorations.

Indeed, the notion of replacing one human limb with another pushed so far beyond the limits of surgeons' abilities it was considered miraculous. It was not natural, but supernatural. At the turn of the sixteenth century, most German medical practitioners would have been familiar with the story of the leg transplantation miracle of the brothers Cosmas and Damian, the patron saints of medicine martyred c. 300. In 1517 they appeared on the title page of Gersdorff's *Feldbuch* to embody medicine broadly.[95] They were celebrated as the patrons of barber-surgeon and bath master guilds from the Middle Ages into the eighteenth century, though their cult of devotion increasingly concentrated in southern German-speaking lands after the Reformation.[96] In 1649, Munich—in Counter-Reformation Bavaria—welcomed the saints' relics in an elaborate translation after the Protestant town of Bremen sold them and the medieval reliquary that housed them.[97] The leg transplantation was one of two miracles depicted on the interior of the reliquary doors that opened for public display on special days of veneration.

The version most widely known in the Holy Roman Empire came from the saints' hagiography in the *Legenda aurea* of Jacob de Voragine from the thirteenth century. A man in Rome suffered from a leg consumed by cancer. According to the account:

> While he was asleep, the two saints appeared to their devoted servant, bringing salves and surgical instruments. One of them said to the other: "Where can we get flesh to fill in where we cut away the rotted leg?" The other said: "Just today an Ethiopian was buried in the cemetery of Saint Peter in Chains. Go and take his leg, and we'll put it in place of the bad one." So he sped to the cemetery and brought back the Moor's leg, and the two saints cut off the sick man's leg and inserted the Moor's in its place, carefully anointing the wound. Finally they took the amputated leg and attached it to the body of the dead Moor.[98]

Waking without pain, the man discovered he was healed. Others who heard his story investigated the Moor's tomb and "found that his leg had indeed been cut off and the aforesaid man's limb put in its place in the tomb."[99] Early modern images in Western Christianity follow Voragine's account, which was the first to claim the corpse was a recently deceased Moor.[100] European artists, working within a long (and problematic) iconographic tradition of portraying black bodies, used contrasting colors to visually heighten the drama.[101] The saints' patient typically appears as a white man with one black leg, or with one black lower leg attached to a white thigh. Viewers are left without doubt that the pious man's cancerous leg was not simply healed of its affliction but replaced with that of another person.

Most images depict the transplantation as a divine amputation that removes the diseased limb and creates a stump to which the saints affix the Moor's leg. By contrast, a sixteenth-century painting in Vienna interprets the operation as a skin graft (figure 4.2). Originally created as part of an altarpiece, it relates what came after the procedure, with the saints notably absent. The artist depicts three scenes, from left to right. First, the afflicted man examines his thigh with a candle, discovering his cancerous parts replaced by the Moor's flesh. Concentrating the site of the operation on the upper leg emphasized the severity of the man's condition, and in doing so enhanced the wonder of the miracle. He lifts his clothing in the next scene to reveal the transformation to others. In the final tableau, a crowd gathers around the Moor's grave, some covering their noses from the smell of the decaying body. Together the scenes emphasize that the miraculous transplantation is not of an *entire* leg but of *parts* of the leg above the knee. The healed man stands with a black thigh and white shin. Meanwhile the artist's depiction of the deceased Moor implies a dissection of the leg rather than its removal. A large portion of the thigh has been removed, but the bare femur and the back of the thigh remain intact.

At first glance, this appears to suggest an exchange of flesh closer to the scenario Gehema puzzled over in his seventeenth-century surgical observations. But when Gehema, a Cartesian medical reformer,[102] speculated about using another person's flesh to refill a deep wound in a patient, he focused on the nose. He did not address arms or legs. To achieve the true restoration of an entire limb—or even a large portion of a limb—that had been surgically removed remained beyond the realm of the natural in early modern Germany. This was precisely why a leg transplantation was an appropriate subject for religious artwork.

If a true restoration replaced human parts with human parts, a false one replaced them with anything else. A historian of early modern medicine might expect us to turn now to Ambroise Paré's influential book of artificial body parts. But I am going to address this work in Chapter 6, at a point in our story when we are well versed in craft practices among artisans and prepared to examine Paré's book in light of them. Here we will draw from it alongside the works of other authors to learn about false restorations. Wood, metal, leather, and cloth, all considered artificial in this context, could conceal a missing or damaged part, assist the physiological function of a part, or both. Tubes of wood or metal facilitated urination.[103] Artificial teeth of bone or ivory allowed

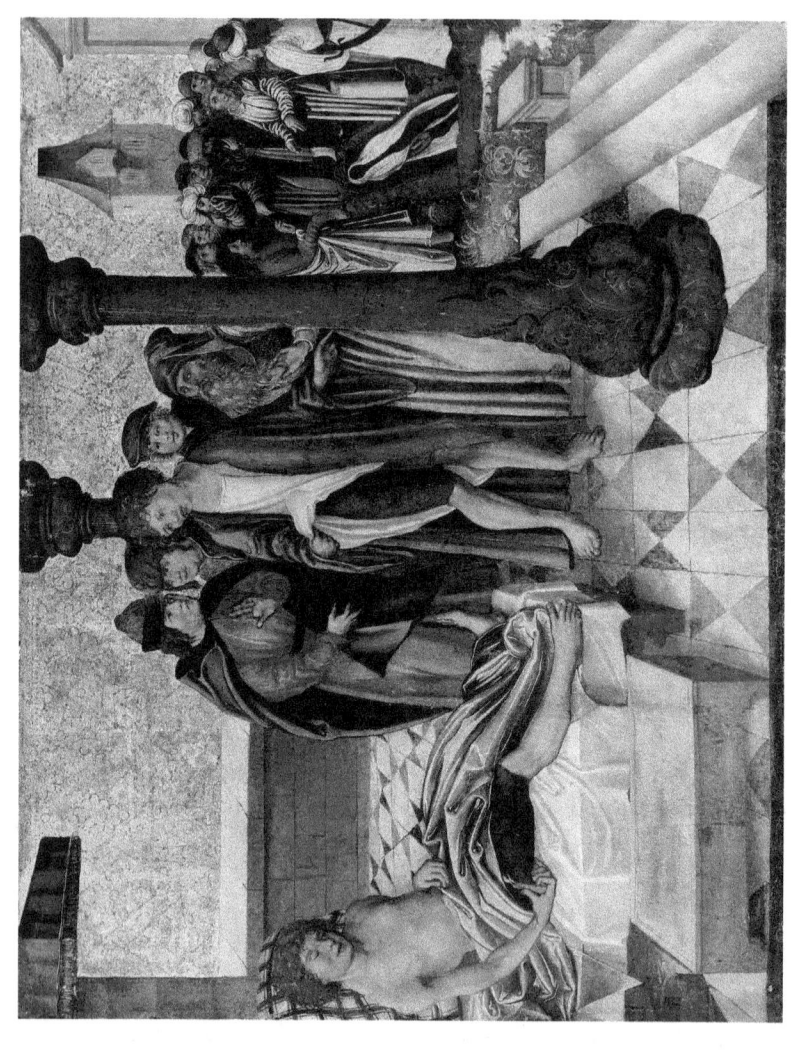

4.2 Master of the legend scenes, *Wunderbare Beinheilung durch die Hll. Cosmas und Damian*, early sixteenth century. Painting formerly on wood, transferred to canvas. 68 × 86 cm. Inv.-Nr. 4968.

patients to eat, while artificial palates enabled them to drink and speak.[104] The surgeon Francisco de Arce (1493–c. 1573), for instance, recounted the case of a patient who was gored in the face by an ox. Although the exterior of the patient's face healed, a hole remained in the roof of his mouth the size of a man's thumb. Arce plugged it with a delicate rind covered with a linen cloth, which allowed the patient to speak, drink, and eat.[105] Prosthetic palates also appear in the writings of Joseph Schmid, who used a little metal plate of white tin, copper, or silver—depending on the patient's pocketbook.[106] Franz Renner, who practiced in Nuremberg, preferred to use leather fixed on sponge pieces rather than metal, which he considered too painful to take in and out.[107] Furnishing prostheses was not a service every surgeon or barber-surgeon provided. But particularly in the case of small, practical supplements, there were practitioners who not only had experience designing or procuring them, but did so on a regular basis.

Artificial eyes, ears, and noses disguised and concealed. "As a nose, when it is well formed and whole, gives an ornament to the entire face," wrote Johann von Jessen, "one must create and devise another in the place of a mutilated one to disguise such blemishes."[108] One could use silver, wood, paper, or a small cloth shaped and painted the color of a nose, which one attached with small cords behind the head.[109] In the case of a patient whose upper lip was damaged along with the nose, surgeons suggested adding an artificial moustache.[110] (They offered no advice regarding the concealment of damaged upper lips for female patients.) Artificial ears and eyes could also be made of a variety of materials and tied behind the head. "One can suggest a real ear," Jessen explained, "from something devised from glued paper or painted leather."[111] For artificial eyes, he recommended using a thin and flexible iron wire— similar to the ones "with which noblewomen straighten their hair"—that could reach from under the ear and cross the head with a broad section over the eye socket that could be covered with white silk, "so that in it the lost eye can be depicted by the painter with his colors."[112] If one could not obtain a prosthesis, surgeons suggested other options, including growing one's hair long or donning a hat.[113] These facial prostheses, Jessen admitted, were "only a false restoration, but not so bloody and troublesome" as reconstructive surgery.[114]

Surgical treatises consider the desire to conceal certain blemishes as universal. The source of an injury—whether it was inflicted as punishment, the result of a duel, or a symptom of disease—made no difference when it deformed an eye or nose.[115] The notion of a scar as a badge of honor, indicating a heroic deed, does not appear in the surgical literature. After all, surgeons and barber-surgeons were in the business of minimizing and masking perceived defects.[116] Their treatises reflect their care for the body's appearance, including instructing on how to sew wounds of the head and face without leaving scars.[117] Felix Würtz emphasized that when treating the face, one must use as few stitches as possible and remove them the very moment the skin begins to heal. To leave the stitches in would cause "very ugly, deforming scars."[118] He also gave tips to "good womenfolk" and others to prevent facial scars at home using a secret recipe.[119] In fact, practitioners tailored many recipes to meet cosmetic concerns. Jessen, for example, promised ones to grow luxurious hair and beards.[120] Surgeons approached false restorations with an attitude consistent with this broader concern for patients' appearances.

False restoration described and treated the human body as a composite of natural and artificial parts. It offered an answer to the limitations of the body's ability to heal and of surgery's ability to graft or transplant. Jessen's description of an artificial eye made of precious metals alludes to these limits, which were at the heart of the early modern surgeon's understanding of prostheses:

> We can hide the injury—from whatever cause—of a missing eye (since an eye that has been removed does not grow again for man in the manner that several relate of the *Fisch Myro*), when we heal the injury, and insert a second in its place made from silver or gold, also from enameled work, painted and polished, so that it seems like a real eye. A goldsmith from Florence has similar false eyes—fashioned with astonishing subtlety—for sale in Venice for six or seven *Cronen*.[121]

A human eye, once removed, could not be regrown. Restoring it required an artisan to craft an object from silver, gold, or glass with the shape and appearance of the lost eye.[122]

Jessen characterized the creation of artificial limbs as art imitating nature. "Necessity," he wrote, "is an inventor of the arts: she also invented how one might replace severed limbs, almost imitating nature in this."[123] In contrast to his descriptions of false eyes and ears, he did not mention appearance. "Many of those with fabricated legs," he explained, "manage the task to walk [and] stand; [those with fabricated] arms somewhat to grasp and hold."[124] "Imitating nature" in this context meant performing certain physical tasks. This description is revealing on multiple levels. Jessen made explicit the project of false restorations as the use of art to mimic nature. Recent scholarship situates discussions of reconstructive surgery within a broader exploration of the boundaries between art and nature manifested in many different areas of early modern science.[125] Jessen's observation suggests that conversations surrounding false restorations in vernacular literature offered another avenue of engagement with this wider cultural and intellectual debate. This presents a strain of thought distinct from the way surgeons discussed their own mediating role. Authors such as Paul Barbette characterized surgical treatment this way: "through art the obstructions to the cure are moved out of the way, however nature itself heals the damage."[126] In an operation, the surgeon used art to enable nature to perform a cure. But nature had limits; it could not replace a limb. A false restoration of a limb involved someone else using art to do what nature could not, imitating nature rather than aiding its healing process. Jessen lauded a locksmith reported by Paré as a "clever and artful inventor" because of the iron hands he crafted.[127] False restorations both reinforced and blurred distinctions between art and nature. Surgeons defined artificial parts in opposition to natural ones, yet the result was a conception of the human body as an amalgamation of natural and artificial parts working together.

On another level, Jessen's remarks reveal that surgeons measured the achievement of a false restoration of an amputated arm or leg in the recovery of physical function—walking, standing, grasping, holding. Limb prostheses rarely appear in surgical treatises. Like Jessen, many authors referred readers to Paré because his work uniquely provided a locksmith's designs for mechanical limbs. When treatises do refer to these objects, it is more likely to occur within instructions on amputation to explain the proper length and treatment of a stump capable of bearing a prosthesis.[128] Descriptions of amputees often, but not always, appear in connection to these remarks in the form of anecdotes or references to other works. They focus on the presence (or absence) of an artificial replacement for what a surgeon had removed. As Jessen's example suggests, these authors evaluated the success of limb prostheses through signs of physical utility.

Evidence of an effective false restoration influenced the emotional and moral valences of these accounts. Positive depictions emphasize an individual's artful ability to physically maneuver and perform tasks. Jessen referred to a nobleman who lost both hands and used two iron ones to take his hat on and off, fasten his belt, and even write his name.[129] He was citing a famous example from Giovanni Tommaso Minadoi's *De humani corporis turpitudinibus cognoscendis et curandis* (Pavia, 1600), a treatise that does not appear to have circulated in German yet entered the corpus of vernacular literature through passages like the one found in Jessen. Jan Muys recounted the case of a youth in Rotterdam "who—using in place of his lower leg, amputated a little below the knee, one of wood—could move on the ice as swiftly with skates as any other."[130] The image of a leg prosthesis in Pieter Adriaanszoon Verduyn's *Neue Methode, die Glieder abzunehmen* (1697) is a powerful illustration of how surgeons envisioned the rehabilitated patient: the figure of a man equipped with a prosthesis that can be hidden from sight under his clothes, and that allows him to move at an easy gait (figure 3.4). These contrasted with negative portrayals depicting individuals who either cannot acquire or are incapable of using prostheses effectively: those experiencing chronic pain from complications in their stumps, those who required a crutch in addition to a wooden stilt, and those who must beg because they cannot resume their previous employment.[131]

Placed within the conceptual framework of true and false restorations, this rhetorical pattern points to two interrelated aspects of how surgeons viewed amputees. First, they connected artificial limbs to social adjustment. This perspective aligns broadly with Klaus-Peter Horn and Bianca Frohne's thesis on the fluidity of premodern "disability" in Europe. Keeping in mind that "disability" is the product of modern discourse, they argue that the status of bodily difference was "neither a static social attribution nor does it refer to a permanent or irrevocable medical condition."[132] It applied only to a period during which individuals and their families could not find practical solutions to overcome various challenges to social adjustment.[133] For surgeons, an effective false restoration was the best solution for any physical impairment that resulted from an amputation. During post-operative convalescence, they treated a body that might eventually bear an artificial limb. Once the patient transitioned out of the surgeon's care, this potential remained. It could only be truly extinguished if the stump proved unable to bear the weight and friction of a prosthesis.

Second, surgical treatises imply that the onus of achieving this false restoration fell largely upon the amputee. Surgeons did not share in this responsibility. They did not present themselves as active participants in the process beyond shaping and healing a patient's stump. Even in the extraordinary examples of treatises that illustrated designs for artificial limbs, the authors offered no case histories suggesting their involvement in designing, fabricating, or obtaining them.[134] Depictions of amputees with prostheses in anecdotal asides or case histories gloss over the process of false restoration by simply declaring the individuals acquired prostheses or already possessed them before describing what tasks they could perform.[135] Once again Horn and Frohne's notion of fluidity appears compatible with this medical perspective: it emphasizes the responsibility of persons with physical impairments and their families to find solutions to challenging situations.[136] The analogy of the open door in Amman's woodcut takes on another, deeper meaning. Amputees—individuals who recovered and were no longer patients—are beyond the vanishing point in the image because they are beyond the surgeon's supervision and agency over the body.

The arc of an amputee's story of "successful" assimilation presented in surgical literature is a play in three acts. It begins with the amputation, including the circumstances leading to it. Next is the recovery, defined as the healing of the stump and any complicating issues from the procedure. Then surgeons exit stage left for the final act, in which it is up to the amputee to achieve an effective false restoration. Anyone who succeeds in this effort is depicted in positive terms. In this context, surgeons did not just conceive of the body as a mixture of natural and artificial parts. They embraced it.

They were not the only ones. Consider the case of Christian the Younger (1599–1626), the duke of Braunschweig-Lüneburg and a prominent Protestant commander under contract with the Dutch Republic in the early stages of the Thirty Years' War.[137] During a pitched battle at Fleurus in August of 1622, a bullet struck his left arm. Surgeons amputated it three days later. Descriptions of his injury, convalescence, and return to society in the autumn and winter of 1622–1623 not only reinforce how surgical treatises depicted the role of surgeons, but also suggest that the medical imaginary surrounding false restorations held a wider cultural resonance.

An unsigned *Relatio* in the Wolfenbüttel Staatsarchiv describes his treatment from August to December of 1622.[138] The report, written in the first person along with additional (unsigned) annotations by others, refers to at least seven medical practitioners involved in his operation and post-operative care.[139] It begins with his injury, though the author notes that he did not arrive until the patient's convalescence. The practitioners explain both Christian's condition and their decisions. The gunshot wound, located four fingers above the elbow, caused pieces of bone and debris to crush the blood vessels and block the flow of nourishment. The cold fire took root the next day. By the third day it was clear to the three surgeons attending the duke that "the entire arm was dead."[140] They agreed that Christian would die if they did not amputate immediately. During the procedure, they found a bullet blocking the brachial artery and determined this had saved him from exsanguination on the battlefield. Afterward, he traveled "day and night" with his army to Breda.[141]

The report's focus shifts to healing the stump. A series of complications kept the growing number of surgeons, physicians, and assistants busy over the next three months.[142] They removed more dead flesh, battled inflammation, and watched the damaged blood vessels closely. The patient was in such agony that the surgeons reduced the frequency of their dressings because Christian "had a loathing for the great torment."[143] Around the fifth week, the *Relatio* notes that he became frustrated, incensed that the stump had swollen two fingers' thicker than before. Some developments were expected: the wound expelled dead material over a long period of time, with a splinter of dead bone finally emerging during the sixth week of treatment. Other issues were dangerous discoveries uncovered while surgeons continued to shape and treat the stump. In late October, while filing the bone to help the flesh grow around the brachial artery, three surgeons found the bone was rotting and removed pieces of it while attempting to preserve the nearby flesh. The wound also emitted a putrid odor: a month after the amputation, when the thread was removed from the brachial artery, a black liquid leaked from the vessel for three weeks, producing a terrible stench that did not abate until well into November. In December, when the *Relatio* ends, Christian was suffering from pain in his shoulder blade and back.[144] This report reflects the activities and concerns that surgeons described in their treatises. It also ends when treatises envisioned the role of the surgeon ending: when the stump and the patient were stable, if still experiencing pain.

Non-medical accounts of Christian's experiences diverge sharply from the *Relatio*, weaving dramatic narratives in which an artificial limb plays a key role. His fate following his injury generated great interest during the ongoing war between Catholics and Protestants. One contemporary recorded news of Christian's death in his diary three different times between September and December of 1622.[145] Another claimed in his memoirs that the greatest loss of the Battle of Fleurus was Christian's left arm.[146] Most accounts explained that the injury resulted from heroism, though a less sympathetic (Catholic) author in Cologne called it divine punishment for using gold and silver stolen from a church to mint coins with the taunting inscription "God's friend and priests' enemy."[147] Popular accounts condense his convalescence in Breda—a painful period of messy procedures in the *Relatio*—to a theatrical message he sent opponents from his sickbed. In the *Theatrum Europaeum*, he orders a Spanish trumpeter who was being held prisoner to convey his words to Ambrogio Spinola, the general of the Spanish Army of Flanders: "the *tolle Hertzog* [the mad duke] may have indeed lost his one arm, but keeps the other to take vengeance on his enemies."[148] "An artful Dutch craftsman from Maasland," the chronicle continues, "thereafter fashioned for him an iron arm, which can manually bend and move, [and] also govern and grip everything, to be affixed to him with gold."[149] Allusions to an artificial arm repeatedly appear in accounts of the Battle of Fleurus and its aftermath. The poet Georg Greflinger memorialized the story of Christian's ordeal in his verse chronicle of the Thirty Years' War in 1657:

> In this hot fight was Duke Christian
> In the left hand injured/ and because the young man
> Bothered not with his wound in his fervor for battle/
> Since the glory of war more than life for him mattered/
> Caught fire from delayed attention his hand
> and the arm also following into a *kalten Brand*/
> It then from his body/ to keep the worst at bay/
> Because better half to lose than whole/ was cut away.
> Thereafter he instead an iron one carried/
> and yet still did enough to keep his enemy harried.[150]

Christian's adoption of a prosthesis provided a satisfying conclusion to his story in widely circulated publications. Any further details concerning its appearance and construction were apparently unnecessary. Its importance rested in what it enabled Christian to do: symbolically signal his full recovery and return to society.

Indeed, despite reports from individuals who claimed to have seen the object after his death, there are no detailed descriptions or drawings of Christian's artificial arm. In 1674, the physician and naturalist Friedrich Lachmund reported seeing in Duke Anton Ulrich's *Kunstkammer* an artificial arm of silver that Christian the Younger used to replace what he had lost in battle.[151] In 1705, Leonhard Christoph Sturm, a mathematician and engineer, remarked in his book of rarities and cabinets of nature that "the wooden arm which Duke Christian of Braunschweig used in place of his lost left arm" was in the *Kunstkammer* in Wolfenbüttel.[152] Rehtmeyer's *Chronica* of 1722 confirmed for readers that Christian's silver arm was kept there.[153] Another physician and naturalist, Franz Ernst Brückmann, remarked in a letter that he saw the artificial arm in 1753 and noted that it was made of wood, not silver.[154] One nineteenth-century source claimed that until the end of the previous century the "metal arm" was kept in Wolfenbüttel, "just like a relic of the bold *welfischen* Prince." But then it was sold to a local count, who put it on display in his castle.[155] Whether the object Christian's descendants exhibited was the same one chronicles described is immaterial for our present purpose. Indeed, whether the artificial arm of popular accounts accurately represented the reality of his experience is immaterial, too. What matters is that a cultural narrative developed around the figure of Christian that celebrated interventionism and feted activities blurring the boundaries of natural and artificial in the human body. Surgical perspectives of amputees resonated with this form of early modern cultural narrative. The *Theatrum Europaeum*, which contained the account most widely disseminated and copied in other chronicles and sources, emphasizes above all the physical tasks that Christian's artificial arm supposedly could perform. It bends, moves, grips, holds. These were the features that surgeons considered fundamental to a successful false restoration. The rehabilitated Christian the Younger of popular accounts resembled the rehabilitated amputee of surgical treatises—a composite of natural and artificial parts.

Surgeons think through questions

Through the writings of early modern surgeons, we have returned time and again to the language of "false"—false imaginations, false restorations. Each context conveyed a different meaning. In phantom sensations, surgeons described a confusion of the internal and external senses that communicated pain in a limb that was no longer there. False, here, was an inadvertent deception of the patient by the movement of animal spirits or the symptoms of injured nerves. Prostheses, by contrast, referred to very real material objects intentionally made and worn. On one level, they were false because they concealed bodily damage from others rather than healing it, particularly in the case of small and primarily aesthetic devices such as leather ears. On a deeper level, they were false because they were not made of flesh and bone, but instead from non-human materials attached to human bodies. False in this sense might better be read as *artful*.

The distinctions between kinds of "falseness" point to larger conceptual frameworks surgeons drew upon and the notions they developed around phantom limbs and limb prostheses. Both subjects dealt with responses to the radical physical alteration an amputation created. In one, surgeons' discussions focus on the reaction of the body, describing it as resilient, self-regulating, and capable of adapting to change but also as dangerous to itself. Surgeons must, according to Fabry and Döring's accounts, convince patients to persevere in stillness and calm while their bodies heal. False imaginations drew from a medical and intellectual discourse about the body and the embodied mind. Ideas about human cognition, understandings of the emotions and health, and the power of the imagination contributed to their interpretations of patients' experiences.

False restorations, by contrast, implicitly focused on human responses—on individuals who obtained and used prosthetic limbs. Surgeons' discussions of prostheses expressed expectations that a material intervention was desirable. The meaning of false restoration derived from its contrast to the medical concept of true restoration, of those manual operations surgeons performed to reconstitute what they perceived as lacking in a body. The conceptual framework was one inherently about the surgeon's craft, distinguishing between the "natural" operations of the surgeon and the "artful" work of artisans. Amputees were responsible for obtaining artificial limbs because the surgeon's primary task lay in aiding nature to heal the body, at times even moving the natural material of human flesh from one part to another to do so. Surgeons could incorporate smaller prostheses into their repertoire of services, and some certainly did. But artificial limbs, in our surgeons' writings, seem to be objects not only larger in design, but potentially more complex and, above all, useful for performing physical activities. We can detect surgeons' notions of a hybrid form of embodiment, one that incorporates the artificial into the natural, developing through a critique of art's role in providing what nature could not.

Our exploration of how surgeons thought through questions reveals a dynamic interplay between experience and surgical activities, on the one side, and structures of knowledge found within a growing corpus of surgical literature, on the other. This interaction was crucial to the ways surgeons constructed medical ideas about how to treat convalescing patients and how to view amputees. The relationship worked differently in each context. Fabry and Döring corresponded about a symptom they encountered firsthand. To return to the analogy of Amman's woodcut, they write from the perspective of a practitioner treating a patient inside the sickroom. Fabry's approach reveals that he is willing to accept more than one explanation, drawing from multiple authors, while prioritizing treatment. By characterizing phantom pain as an experience that rarely happens outside the transitional period of convalescent care and recovery, Fabry implicitly situates his understanding of its cause and treatment within his own context of encountering the symptom. Fabry's experiences treating the condition directly influence his understanding of it.

The false restoration of a limb reveals another kind of dynamic between experience, textual knowledge, and the construction of medical views. Here, practitioner-authors for the most part reflect upon passersby they glimpse through the door of Amman's sickroom. Discussions of artificial limbs are not drawn from surgeons' own experience. Instead, they relied on practical knowledge they gained in other areas as well as the medical framework of surgical restoration. Positive attitudes toward prosthetic limbs reflected their views on disguising perceived blemishes and providing small artificial parts to aid bodily functions. They drew on notions from their everyday activities related to facial scarring, artificial eyes, and urination tubes and applied them to a much larger part of the body. The result was a medical construction for viewing amputees as individuals who should, if their stumps allowed, artificially restore what the surgeon removed—albeit with the understanding that the more artificial the body became, the less power or responsibility surgeons could exert over the form it took. The broader implication was a human body that could become a hybrid of artificial and natural parts.

Our discussion has focused on how surgeons constructed medical views. This was not simply a projection of established medical ideas onto amputees' bodies—there was a give-and-take in the way one influenced notions of the other. And amputees played an active role in providing information that surgeons pondered and interpreted through their various analytic filters. In contrast to many other complications that occurred during convalescence, phantom pain was invisible to the naked eye. Without the words of amputees who decided to express their experiences, practitioners could not detect it. Likewise, considering amputees within the framework of false restorations was more than an abstract extension of surgeons' experiences with small prosthetic devices. Allusions to iron hands and wooden legs in their treatises signified the impact on medical thinking of real material practices with which amputees engaged. The following chapter turns to these practices.

Notes

1 Paracelsus, *Opus Chyrurgicum*. See also Herrlinger, "Die Anatomie des Jost Amman"; Seelig et al., *Jost Amman*, 1:222–226.
2 Scholars have examined attitudes toward perceived disability or infirmity in medical sources and among medical professionals in a variety of contexts: e.g., Niiranen, "Sexual Incapacity"; Bernstein, "Rehabilitation Staged." For examples that explore attitudes toward amputees: Linker, *War's Waste*; Heide, *Holzbein und Eisenhand*.

3 E.g., essays in Mendelsohn et al., *Civic Medicine*; Murphy, *New Order of Medicine*, esp. 14–16; Pomata, "Sharing Cases."
4 Hildanus, *Gründlicher Bericht*, 156, 164.
5 Gehema, *Feld-Medicus*, 57.
6 Hildanus, *Gründlicher Bericht*, 152.
7 Ibid., 153: "er sich nicht bewegt, nicht hustet, niest, überlaut schreit, lacht, zuviel redet, hitzige Speisen und Getränke genießt oder sich den Leib zu schwer, besonders mit warmen Tüchern, decken läßt, sondern daß er sich gut still hält."
8 Ibid., 154–155.
9 Ibid., 139.
10 Allusions to cases of amputees who felt pain in missing limbs appear in *Principia philosophiae* and *Meditations on First Philosophy*: Descartes, *Philosophical Writings*, 1:283–284, 2:53.
11 Crawford, *Phantom Limb*, 6.
12 Ibid., 108–109; Finger and Hustwit, "Five Early Accounts of Phantom Limb."
13 Louis and York, "Weir Mitchell's Observations on Sensory Localization," 1242; Finger and Hustwit, "Five Early Accounts of Phantom Limb." For modern medical debates: Crawford, *Phantom Limb*, 73–106.
14 Crawford, *Phantom Limb*, 212.
15 Hintzsche, Introduction, 12.
16 Hildanus, *Wund-Artzney*, 304: "was in deß Herrn Buch/ vom heissen und kalten Brand gelesen wird."
17 Ibid.: "Aber was thun die Wundärtzt? Erstlich verachten sie meinen rath."
18 Ibid., 252–253: "über nichts mehrers sich beklagt/ als daß ihm einig und allein der grosse Zehe wehe thut."
19 Ibid.: "hat er mit den Fingern in der Bettladen/ wo alle Zeit der Fuß zu seiner Ruhe hingelegt war/ gedeutet/ als wolte er dardurch den umbstehenden solches zu glauben desto ehender bereden."
20 Ibid., 253: "der längst hinweg geschnitten."
21 Ibid., 303.
22 Ibid., 253: "Welches weil ich gehört/ daß es der Krancke so beständig bestreiten wollen/ ist mir zu guter Gelegenheit ein Geschicht zu gefallen/ die mir mein günstig. Herr/ wann mir recht ist/ selber erzehlet. ... Als nemblich einer als ihme das Bein abgenommen gewesen/ nicht anderst vermeint/ als hätte er dasselbige noch nicht verlohren/ unnd deßwegen vom Bett auffstehen wollen/ aber als er zu Boden gefallen/ habe er mit seinem Schaden und nicht ohne Gefahr erfahren/ daß er den Schenckel nicht mehr habe. Darumb als ich dem Krancken solches erzehlet hat er alsbald angefangen außzubrechen: er förchte gar sehr/ es möcht ihm eben das auch begegnen."
23 Ibid., 252: "was nemblich für ein wunderbare Krafft seye in der Einbildung und der allgemeinen Empfindligkeit."
24 Roodenburg, "Senses," 42.
25 Hildanus, *Wund-Artzney*, 252: "entweder überlästig/ oder deren man gewohnt gewesen/ als wann sie noch gegenwärtig," "entweder hassen oder lieben."

26 Ibid., 252–253: "Von falschen Einbildungen/ welche denen zubegegnen pflegen/ welchen ein Gleid abgenommen worden," "Von falschen Einbildungen die denen begegnen welchen ein Glied abgeschnitten worden."
27 E.g., Hildanus, *Wund-Artzney*, 251, 255.
28 Ibid., 304.
29 Clark, *Vanities of the Eye*, 42; Rather, "Imagination," 352. For historiography of imagination in early modern Europe, see Clark, *Vanities of the Eye*, 42–43.
30 Haskell, "Introduction," 6; Swan, "Eyes Wide Shut," 561; Rather, "Imagination," 352; Gowland, "Melancholy, Imagination, and Dreaming," 59.
31 Clark, *Vanities of the Eye*, 43. See also Park, "Imagination in Renaissance Psychology."
32 E.g., the essays in Haskell, *Diseases of the Imagination*; Schott, "Paracelsus and van Helmont on Imagination" and "'Invisible Diseases'"; Rather, "Imagination"; Paré, *Wundt-Arztney* (1601), 1064–1066; Purmann, *Wund-Artzney* (1692), 1:335–344.
33 Carrera, "Anger," 96.
34 Herls, *Examen*, 405: "traurig/ schwermüthig/ verdrießiich/ fortchtsam."
35 Lindemann, *Medicine and Society*, 14.
36 Carrera, "Anger," 96.
37 Barbette, *Schrifften*, 397.
38 Carrera, "Anger," 120; Roodenburg, "Senses," 43.
39 Paré, *Wundt-Arztney* (1601), 42–43. See also Carrera, "Anger," 124.
40 Gowland, "Melancholy, Imagination, and Dreaming," 63–64.
41 E.g., Hildanus, *Wund-Artzney*, 1010, and *Gründlicher Bericht*, 162; Muys, *Praxis*, 319.
42 Hildanus, *Gründlicher Bericht*, 148–150.
43 Solingen, *Hand-Griffe*, 376.
44 Hildanus, *Gründlicher Bericht*, 148: "einen mutigen und redegewandten Mann."
45 Ibid., 163.
46 Ibid.: "Ist aber der Kranke traurig, voll schwerer Gedanken und hat er Verstimmungen des Gemüts, was bei Amputierten fast regelmäßig der Fall ist, so soll man alle Mittel und Wege suchen, ihn zu erheitern und mit kurzweiligem Gespräch und ehrbarer Gesellschaft zu erfreuen." See also Hildanus, *Wund-Artzney*, 202, and *Gründlicher Bericht*, 164–165.
47 See the Introduction for Götz's account.
48 *MFH*, 75–77.
49 Ibid., 75: "Und khamen sunst vill annderer mehr gesellenn zu mir, also das ich inn zweyenn oder dreyenn tagen nit vill ruhe hett, es wahr gleich ein walfart zu mir. Und khamen viell gutter leutt, die mich kanthen unnd besahenn, wie mirs giennng."
50 Hildanus, *Wund-Artzney*, 254: "sich eingebildet/ er leide überauß grosse Schmertzen umb den Reyen/ Versen und Zehen."
51 Ibid.: "Aber/ welches zu verwundern/ zu End der Heylung/ als er auff ein Zeit vom Schlaff erwacht/ und zu Stuhl gehen wollen/ hab er bey sich selbst (dann es war niemand sonst umb ihne) zu zweiflen und zu berathschlagen angefangen; ob er allein auß dem Bett auffstehen könne/ oder seine beede Füß noch habe oder

nicht; Endlich/ als er bey sich selbst beschlossen/ er hab in allweg seine beede Füß noch/ unnd fehl ihme nichts/ hab er versucht von dem Bett auffzustehen: aber er hat sich heßlich betrogen befunden: Dann er gleich alsbald über das Bett herunder gefallen/ unnd den Stumpff übel verletzt."

52 Scultetus, *Wund-Artzneyisches Zeug-Hauß* (1666), 1:206.
53 Ibid.: "als solches der Patient nicht wahr genommen/ ja nichts davon wuste."
54 Ibid., 1:207: "Den dritten Tag/ nach abgenommenem Schenckel beklagte sich der Patient, was für grosse Schmertzen er an der grossen Zäen deß rechten Fusses erleidete. Deme der Chirurgus lächlend darüber geantwortet/ er verwundere sich nicht wenig/ wie er/ der Patient über sein grosse Zäen klagen könte/ als welche bereits vor dreyen Tagen begraben worden seye. Als solches der Patient vernommen/ ist er dermassen darüber erschrocken/ daß er alsobalden in ein schwäre Ohnmacht gefallen."
55 Joubert, *Traitté des arcbusades*, 117–120.
56 Hildanus, *Wund-Artzney*, 254: "Dann der Sinnliche Geist der durch die Nerven fliesset/ stellet gleichsam dar die Empfindligkeit deß abgenommenen Glieds/ in welches er hat sollen einfliessen: Weil er aber nicht weiter kommen kan/ so gehet er wider zuruck zu der allgemeinen Empfindligkeit/ daselbst wird ein falsche Einbildung verursachet." Compare with Joubert, *Traitté des arcbusades*, 118.
57 Hildanus, *Wund-Artzney*, 254: "Sonsten daß diejenige welchen ein grosses Glied/ als Arm/ oder Schenckel abgenommen worden/ in dem der Stump noch Schmertzen/ Entzündung oder andere Zufäll leidet/ sich einbilden es thue ihnen der Finger oder Zehen wehe/ ist sich nicht zu verwundern. Dann desselbig begegnet schier allen/ denen dergleichen Glied abgeschnitten ist."
58 Ibid.: "Wann aber die Heylung fürüber so geschehen dergleichen Einbildungen gar selten mehr."
59 Ibid.: "Dann zwey Jahr nach vollendter Heylung hat er selbsten vor dem Herrn Merula, Diener am Wort Gottes/ unnd vor andern mehr ... bekennt/ und bezeuget/ er meine offt er habe noch Schmertzen am Fuß/ Reye und Schönbein."
60 Ibid.: "hat er sich wol befunden/ unnd hatte weder Fieber/ noch einigen Schmertzen."
61 Ibid.: "kam nicht her auß einer Wahnsinnigkeit/ oder Verruckung deß Verstands." Compare with Joubert, *Traitté des arcbusades*, 118.
62 Paré, *Wundt-Arztney* (1601), 530: "sie auch etliche Tage/ ja wol etliche Monat hernach uber das allbereit abgeschnittene Gliedt klagen/ als ob es noch zugegen unnd ihnen wehe thue/ welches den ein wunderbarlich unnd fast unglüblich Ding ist/ wo ichs nicht selbst mit Augen gesehen/ unnd von den Patienten gehöret hette."
63 Paré, *Wund-Artzney* (1635), 424.
64 Ibid.: "spa[n]näderichen Glieder."
65 Ibid.: "welches denn meines Erachtens/ nirgend anderst wo herkömpt/ denn dieweil die abgeschnidenen Nerven/ sich zurück und ihrem Ursprung zu ziehen unnd also einen Schmertzen dem Krampff gleich erregen."
66 E.g., Paré, *Wundt-Artzney* (1601), 372–373, 617.
67 Ibid., 457.

68 Ibid., 373: "zu ihrem Ursprung dem Hirn/ und begeren gleichsam von demselbigen/ als von ihrem Gebärer Hülff und Beystand."
69 Ibid., 26.
70 Hildanus, *Gründlicher Bericht*, 166–167.
71 Ibid., 168: "weil die Geister des Gehirns (Spiritus animales genannt), wenn sie bis zu dem Stumpf hinab ziehen und dort nicht weiterkommen, ungestüm und widerwillig zurückdrängen."
72 Ibid.
73 Ibid., 168–169.
74 Hildanus, *Wund-Artzney*, 254: "er im dritten Tag in meinem Abwesen den Arm (dann er ihm einbildet/ daß er ihne noch habe/ unnd nicht abgeschnitten seye) außstrecken/ und weiß nicht was mit der Hand langen oder ergreiffen wollen."
75 Ibid.: "Mir ist genug wann ich die angehende Wundärtzt dardurch erinnere daß sie fleissig unnd wachtsam seyen/ daß ihre Krancken/ wegen solcher falschen Einbildung den Stumpff nicht bewegen/ unnd dardurch ein Erbluten unnd sehr grosse Schmertzen verursachen."
76 Solingen, *Hand-Griffe*, 414: "so ist es ofters sehr nöthig/ daß bey den Patienten ein Balbier-Geselle wache/ weilen der Patient wohl zuweilen falsche Einbildungen in den Schlaf bekommet/ wodurch der Strunck von den Fuß beweget wird/ und eine neue Blutstürzung drauf folget."
77 Wunderlich, *Paradoxa Sensatio, sive Dolor Membri Amputati*.
78 Ibid., 5–7.
79 The instance that perhaps comes closest to a discussion of everyday tasks is a one-sentence description of a leather or paper hand with a quill to facilitate writing: Paré, *Les Oeuvres* (1585), 917. It first appeared in the 1585 French edition of Paré's collected works but did not appear in German editions. See also Lamzweerde, *Appendix*, 18–19.
80 E.g., Perry, *Recycling the Disabled*; Linker, *War's Waste*.
81 Barbette, *Schrifften*, 1, 86.
82 E.g., Barbette, *Schrifften*, 86.
83 Gadebusch Bondio, "Function, Utility, and Fragility of the Nose," 35, 40–41; Savoia, *Tagliacozzi*, 123.
84 See Gadebusch Bondio, *Medizinische Ästhetik*; Savoia, *Tagliacozzi*; Cock, *Rhinoplasty*.
85 Jessen, *Wund-Artznei*, 201–204; Purmann, *Wund-Artzney* (1692), 1:230–242.
86 Gehema, *Observationes*, 51.
87 Ibid., 52: "Einem Polnischen vom Adel wurde von einem andern Edelmann mit einer Säbel die Nase abgehauen/ man *persuadir*te einen seiner Unterthanen/ mit *promessen* einer nicht gereuenden Belohnung/ er solte sich auß dem Arm ein Stück Fleisch schneiden lassen; Der arme Unterthan *resolvir*et sich darzu/ des Edelmanns Angesicht ward auff des Bauren Arm gebunden/ und darauß eine Nase dermassen künstlich geschnitten/ als wann sie von einem Bildhauer wäre *formir*et worden/ es wolte aber diese *curieuse invention* nicht wol glücken/ sondern die angemachte Nase faulete bald wieder ab/ und muste sich der unglückliche Edelmann nur einer hölzernen Nasen bedienen/ welcher von einem Mahler eine natürliche Farbe gegeben ward."

88 Ibid., 54: "im menschlichen Cörper aber/ sind solche *tubuli* dermassen zart/ subtil und weich/ daβ sie von der geringsten Verletzung gantz und gar verwirret und verschoben werden können/ wodurch dann die *circulation* des Bluts und der Säffte verhindert wird/ und kein Anwachs geschehen kan."
89 Muys, *Praxis*, 79–80; Purmann, *Wund-Artzney* (1692), 1:231. See also Paré, *Wund-Artzney* (1635), 740. On medical discussion of plant-grafting: Savoia, *Tagliacozzi*, 140–174.
90 Van 'T Land, "Sperm and Blood."
91 E.g., Purmann, *Wund-Artzney* (1692), 3:7.
92 Paré, *Wundt-Artzney* (1601), 96.
93 Ibid., 366: "ein harte und dicke Schwüle." Compare with Renner, *Handtbüchlein* (1559), 104v.
94 Gadebusch Bondio, "Function, Utility, and Fragility of the Nose," 38.
95 Panse, *Feldbuch der Wundarznei*, 93–95.
96 Wittmann, *Kosmas und Damian*, 137–143.
97 Ibid., 73, 75, 212.
98 Voragine, *Golden Legend*, 584.
99 Ibid.
100 By contrast, no mention or depiction of an Ethiopian or Moor appears in the Greek Orthodox tradition: Zimmerman, "Introduction," 12.
101 Devisse and Mollat, *Africans in the Christian Ordinance of the World*, 101, 229–233. European depictions of the Moor were shaped by regional inflections and meanings, as Carmen Fracchia demonstrates by linking images of the miracle to the context of slavery in early modern Spain: "Spanish Depictions of the Miracle of the Black Leg."
102 Munt, "Dutch Cartesian Medical Reformers."
103 E.g., Stein, *Negotiating the French Pox*, 126.
104 Jessen, *Wund-Artznei*, 205–206; Paré, *Wund-Artzney* (1635), 741–742. Jessen follows Paré's work closely, and both cite Hippocrates.
105 Arcaeus, *Fraxinalensis*, 56–57.
106 Schmid, *Bericht*, 298–299.
107 Renner, *Handtbüchlein* (1559), 86r.
108 Jessen, *Wund-Artznei*, 200–201: "Eine Nase/ als die dem gantzen Angesicht/ wann sie wohl formirt und gantz/ eine Zierd gibt/ muβ man/ an statt einer abgestümmelten/ eine andere bilden und anmachen/ um solchen Schandfleck zu verstellen."
109 Ibid.; Paré, *Wund-Artzney* (1635), 740; Purmann, *Wund-Artzney* (1692), 1:231. See also Petraeus, *Encheiridion Cheirurgicum*.
110 Paré, *Wund-Artzney* (1635), 740; Schmid, *Bericht*, 362.
111 Jessen, *Wund-Artznei*, 200–201: "aus etwas/ von zusammen geleimten Papier/ oder gemahltem Leder angemachet/ ein rechtes Ohr vorstellen."
112 Ibid., 205: "lässt/ gleich einem solchen/ damit die Edel-Damen ihre Haare schlichten," "damit darinnen das verlohrne Aug von dem Mahler mit seinen Farben könne dargestellt werden."
113 Paré, *Wund-Artzney* (1635), 744.

114 Jessen, *Wund-Artznei*, 200–201: "nur eine falsche Ersetzung/ aber nicht so blutig und beschwerlich."
115 On the stigma surrounding mutilated noses: Groebner, *Defaced*, 67–86.
116 E.g., Cavallo, *Artisans of the Body*, 38–57; Savoia, *Tagliacozzi*, 127–132.
117 Paré, *Wund-Artzney* (1635), 348–349.
118 Würtz, *Practica* (1639), 174: "sehr heßliche ungestalte Schrammen oder Narben."
119 Ibid., 186–187: "ehrlichen Weibs-Personen."
120 Jessen, *Wund-Artznei*, 193–196.
121 Ibid., 204–205: "Eines/ von was Ursach es wolle/ ermanglenden Augs Unform (sintemahln dem menschen ein ausgestossen Aug nicht wieder wächst/ wie etlich von dem Fisch Myro vorgeben) können wir verstellen/ wann wir den Schaden heilen/ und ein anders gebildtes/ an des ausgestossenen statt/ ein von Silber/ oder Gold/ auch von geschmältzter Arbeit/ gemahlt/ und ausgepolirtes/ daß es einem rechten Aug gleich sehe/ einschieben. Dergleichen/ mit verwunderlicher Spitzfindigkeit gemachte/ falsche Augen/ zu Venedig/ ein Goldschmied von Florentz/ um sechs oder sieben Cronen feil hat."
122 Purmann, *Wund-Artzney* (1692), 1:243; Fabricius ab Aquapendente, *Wund-Artznei*, 1:273.
123 Jessen, *Wund-Artznei*, 208: "Die Noht ist eine Erfinderin derer Künste: die hat auch erfunden/ wie man die abgehauene Gliedmassen ersetzen möge: der Natur hierin fast nachäffend."
124 Ibid.: "ihrer etliche mit gemachten Schenckeln das Ampt zu gehen/ stehen/ mit den Armen/ etwas zu ergreiffen und zu fassen/ verwalten."
125 E.g., Savoia, *Tagliacozzi*, 143.
126 Barbette, *Schrifften*, 161: "Durch die Kunst werden die Hindernüssen der Heilung auß dem Wege geraumet/ aber die Natur selbsten heilet den Schaden."
127 Jessen, *Wund-Artznei*, 208: "scharffsinn-und künstlichen Erfinder."
128 E.g., Hildanus, *Gründlicher Bericht*, 118.
129 Jessen, *Wund-Artznei*, 208.
130 Muys, *Praxis*, 319–320: "ein Jüngling/ welcher an stat des ein wenig unterm Knie abgenommenen Schenckels ein hölzernes brauchend/ eben so geschwinde mit Schrittschuhen auff den Eise lauffen kunte als ein anderer."
131 E.g., Paré, *Wund-Artzney* (1635), 421; Gehema, *Feld-Medicus*, 25. See chap. 3.
132 Horn and Frohne, "Fluidity," 40.
133 Ibid.
134 E.g., Paré, *Wundt-Arztney* (1601); Verduyn, *Neue Methode*.
135 Jessen, *Wund-Artznei*, 208; Muys, *Praxis*, 319–320.
136 Horn and Frohne, "Fluidity," 38.
137 Bok, "Christian von Braunschweig in den Niederlanden," 27.
138 NLA-WO, 1 Alt 22 Nr. 103, fol. 198–199 [hereafter, NLA-WO-103].
139 Although the author's identity remains unknown, there is evidence to suggest the writer was employed by Count Ernst Casimir I (1573–1632), Christian's brother-in-law.
140 NLA-WO-103, fol. 198r: "der gantze arm todt wahr."
141 Ibid.: "tag und nacht."

142 Christian did not spend this entire period in Breda: Dudley Carlton to Thomas Roe, 14 October 1622, in Roe, *Negotiations*, 96; NLA-WO-103, fol. 199r.
143 NLA-WO-103, fol. 198v: "vor der vorgehanden gehalten grossen Pein, ein abscheus gehabt."
144 Ibid., fol. 198v–199r.
145 Christian II (of Anhalt-Bernburg), *Tagebuch*, 54, 68.
146 Baudaert, *Memorien*, 154.
147 Brachelius, *Historia*, 29: "Gottes Freunde und der Pfaffen Feynde."
148 Abelinus, *Theatrum Europaeum*, 668: "der tolle Hertzog hätte zwar seinen einen Arm verlohren/ aber den andern behalten/ sich an seinen Feinden zu rächen." See also Baudaert, *Memorien*, 154; NLA-WO-103, fol. 143v.
149 Abelinus, *Theatrum Europaeum*, 668: "Ihme hat hernacher ein Holländischer kunstreicher Baur auß dem Maasland ein eysern Arm/ der sich mit der Hand rühren und bewegen/ auch alles regieren und fassen können/ gemacht/ so ihm mit Gold angehefftet worden." See also Rehtmeyer, *Braunschweig-Lüneburgischen Chronica*, 1261; Gottfried, *Fortgesetzte Historische Chronick*, 139; NLA-WO-103, fol. 143v.
150 Greflinger, *Der Deutschen Dreyßig-Jähriger Krieg*, 24:

> In dieser scharffen Schlacht wurd Hertzog Christian
> In lincker Hand verletzt/ und weil der junge Mann
> Aus Eiffer auf den Krieg nichts nach dem Schaden fragte/
> Weil ihm des Krieges Ruhm mehr als sein Blut behagte/
> Geriethe durch Verzug der Auffsicht seine Hand
> und folgends auch der Arm in einen kalten Brand/
> Der ihm hierauff vom Leib/ umb ärgers zu verhütten/
> Dann bässer halb verlohrn als gantz/ wurd abgeschnitten.
> An dessen statt hernach Er einen eisern trug/
> und that doch gleichwol noch vor seinem Feinde gnug.

151 Lachmund, *De Ave Diomedea Dissertatio*, 11.
152 [Sturm], *Des geöffneten Ritter-Platzes*, 142: "der Höltzerne Arm/ welchen Hertzog Christian von Braunschweig an statt des ihm abgeschossenen lincken Arms gebrauchet."
153 Rehtmeyer, *Braunschweig-Lüneburgischen Chronica*, 1261.
154 Brückmann, *Centuriae Tertiae Epistolarum Itinerariarum*, 974.
155 Spehr, *Braunschweigischer Fürstensaal*, 291: "gleichsam als eine Reliquie des kühnen welfischen Fürsten."

5

Mechanical hands

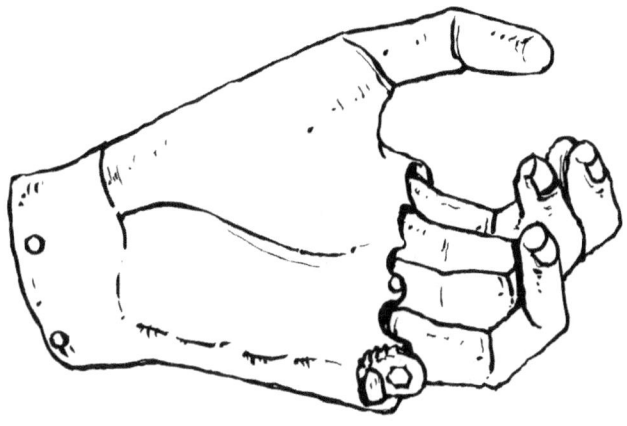

Most early modern hand prostheses sit unnoticed in the shadowy corners of armor exhibits, in museum storerooms, or in private collections. Over the last several decades, some have occasionally cropped up in exhibition catalogs or sourcebooks, which describe them as the curious precursors of modern artificial limbs.[1] Only recently have scholars begun to look more closely at these objects.[2] They pose as many challenges as they do opportunities for the study of the early modern world. The scarcity of textual sources concerning them opens no direct path to reconstructing their social and cultural meanings. Indeed, without artifacts, there would be scant evidence the images of mechanical limbs that the surgeon Ambroise Paré first published in the sixteenth century, and which were copied and circulated in the Holy Roman Empire through the seventeenth, were anything more than literary fantasy.[3] Artifacts point to the material practices underlying surgeons' brief asides to "iron hands" in their treatises, and which colored their sparse discussions of limb prostheses.[4] Yet surgeons had little to do with their creation.

This chapter examines the material culture of mechanical hands as evidence of the crucial role that amputees played in expanding the pliability of the early modern body. These were singular objects of artifice designed to supplement the natural body. With moveable fingers and flesh-toned paint, they incorporated practical and aesthetic functions in ways impossible with other kinds of prostheses. After all, silver noses could not smell, nor enameled eyeballs see.

Mechanical hands, by contrast, could hold things. Rare examples of iron legs with locking joints had limited utility for walking, and their weight would have made it difficult to propel them forward.[5] Artificial legs needed to be lightweight, but also sturdy enough to support the wearer's body. This made a wooden shaft ideal.[6] For this reason, a lower limb prosthesis was commonly referred to as a *Stelzfuß*, which indicated a wooden shaft with either a fitted socket for the wearer's stump or a wide trough to rest a long lower leg stump horizontally. While exceptions existed, on the whole it was artificial hands that provided amputees and artisans with the most opportunities for exploring combinations of articulation and ornamentation.[7]

Consider three examples. In 1836, a left iron hand with an attached forearm casing was found in the bed of the Rhin river near Alt-Ruppin in northeastern Germany (figure 5.1).[8] The object, which dates to the late fifteenth or early sixteenth century, is heavily corroded and no longer functions.[9] It has two finger blocks along with a moveable thumb. A "finger block" indicates two or more artificial fingers attached at their base, which move together. On the Ruppin Hand, these were once capable of locking in multiple positions through internal springs designed to catch toothed wheels at the joints where the fingers meet the hand. Wearers operated objects like this passively, using their other hand to press down on the prosthetic fingers from the outside until they locked in the desired position. Pressing the two exterior release buttons located on the wrist, beneath the palm, relieved the tension of the springs and allowed the fingers to move freely. The internal mechanisms are hidden by a plate secured over the wrist opening where the hand attaches to the forearm casing. The object's surface is too damaged to determine whether it was originally painted, but the engraved fingernail details remain prominent (figure 5.2). A precise pattern of increasingly long and narrow rectangles in the forearm casing reveals a form of "openwork." This was a decorative technique for armor that involved cutting out patterns, often to reveal a layer of textile or metal beneath.[10] Applied to a prosthesis, it reduced the object's weight. A bump at the side of the wrist, created by a small expansion in the interior of the forearm casing, appears to have been made after the arm was complete.[11] This may suggest someone performed an alteration—as a tailor might do to the cuff of a sleeve—to adjust the fit. Today the artifact is in storage at Museum Neuruppin.

Even more battered are two fragments of a left arm prosthesis discovered in 1908 during the renovation of a church in Balbronn, located in the Alsace region of present-day France (figure 5.3).[12] The artifacts were found along with human bones under the decorated grave plate of Hans von Mittelhausen, a figure known only from the funerary inscription referring to him as a nobleman and town official who died in 1564.[13] Balbronn, twenty-five kilometers from the imperial city of Strasbourg, was in German-speaking lands during Hans's lifetime. Smiths in Strasbourg made three identical reconstructions of

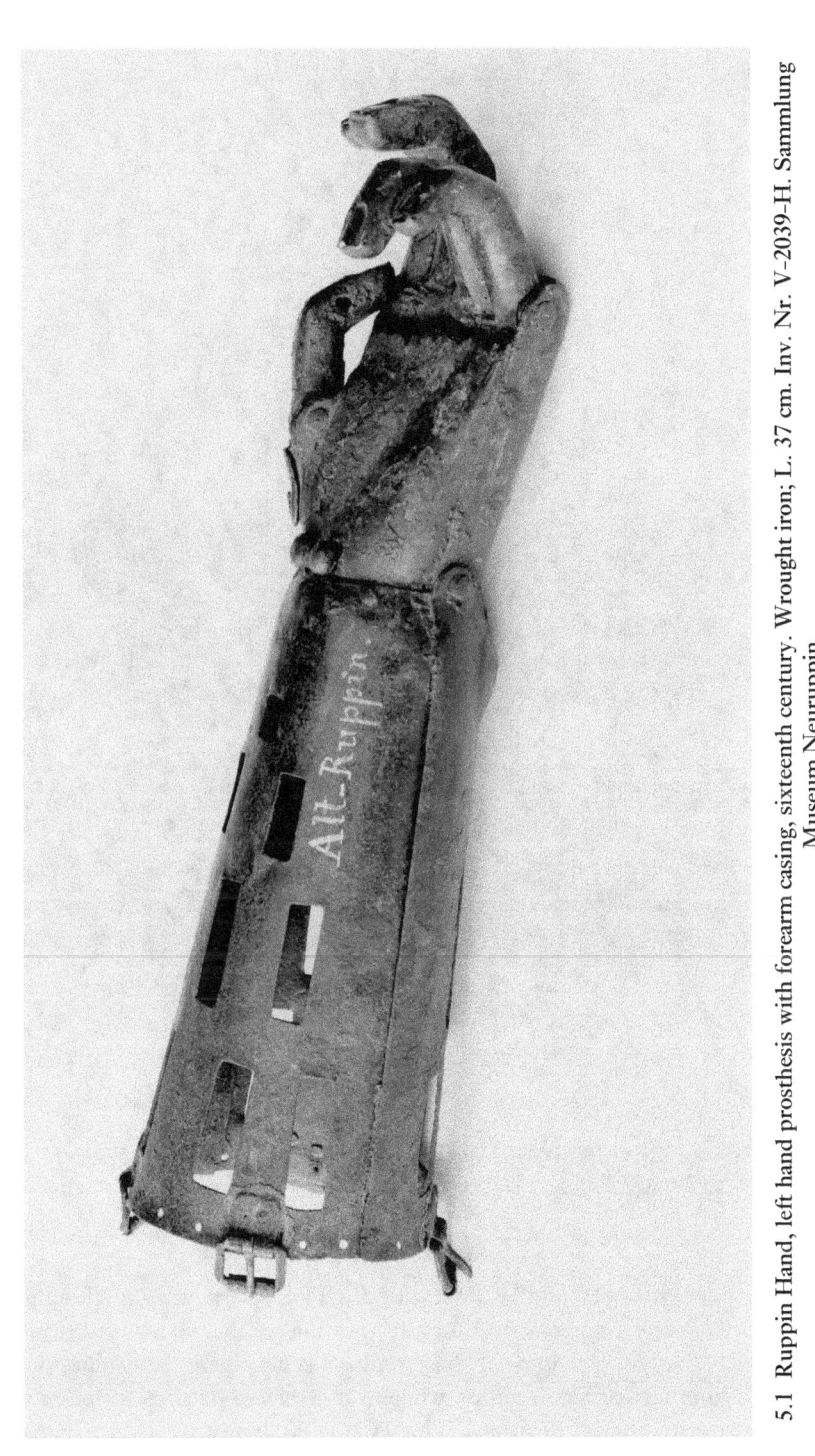

5.1 Ruppin Hand, left hand prosthesis with forearm casing, sixteenth century. Wrought iron; L. 37 cm. Inv. Nr. V-2039-H. Sammlung Museum Neuruppin.

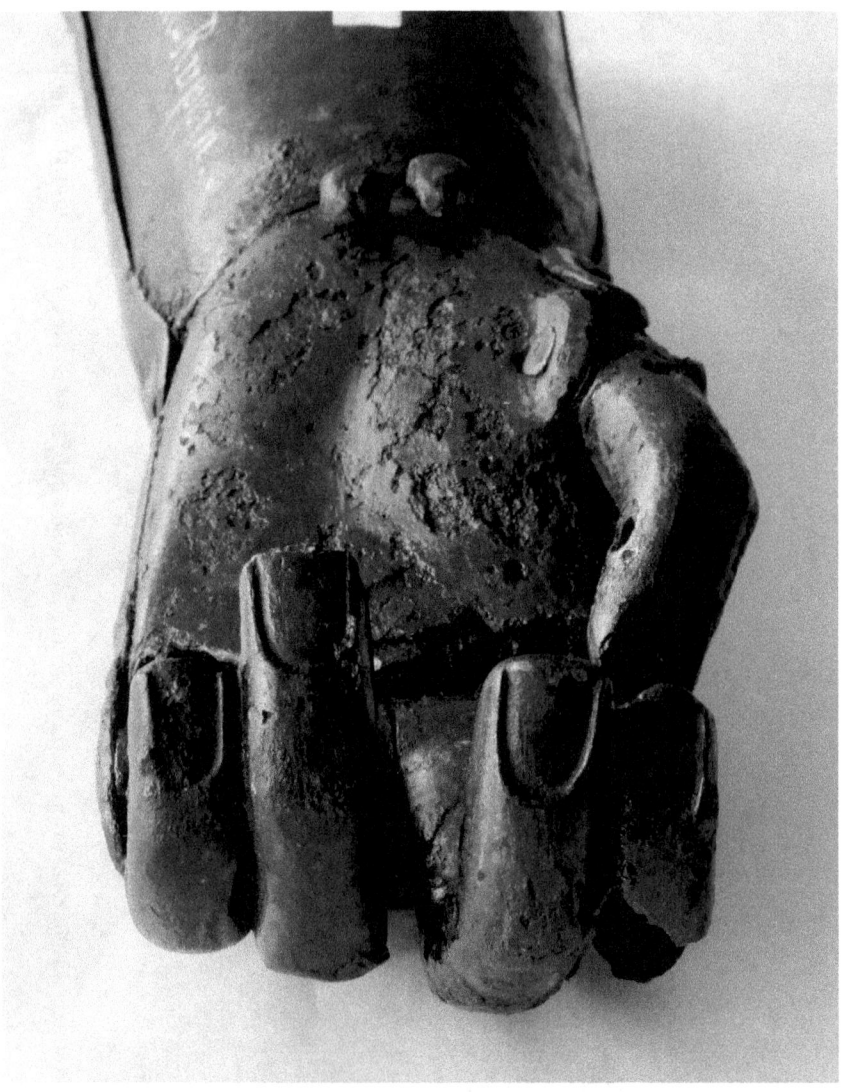

5.2 Ruppin Hand (detail), left hand prosthesis with forearm casing, sixteenth century. Wrought iron; L. 37 cm. Inv. Nr. V-2039-H. Sammlung Museum Neuruppin.

the artifact between 1908 and 1918 (figure 5.3). These were probably designed with the aid of early nineteenth-century diagrams of another sixteenth-century prosthesis.[14] Every finger joint of these replicas is articulated and relies on a system of internal springs, toothed wheels, and release buttons to lock into an impressive number of positions. The wrist and elbow are also articulated.

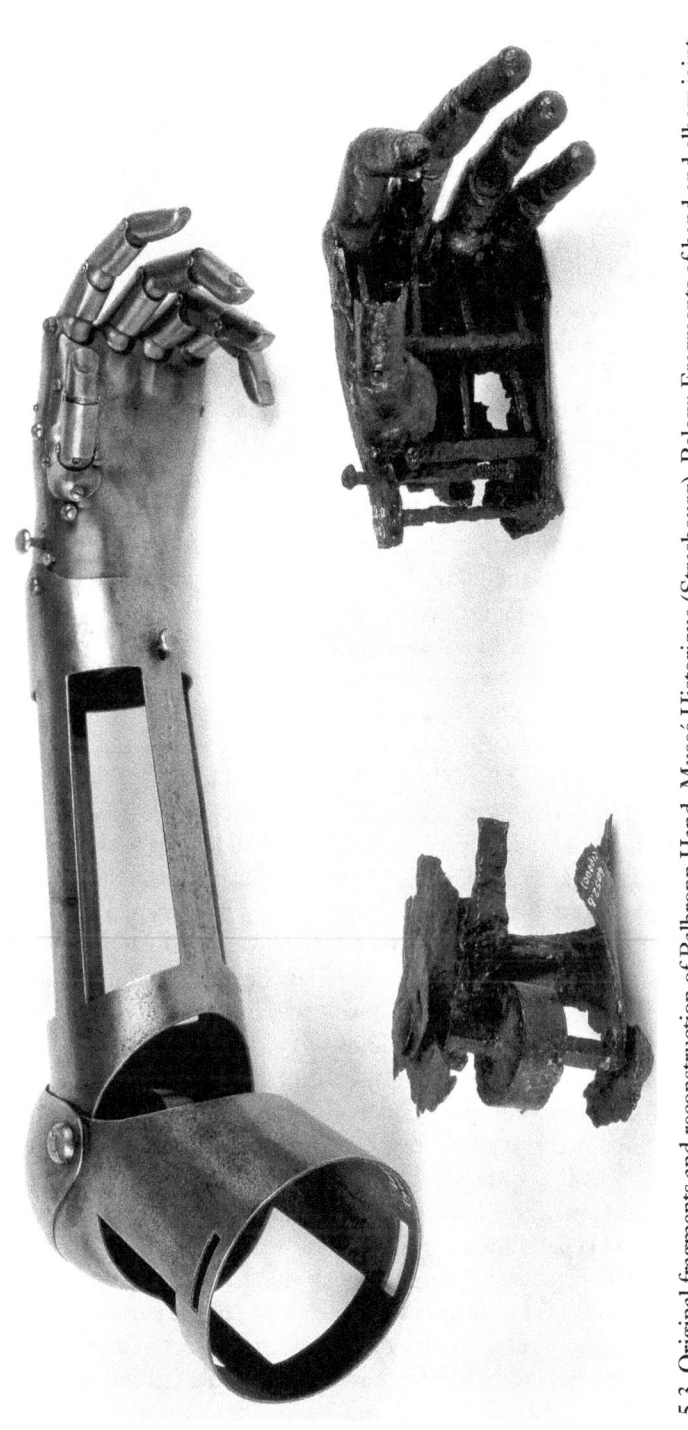

5.3 Original fragments and reconstruction of Balbronn Hand, Museé Historique (Strasbourg). Below: Fragments of hand and elbow joint from a left arm prosthesis, c. 1550. Wrought iron; hand: L. 16 cm; elbow joint: L. 9 cm. Inv. Nr. MH 4052 a–b. Above: Reconstructed left arm prosthesis by Zschokk, c. 1918. Wrought iron; L. 47 cm. Inv. Nr. MH 4053.

The original fragments and one of the 1918 reconstructions are currently on display in a dimly lit exhibit labeled "Armor" in the Historical Museum in Strasbourg.

The original provenance of a right arm prosthesis at the Deutsches Historisches Museum in Berlin is a forgotten family secret (figure 5.4). It has been dated to the sixteenth century, but no mention of it appears in textual sources until the Hornstein family history of 1911, which states only that the object had been kept as an heirloom since living memory.[15] The artifact, which is in remarkably good condition, consists of an upper arm casing, a wooden forearm, and an iron hand—all of which can still be disassembled. The hand is decorated with flesh-toned paint and has grooves imitating fingernails, as well as wrinkles on the knuckles. Like the Ruppin Hand, it has two finger blocks, which could be positioned and released separately by two buttons on the top of the hand. The thumb is rigid, and the elbow can be locked into six positions. A piece of leather that was probably used to fasten the arm to its wearer is still attached to the proximal end of the upper arm casing, or the part closest to the point of attachment to the body. It appeared in a display cabinet with other family treasures in a private collection at Schloss Grüningen, in southwestern Germany, until its sale to the museum in 2016.

What do these objects have in common? Mechanical hands like these have survived when early modern upper limb prostheses primarily made of wood or leather—options more affordable for the majority of the population—have not.[16] Most are made entirely of iron. The Ruppin Hand, discovered in a riverbed, attests to the durability of their materials. Some were buried with wearers of high social status in well-preserved tombs, like the Balbronn Hand. Still others were held as keepsakes, passed from one generation to the next, as with the Grüningen Hand. Each offers a glimpse into experimental practices with technology and the body, forged from a discursive partnership between individual amputees and artisans. These material responses to amputation reveal another way in which early moderns explored, questioned, and manipulated the form, movement, and texture of limbs.

There is no comprehensive list of extant early modern European artificial hands. I am familiar with approximately thirty-five objects, some of which, although documented and photographed, were lost in the first half of the twentieth century. Thanks to the generosity of several museums and their staffs, as well as private owners, I have examined fifteen of them. Twelve fall within the temporal and geographic scope of this study: eleven early modern artifacts, as well as a modern reconstruction of one of these. The following draws from direct examinations of the objects and the expertise of the curators and conservationists who preserve and care for them. They represent a form of prosthetic technology—the mechanical hand—that first appeared in the late fifteenth century and continued into the sixteenth and seventeenth centuries. The examples

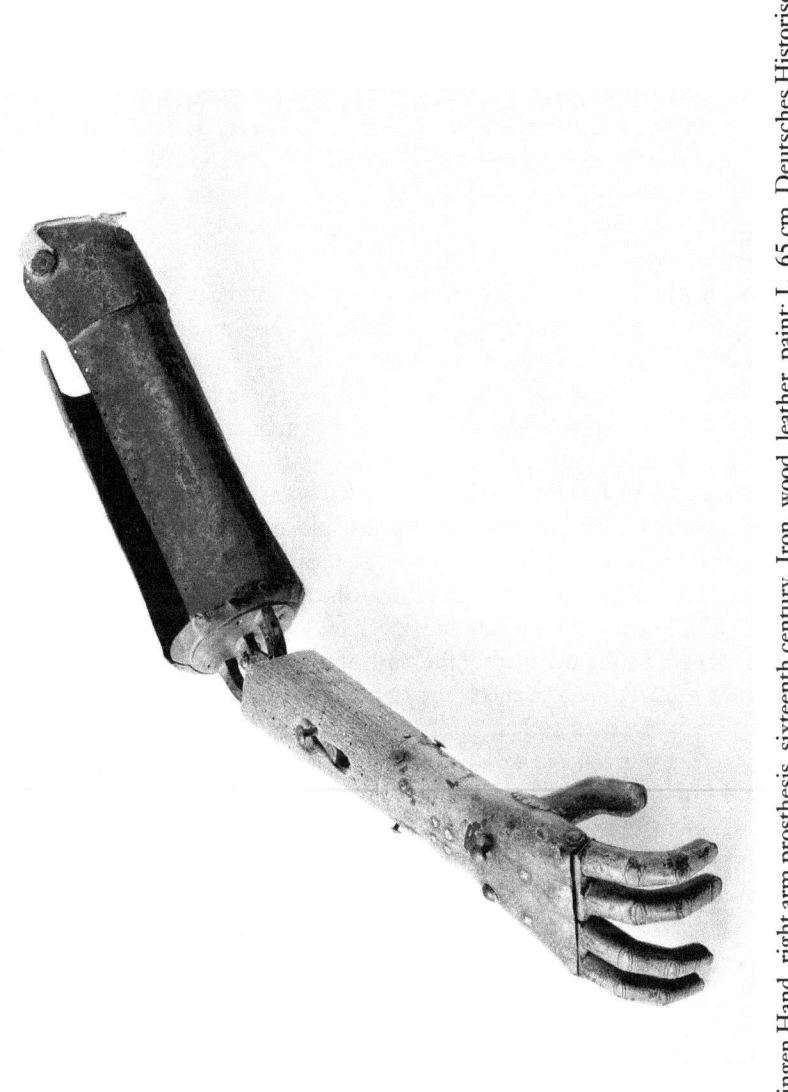

5.4 Grüningen Hand, right arm prosthesis, sixteenth century. Iron, wood, leather, paint; L. 65 cm. Deutsches Historisches Museum (Berlin).

in my source pool date between 1500 and 1700. They were either discovered in the German-speaking lands of Central Europe or are objects of unknown provenance currently held in German collections.

Our investigation will delve into objects like the Ruppin Hand and the Balbronn Hand, examining their histories, their production, and their many functions. After briefly contextualizing their modern reception, we will learn how their mechanisms worked, and what this can tell us about how they were made. Then we will apply this knowledge to a deeper exploration of their decorations and forms to learn what they can reveal about their makers and wearers. Through these objects, we find glimpses of the ongoing material activities amputees sponsored, and in which they participated, as they shaped their limbs and the meanings of bodily change.[17]

This chapter contends that careful analysis of mechanical hands recovers not only a vital dimension of the experiences of early modern amputees, but also sheds new light on the impact they made on the development of prosthetic technology and medical views of prostheses. The argument is built on the convergence of three major areas of intervention: our interpretation of the artifacts, the artisans who made them, and the amputees who commissioned them. Contributing to recent efforts in the history of science, technology, and medicine to engage with objects, I employ the interdisciplinary methods of material culture studies and disability history to approach each artifact as a starting point from which I build outward.[18] Rather than the battlefield, my study reframes the cultural context for understanding mechanical hands as the art cabinet and craft workshop. I also push further the work of scholars who have broadened our definitions of early modern medical practice and practitioners.[19] The chapter explores craft practices and ways of knowing to reveal artisans—locksmiths, clockmakers, armorers, and woodworkers—engaged in work of a medical kind. Finally, I bring together history of medicine and disability history by drawing on notions of "bodywork" in healing, "fluidity" in premodern disability, and the design model of disability to explore the experiences and practices of amputees who commissioned mechanical hands.[20] In contrast to their modern American counterparts,[21] early modern amputees wielded considerable influence in their role as consumers. Indeed, as *patrons*, their commissions drove material practices that produced a new prosthetic technology.

Unraveling the modern reception of early modern objects

Made of metal, wood, leather, and paint, early modern mechanical hands have sparked modern imaginations since the nineteenth century. Pseudo-historical accounts of their origins arose in this period, describing them as the possessions of injured knights. Their presentation in museums and print today largely reflects this. Traditionally they have been categorized with arms and armor in museums and private collections.[22] This classification is primarily related to the kinds of craftsmanship the objects display, but it also parallels their prevailing interpretation over the last two centuries. Museum records, local journals, exhibition catalogs, sourcebooks, and recent scholarship describe many as having some connection to combat: the possessor is said to have lost a limb in battle and/or to have used the prosthesis to hold the reins of a horse, often during battle. Even the most nuanced discussions of bodily difference in recent scholarship continue in this tradition. "Iron hands," one scholar writes, "were apparently used in order to maintain horsemanship, an ability of central importance to a knight."[23] Linked to this is the misperception that these prostheses could be used not only to hold reins but also to wield swords.[24]

This chapter's introductory artifacts are typical examples (figures 5.1–5.4). When church renovators found fragments of the Balbronn Hand in Hans von Mittelhausen's grave, Robert Forrer (1866–1947), an archaeologist and antiquarian who oversaw their preservation, suggested Hans lost his left arm fighting in the Peasants' War of 1525, though no evidence linked him to the conflict.[25] Notes from the inventory log of the Musée Historique in Strasbourg dating to its acquisition of the object in 1953 record this supposition as fact.[26] Newspapers advanced a similar conjecture about the Ruppin Hand after its discovery in 1836, speculating that it belonged to a knight who fell from a bridge and into the river during a skirmish.[27] Recent essays and exhibition catalogs continue to describe its purpose as enabling the wearer to hold the reins of a horse.[28]

Written sources provide some contextual evidence for these assertions. In France, an early modern biography of François de la Noue (1531–1591), a Huguenot military leader who lost his left arm after a gunshot wound, explicitly describes his iron prosthesis as holding the reins of his horse when he returned to the battlefield.[29] In the Swiss Cantons, the town council of Fribourg paid an artisan in 1476 to make an artificial hand for Ulrich Wyss, who lost his limb in an explosion while serving as master of artillery.[30] Most significant in the German-speaking context, however, is the example of Götz von Berlichingen.

The routine association between early modern iron arms and warfare today cannot be disentangled from the impact of Johann Wolfgang von Goethe's play, *Götz von Berlichingen mit der eisernen Hand* (1773). Goethe loosely based his drama on the autobiography of the sixteenth-century knight, which had circulated in print since 1731. The fascination and profound cultural pride it generated inspired publications about Götz's life and about two prosthetic artifacts, known today as the Ersthand and the Zweithand (figures 5.5–5.6).[31] The mechanically sophisticated Zweithand received the greatest attention. According to the Hornstein family history of 1911, it passed into their possession through marriage about three generations after Götz's death in 1562. The history recounted that "because of Goethe, *Ritter* Götz had suddenly become a famous man and his iron hand a priceless relic." Marquand von

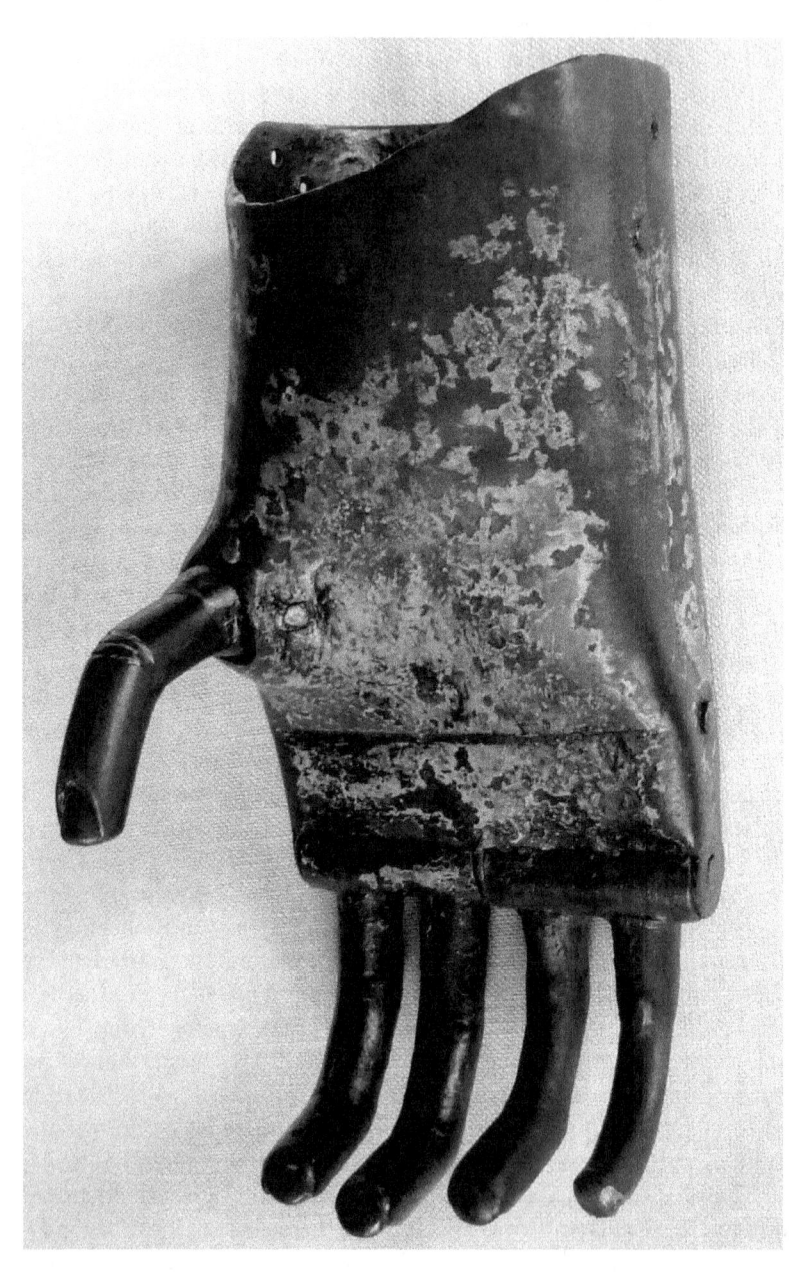

5.5 Ersthand, right hand prosthesis, c. 1510. Wrought iron, paint; wrist to base of fingers: L. 13 cm; fingers: L. 7 cm. Schlossmuseum Götzenburg (Jagsthausen).

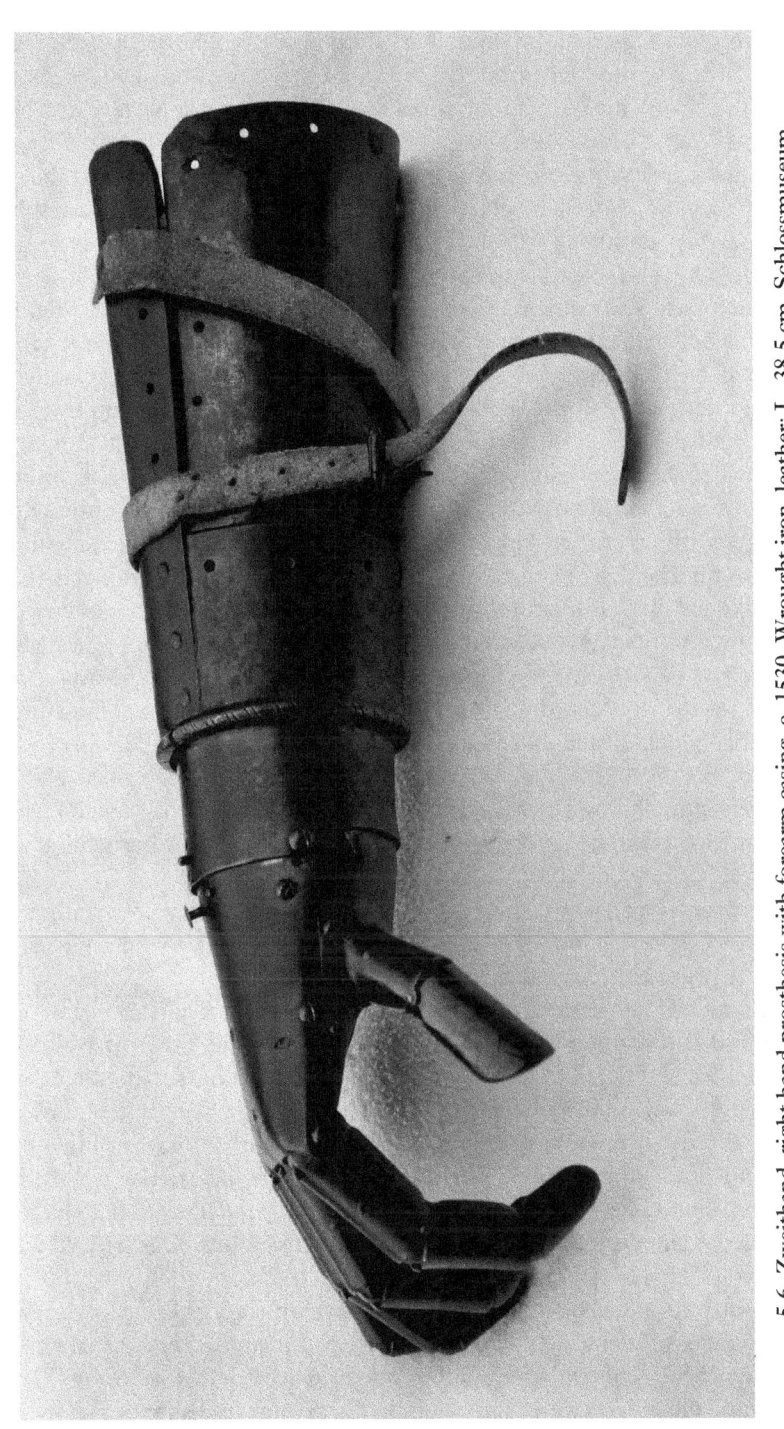

5.6 Zweithand, right hand prosthesis with forearm casing, c. 1530. Wrought iron, leather; L. 38.5 cm. Schlossmuseum Götzenburg (Jagsthausen).

Hornstein reportedly found the publicity dizzying: "'Would that I had never seen the hand,' wrote Marquand, 'so much am I assaulted on all sides about the treasure.'"[32] At the request of Franziska von Berlichingen, he gave it to her family in 1788.[33] Visitors flocked to see it when she put it on display in Vienna and Jagsthausen.[34] When the Zweithand is exhibited in the Götzenburg today, it is kept in a glass case accompanied by a printed copy of Götz's autobiography and Franziska's guestbook, which the museum customarily keeps open to the page with Otto von Bismark's signature.

The notoriety and cultural momentum that developed around the figure of Götz deeply influenced perceptions of early modern iron hands.[35] The survival of many of these objects may to some extent be due to Goethe's continued popularity in the nineteenth century. But this conflation of texts and objects has also led the iconic image Goethe created to overshadow the artifacts. The two iron hands in the Berlichingen collection became archetypes to which all other early modern examples have been, and continue to be, compared. Forrer used Götz as a point of reference in his assessment of the Balbronn Hand, writing that it "obviously" (*ersichtlich*) belonged to a knight who lost his left hand and forearm, and, like Götz's iron prostheses, it was designed to hold a horse's reins in battle.[36] Local newspapers repeatedly referenced Götz's prosthesis when describing the Ruppin Hand upon its discovery in 1836.[37] According to family tradition, the Grüningen Hand once belonged to Götz, although—as the family acknowledges—he lost his right hand and this is an above-the-elbow arm prosthesis.[38] When it was sold in 2016, the auction house advertised it as an object historically associated with Götz that was "produced in the same workshop as the older of Berlichingen's 'hands.'"[39]

This comparison takes a more scholarly form in the use of the informal categories "Ersthand" and "Zweithand" to characterize prosthetic artifacts, a practice as prevalent today as it was in the nineteenth century.[40] These refer to the distinguishing features of the two objects, one of which is mechanically simpler and dated around Götz's injury in 1504, and the other of which is more complex and dated to his later career, c. 1530. Given the attention they have received since the eighteenth century, including published diagrams of their interiors, they provide useful points of comparison for understanding the design and production of other objects.[41] Analytic problems arise when this blurs into using Götz—their supposed wearer—inseparably from the objects, creating a rigid model that leaves little room to discuss anonymous artifacts and their wearers outside of a martial context.

The outsized influence of examples from written sources decidedly skews interpretations of the material culture in one direction. Yet martial cases are likely overrepresented among the few written references we have. They involve individuals who were male, high profile by rank or distinguished by an extraordinary circumstance related to their injury, and were wounded in military service. All of these characteristics made such a figure more likely to appear in municipal records (i.e. the records of the institutional body one served), a biography or autobiography, or printed sources such as popular chronicles. The experiences of injured soldiers and the well-known accounts of figures like Götz should inform our investigation of mechanical hands. However, they should not determine our entire understanding of them. There are more artifacts than there are recorded instances of individuals obtaining iron limbs in archival or printed sources. The masculine, martial interpretive tradition proceeds from a set of assumptions that should be revisited.

Take the example of the Ingolstadt Hand (figure 5.7). This left hand prosthesis dates to the first half of the sixteenth century. The Bayerisches Armeemuseum in Ingolstadt, in southwestern Germany, acquired it in a trade with another museum in 1930. The hand is mechanically simple, but elegantly shaped. Its curved fingers move together on one axis, and the spring mechanism, which locks the fingers into approximately four positions, is located on the outside of the hand. The stiff curve of the fingers forms a hook or "O" when the prosthesis is fully flexed. To release the fingers, the wearer lifts the end of the spring to free the toothed wheel connected to the axis. The object is decorated with flesh-colored paint and engraved fingernails. Perforations on the proximal end of the wrist show where it might be tied to the wearer. The museum has kept the object on display in the same installation of early modern weapons since 1972.[42]

The prevailing interpretation of the object, which has no sources to indicate its original provenance, is strictly martial.[43] When addressing its function, a recent volume notes only that "holding the reins [of a horse] was probably possible," implying that its primary purpose was to serve a horseman.[44] The display label within the showcase at the Bayerisches Armeemuseum indicates that it is an early modern hand prosthesis. In its online digital collection of 2016, however, the museum added the explanation that "presumably the owner lost the left hand in combat and supplemented it with this prosthesis."[45] Modern characterizations of the Ingolstadt Hand rest on three implicit—or sometimes explicit—claims: its wearer was a man, its wearer lost his limb on the battlefield, and its wearer probably used it to hold the reins of a horse. Although none of these claims is implausible, the story they build together does not exhaust the possible meanings of this colorful, delicately curved, and lightweight artifact. Let us briefly examine each claim in turn.

First, women were not exempt from limb amputation, rare though it was. For instance, in 1551 the town council of Munich paid the barber-surgeon Ulrich Welser for removing the arm of a prostitute (*Dirne*), as well as the lower leg of another woman.[46] In his *Observationes*, Fabry von Hilden described

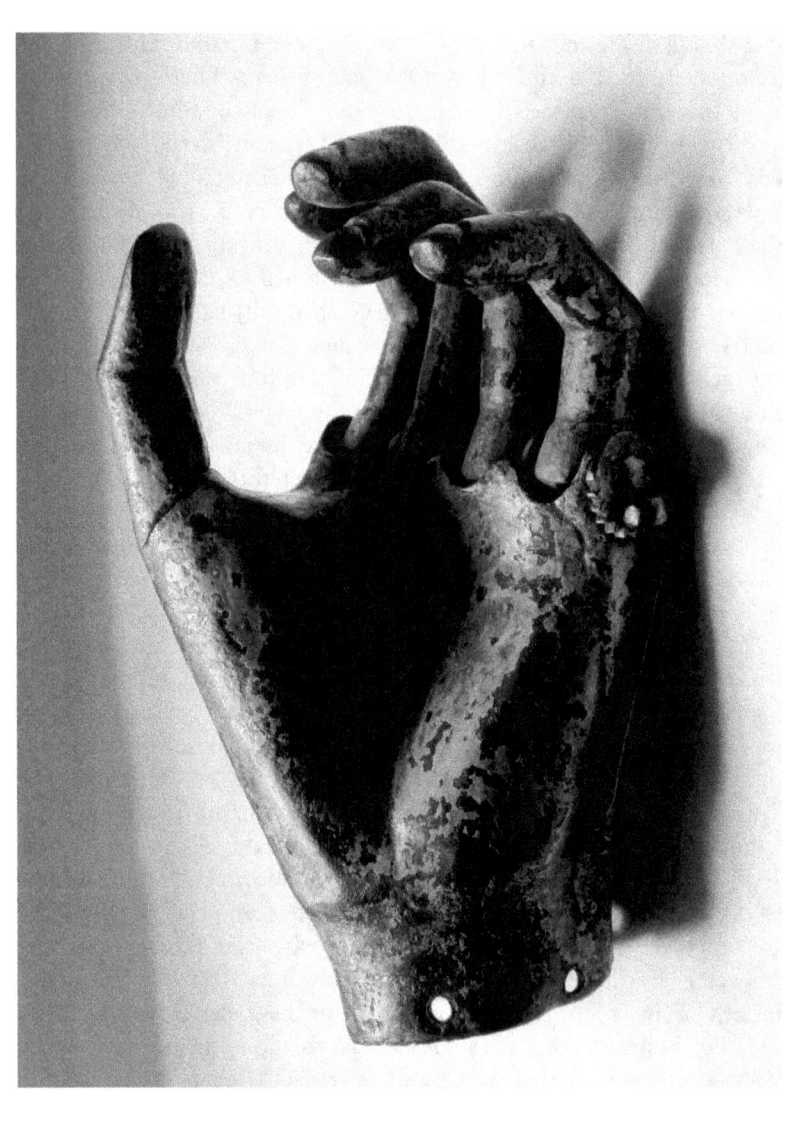

5.7 Ingolstadt Hand, left hand prosthesis, c. 1520. Wrought iron, paint; L. 15 cm. Inv. Nr. 7924. Bayerisches Armeemuseum (Ingolstadt).

the arm amputation of a female patient in 1604. The wife (*Haußfraw*) of Jacob Bagole developed the cold fire in her left hand, turning her fingers black before spreading to her elbow. In the feeble hope that she might be saved, "her husband and kin—also the patient herself—desired that her arm be removed."[47] Fabry performed the procedure in the presence of a pastor, a physician, the Burgermeister of Payerne, and other distinguished members of the community. The patient did not survive, but the number of prominent figures who attended her operation suggests her family may have had the resources to acquire a prosthesis had she lived. Need an artificial arm designed for her have looked very different from examples like the Ingolstadt Hand?

Second, injuries leading to amputation were not confined to the battlefield. Dangerous accidents happened on streets, in workshops, and in homes, from a dyer's assistant falling into a cauldron of hot dye to an innkeeper breaking his leg while gathering wood.[48] Surgeons also discussed putrefaction resulting from diseases like the French pox, botched bloodlettings, bandages wrapped too tightly, and exposure to the elements. Gunpowder warfare and the growing sizes of armies created more contused injuries than before, but early moderns still managed to hurt themselves in other ways, and surgeons used their wartime experiences with amputation on civilian populations.

The third claim raises a particularly difficult question. Can we know that the Ingolstadt Hand was designed with horse-riding in mind? A locking gauntlet adapted to an amputee wearer would have been a sturdier, more reliable, and simpler solution. Locking gauntlets, steel mittens designed to secure the hand of a combatant into an "O" shape around a weapon using a hook and eye-peg, date to the same era as many extant hand prostheses.[49] The design was so effective that it was purportedly banned from some tournaments and has been called the "forbidden gauntlet." The Ingolstadt Hand, with its flesh-colored paint and curved fingers, seems to be doing something *more* than a locking gauntlet. Perhaps it could hold the reins of a horse, but its lifelike appearance and multiple positions of flexion suggest it could have been used in other ways as well. It is because of this danger that we might miss what *more* these artifacts could do that we should examine them individually, without the weight of the martial narrative influencing what we see.

Artifacts like the Ingolstadt Hand have much to tell us all on their own. They offer clues about how and why they were made and give insights into their wearers' experiences.[50] Rather than assume they were injured knights, it is more productive instead to think of their wearers as amputee-patrons. This broadminded perspective emphasizes their role in commissioning hand prostheses—their role in the creation of these objects—without imposing a uniform profile. It allows us to focus on the several kinds of diversity the artifacts display: in the appearance, design, and function of the objects themselves; in the craft groups who made them; and in the levels of skill and quality of materials used. Considering their makers and materiality in turn sheds light on their wearers, undermining one-size-fits-all interpretations that flatten our understanding of human experience. As Katherine Ott argues, "people come back into the story when attention is given to objects."[51]

Craft production and material culture

The techniques evident in artifacts reveal connections to skilled producers, and to places and methods of production. Thus, rather than the battlefield, the first place we should situate these objects is the craft workshop. Most early modern prosthetic hands cannot be linked directly to specific historical persons. They are anonymous. But they can be linked to craft practices, and through these practices to groups of people. We can do this by "reading" these objects. By studying their material components, we can glean information to formulate and answer questions regarding their production, function, and meaning. Direct examination is all the more necessary for studying the objective and subjective functions of mechanical hands because of their relationship to the body—as things designed to attach to it; as things worn, carried, and incorporated into one's routine movements and everyday tasks. Whenever their condition permits, careful handling of the objects, including inspecting and operating their mechanisms, is illuminating. Encounters with the tangible cultivate unexpected insights into the intangible. In what follows, we will closely examine our source pool, reading the objects from the inside out and highlighting ways in which they point to diverse artisans.

We begin on the inside. All surviving upper limb prostheses from early modern Germany have some form of mechanism to lock their fingers into different positions and release them. They are mechanical hands. Two common elements were essential to their operation: ratchets and springs. As we have seen, the Ingolstadt Hand incorporates a single external ratchet—a toothed wheel—that catches on a spring the wearer can lift to release (figure 5.7). Rachets appear in other forms and in greater numbers in other objects, usually as part of internal mechanisms, hidden from view. For example, there are two built into the base of the finger blocks of both the Ruppin Hand and the Grüningen Hand. In the former, each ratchet is a narrow wheel set into the wider base of a finger block (figure 5.1). In the latter, the base of each finger block *is* a wide ratchet with shallow teeth (figure 5.4).

The Zweithand, the right hand prosthesis with a forearm casing in the Berlichingen collection, demonstrates a more complex use of ratchets (figure 5.6).

Its casing has a hinged flap that can be opened, as well as two leather straps to fasten it. The prosthesis is in good condition, with a smooth, unpainted surface. Its only ornamentation is the hint of fingernail impressions. Its fingers and thumb, which can be moved individually, can be released by pressing buttons on either side of the wrist. Franziska von Berlichingen allowed the artist Christian von Mechel to take apart the prosthesis to examine and draw its internal mechanisms. His diagrams, published in 1815, reveal that the interior portion of every joint in each individual finger forms a ratchet that locks through a series of springs (figure 5.8).[52] The further the joint from the base of a finger, the fewer teeth in the ratchet.

A ratchet allows movement in only one direction. In mechanical hands, it also controls the degree of flexion. Each tooth in the wheel creates a fixed position. This is only possible because ratchets lock in place with a spring. Springs appear in countless forms and combinations in mechanical hands from this period. The Ingolstadt Hand has a single long external lever attached near the wrist that stretches up to the ratchet at the base of the little finger (figure 5.7). The wearer lifts the lever up to release the fingers. Other objects whose mechanisms are internal relied on several other kinds of springs, pawls, and levers that often worked together to release ratchets via external buttons. Mechel's diagram reveals that each finger of the Zweithand has a series of three internal locking levers, held at tension by curved springs, which lock into the ratchets of the joints (figure 5.8).[53]

The sixteenth-century Kassel Hand uses different kinds of springs (figure 6.4). The earliest reference to the object in museum records appears in 1874 and does not provide details about its acquisition.[54] Most recently, it has been on display at the Museum Schloss Friedrichstein in Bad Wildungen, where it appears in an exhibition dedicated to early modern military history. The artifact's smooth surface is not a solid color, which could mean the iron is partially discolored, a protective resin is peeling, or that it may have been painted. There are engraved fingernails, but no other decorative details. The wearer likely fastened it to the forearm using two iron rings at the wrist, one of which has broken off. The thumb no longer operates, but the remaining four fingers individually lock into seven positions. The release switch is located on the underside of the wrist. Its mechanisms reveal multiple flat springs: strips of material that store and release energy when deflected by an external load, useful within small spaces. In the Kassel Hand, the base of each finger ends in a ratchet that catches internally on short pawls held at tension by a pair of boot-shaped flat springs (figures 6.5–6.6).

Another form of flat spring appears in the Eisfeld Hand (c. 1525–1550). This left hand prosthesis sits in storage in a castle museum in central Germany. It shows mixed signs of skillful and substandard workmanship. The fingers, which can be locked in four positions, move in two block pairs with a rigid,

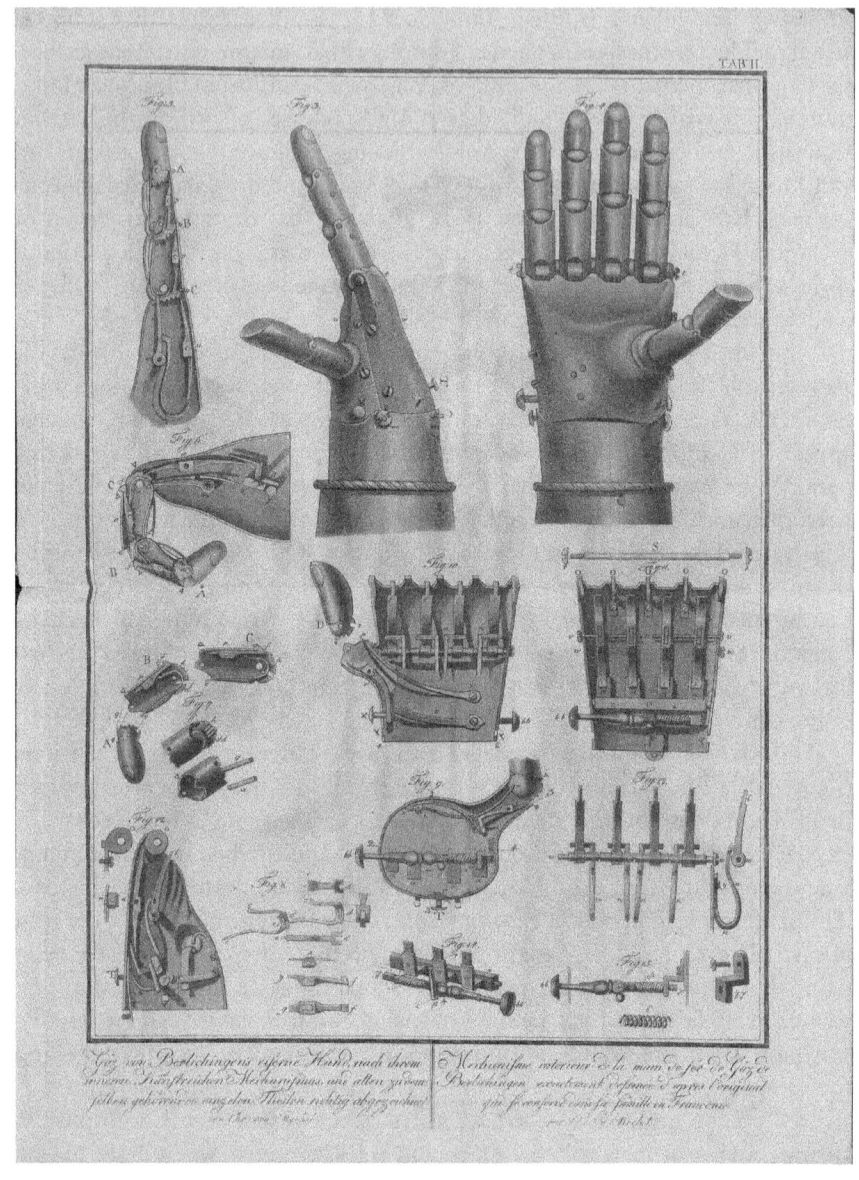

5.8 Zweithand mechanisms in Christian von Mechel, *Die eiserne Hand des tapfern deutschen Ritters Götz von Berlichingen* (Berlin: Decker, 1815), Tab. II.

curved thumb (figures 5.9–5.10).[55] A release button is located at the top of the wrist. The only sign of ornamentation on the heavily corroded surface is engraved fingernails. When the fingers are at full flexion, two bright, untarnished portions of iron become visible at the joints. The shiny metal may be representative of the original condition of the interior, and perhaps even the exterior of the prosthesis. The short wrist casing, soldered to the hand, appears roughly formed and is misshapen at the opening. The internal mechanisms reveal a different caliber of workmanship. They still function despite heavy corrosion, which has fused certain parts and decomposed others. There are at least three axes, or horizontal shafts with connected parts: two are visible from the wrist opening, and another is located at the base of the fingers. The proximal axis is a fixed rod, attached to which are several flat springs (figure 5.11). Three of these are bowed with forked ends that keep pressure on the middle axis while still allowing it to rotate and flex the fingers.

Our brief foray into different forms of ratchets and springs not only suggests the variety of ways common mechanical elements could be fashioned for artificial hands, but also draws attention to the artisans familiar with them. Springs were a basic component in many different kinds of early modern technologies, from furniture and casket locks to spring locks on chamber doors, and from spring-driven clocks to firearms.[56] Ratchets—and various toothed gears—were especially common in clocks but could be found in other technologies as well. These were mechanisms used by locksmiths and clockmakers, the craft groups most likely responsible for those found in artificial hands.

Locksmiths and clockmakers shared deep connections in the evolution of their specialized skills and professional organization during the sixteenth and seventeenth centuries. Clockmakers' guilds were almost always outgrowths of earlier groups of metalworkers who practiced clockmaking among other activities. In Augsburg, clockmakers were part of a smiths' guild that included locksmiths, gunsmiths, ringmakers, and winch- or windlass-makers. In the first half of the sixteenth century, the guild recorded many cases of masters earning double qualifications as clockmakers and locksmiths. This close relationship changed in many cities with large markets when clockmakers were able to establish separate guilds, but in other places the two crafts never officially separated.[57] For instance, the 1577 inventory of the locksmith Jörg Schmidhammer reveals he filled large orders for locks, clocks, and even firearms at the imperial court in Prague.[58] In Ulm during the sixteenth and seventeenth centuries, all metalworkers belonged to the smiths' guild, which was subdivided into goldsmiths, locksmiths, clockmakers, and cutlers. However, signs indicate that the clockmakers were included within the locksmiths' organization rather than comprising a distinct group on their own. The *Zunfttafel* (tablet of arms) of the locksmiths' guild from 1595 displays two types of small clocks along with padlocks and keys. The genealogy of the

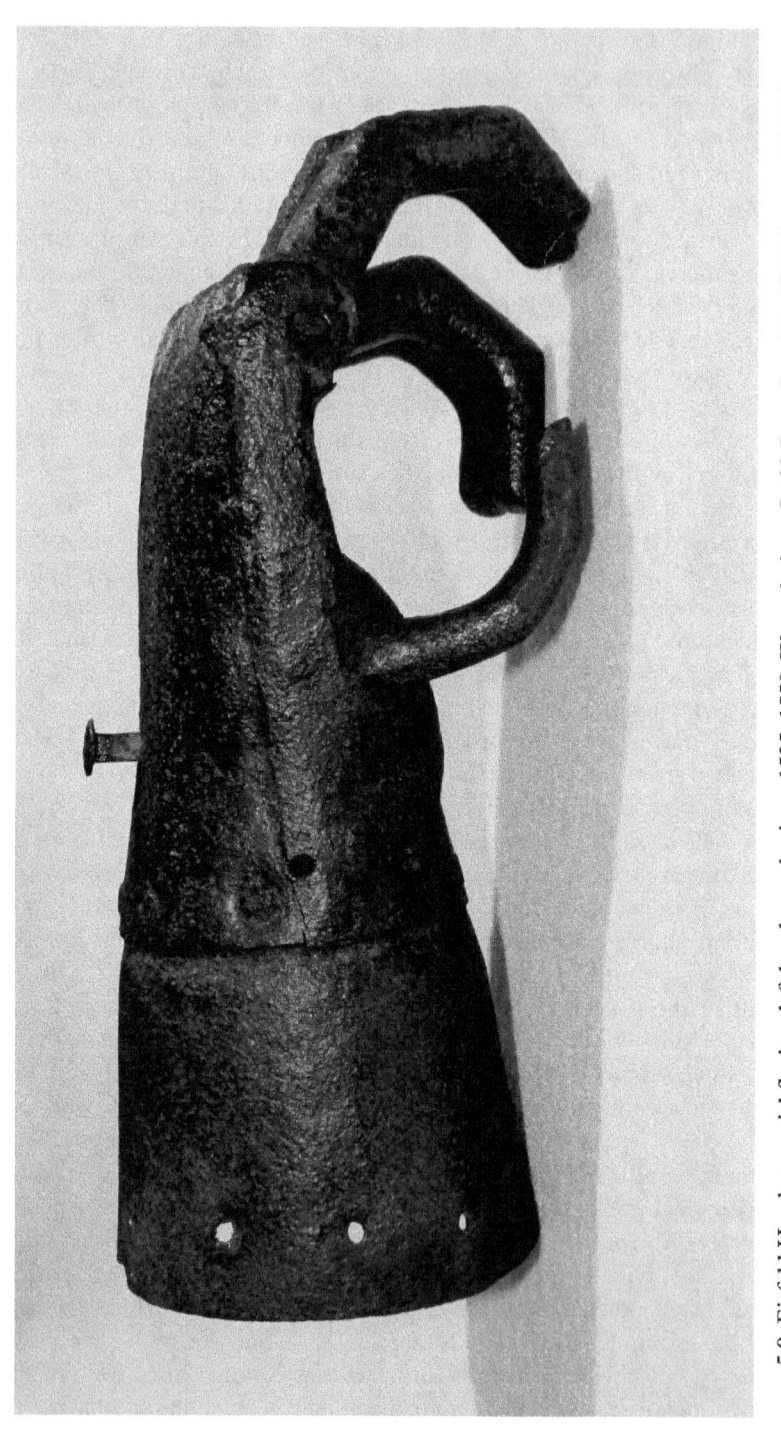

5.9 Eisfeld Hand at partial flexion, left hand prosthesis, c. 1525–1550. Wrought iron; L. 20.5 cm. Inv. Nr. 307. Museum Eisfeld.

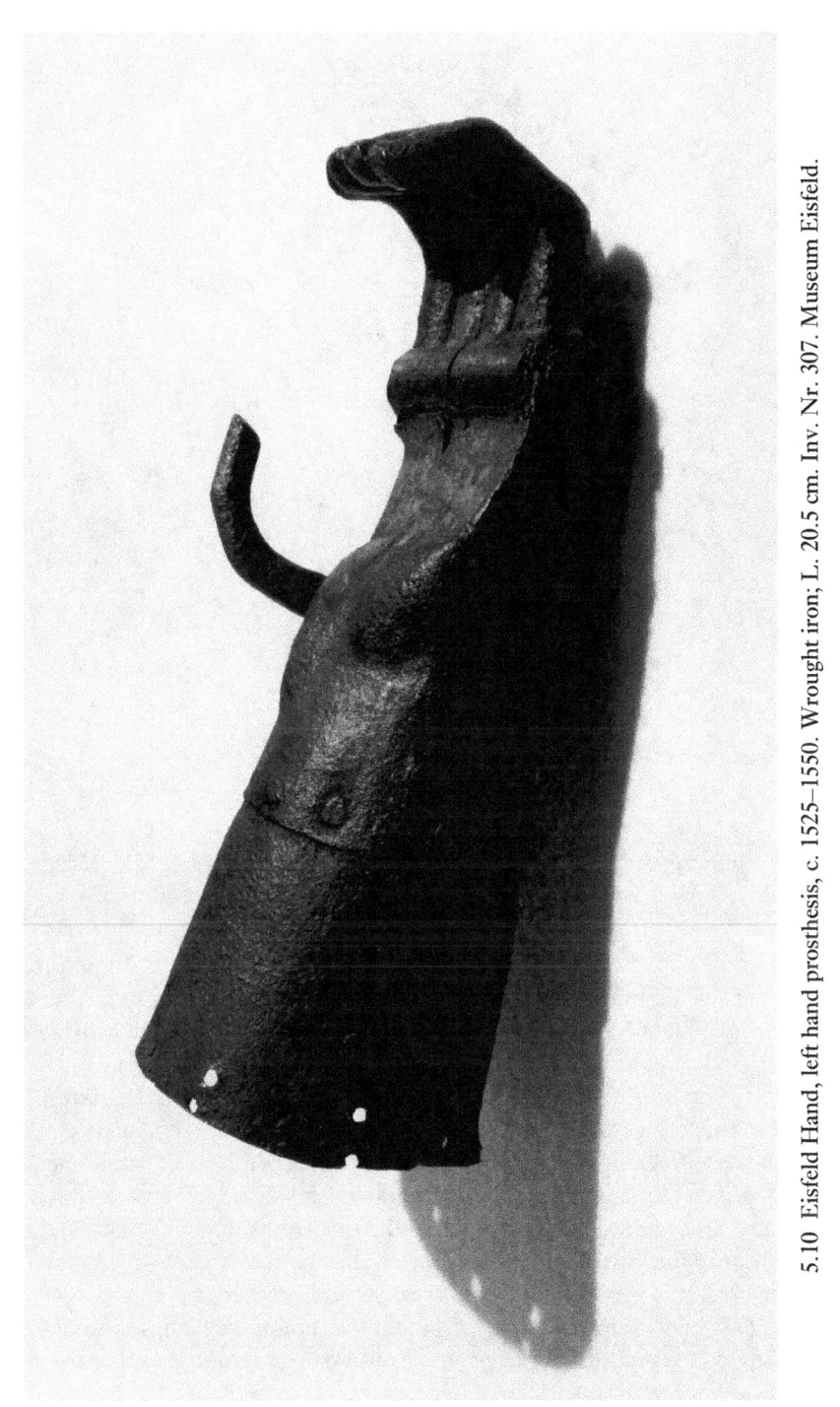

5.10 Eisfeld Hand, left hand prosthesis, c. 1525–1550. Wrought iron; L. 20.5 cm. Inv. Nr. 307. Museum Eisfeld.

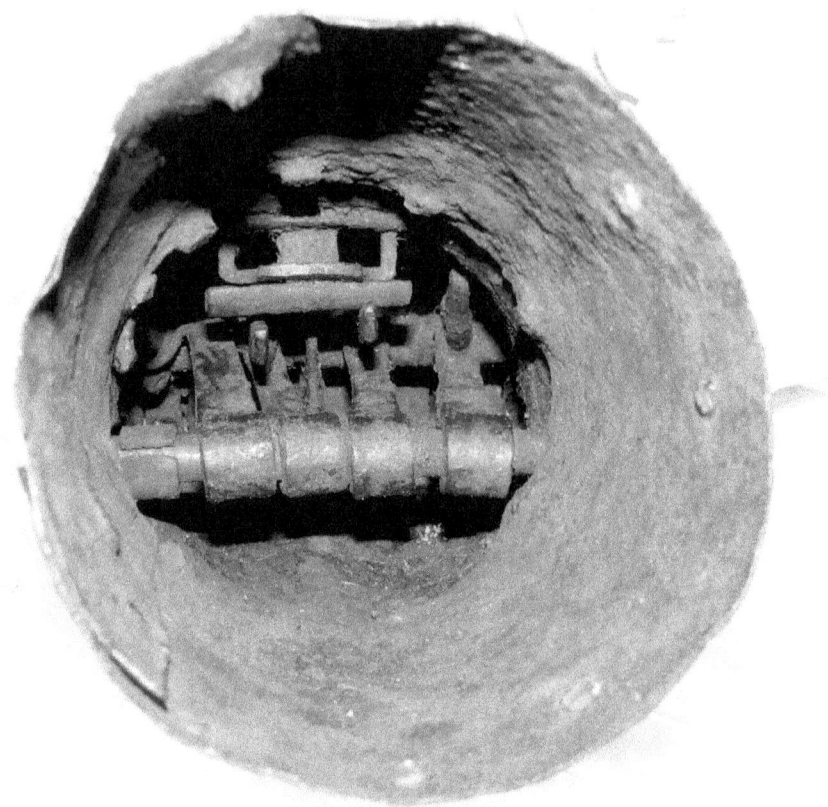

5.11 Internal mechanisms of Eisfeld Hand, left hand prosthesis, c. 1525–1550. Wrought iron; L. 20.5 cm. Inv. Nr. 307. Museum Eisfeld.

Ulm locksmith and clockmaker Johann Wolfgang Gelb (b. 1599) emphasizes the shared skills that enabled fluidity among professions: not only did he come from a line of master locksmiths, but his family included clockmakers, a cutler, and a goldsmith.[59]

The invention of spring-driven clocks around the turn of the sixteenth century transformed clockmaking into a profession. Before 1500, many clockmakers were itinerant and worked in teams to make and repair the immense weight-driven clocks in medieval churches and town halls. Those who were sedentary also worked as locksmiths and blacksmiths, among other trades. With the introduction of spring-driven mechanisms, which could be fitted into smaller objects like table clocks and watches, clockmakers were able to open specialized shops. For over a century, a number of imperial cities in southern Germany dominated the market as master workshops sprouted in Strasbourg, Ulm, Nuremberg, and Augsburg.[60] Augsburg, for example, had between fifty and seventy different shops open in any given year between 1550 and 1650. Each contained at least three workers and could produce a simple clock within two to three weeks, or roughly fifteen to twenty-five a year.[61] Clockmakers used large amounts of prefabricated parts, from metal gears to gilt figurines. They could also collaborate with furniture- and cabinetmakers to make veneered cases and bases.[62]

Metalworkers also devised a variety of custom instruments and machines. The only surviving work of Gelb, the Ulm locksmith and clockmaker, is an exquisitely crafted scientific instrument—a survey and gunnery alidade.[63] Clockmakers also made automata, luxury items often created in coordination with goldsmiths.[64] In the sixteenth century, there was a growing market for small clockwork pieces, especially among the princely courts of the Holy Roman Empire. The master clockmakers of Augsburg and Nuremberg played a key role in the fabrication of these automata.[65] Automaton clocks—clocks with human or animal figures with moving parts—controlled their movements with the mechanisms used to keep time.[66] For example, in one automaton clock depicting the flagellation of Christ (c. 1630), two soldiers whip Christ when the hours strike. Spring-driven mechanisms could be used in all shapes and sizes of automata intended to delight and amaze. A gilt automaton of Diana on a stag (c. 1620), credited to the Augsburg goldsmith Joachim Fries (d. 1620), was used for a drinking game. A mechanism in the base of the automaton propels it forward on a table; whoever is sitting in front of the device when it stops then removes the head of the stag to drink from its body.[67] The Lady Lute Player in the Kunsthistorisches Museum in Vienna is attributed to the clockmaker Gianello Torriano (c. 1515–1585). He reportedly made several figures for the amusement of Charles V during his retirement, including armed soldiers that engaged in battle on the table.[68]

Gunsmiths also crafted small mechanisms comparable to those found in artificial hands. The Braunschweig Hand, located at the Herzog Anton Ulrich-Museum in central Germany, provides an intriguing example (figure 5.12). The above-the-elbow arm prosthesis is made primarily of brass but also contains iron mechanical elements, wood, and cloth. Discovered in several fragments in a tomb in the Domkirche in Braunschweig in 1832, it had deteriorated so much that specialists charged with its restoration in the 1990s could not determine if it was a right or left arm prosthesis.[69] The restorer, who worked on the project between 1989 and 1994, researched literature on the Zweithand and other prostheses from the sixteenth to the turn of the twentieth centuries to consider how its pieces fit together.[70] Museum staff and specialists debated whether a tenable link could be made between the artifact and Christian the Younger (1599–1626), whose left arm was famously amputated four years before his death.[71] When Christian's sarcophagus in nearby Wolfenbüttel was opened for renovation in 1995 and his preserved forearm discovered, measurements of the

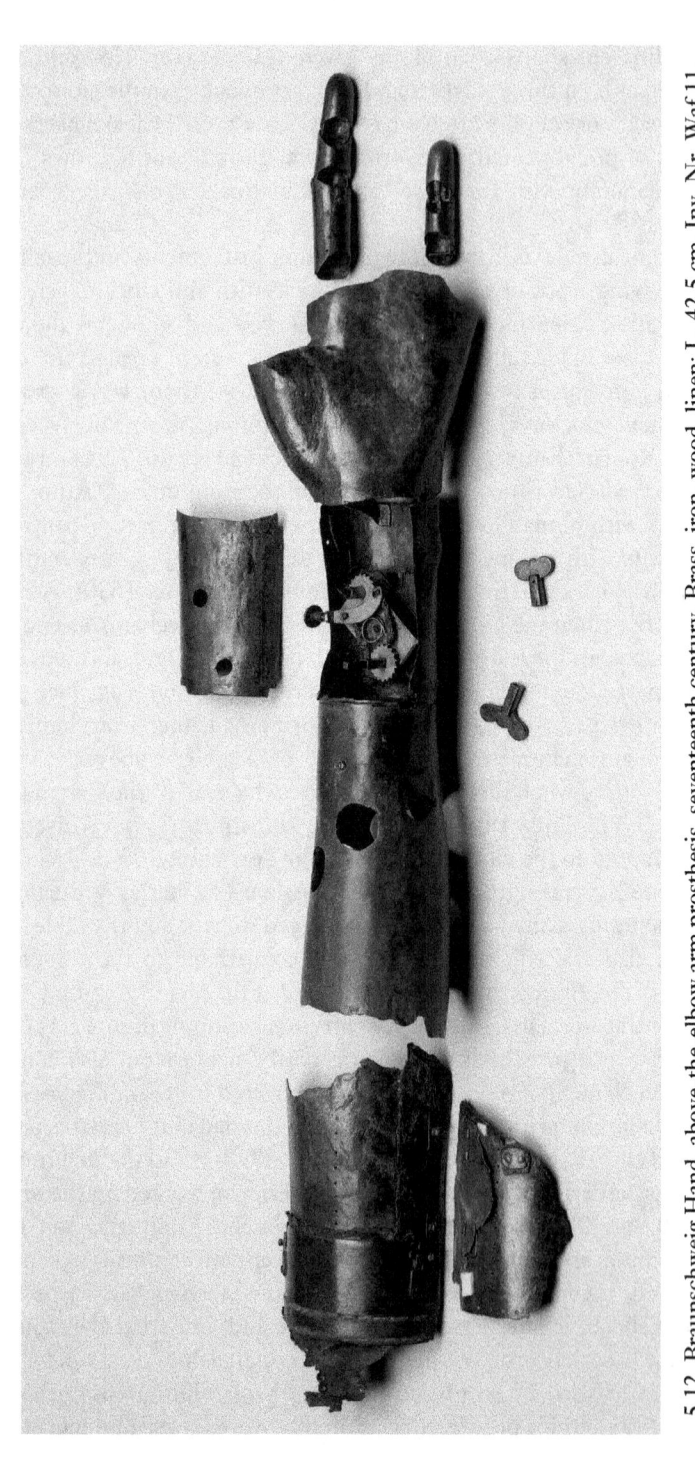

5.12 Braunschweig Hand, above-the-elbow arm prosthesis, seventeenth century. Brass, iron, wood, linen; L. 42.5 cm. Inv. Nr. Waf 11. Herzog Anton Ulrich-Museum Braunschweig.

skeleton and of the museum artifact were taken and scrupulously compared. Although no evidence has been found to connect the object to Christian, the link persists in publications, including a 2002 catalog which labels it as Christian's artificial arm.[72] Estimates placing the object in the seventeenth century have not discouraged speculation, yet these are not based on Christian's biography. Instead, they derive in no small part from comparisons of its mechanisms to the development and use of the wheellock, which was used in self-igniting firearms.[73]

While the delicate outline of the fingernails and the openwork of precise circles on the forearm point to the work of a skilled smith or armorer, it is the mechanism at the wrist that suggests a gunsmith or clockmaker.[74] This sits on a rectangular plate and includes corroded iron chains, a coiled spring, two main shafts, and a curved lever connected to an exterior release button (figures 5.12–5.13). Each shaft has a ratchet (seen on the front of the plate) and a corresponding eccentric wheel (hidden on the back of the plate). The prosthesis once functioned by sliding a spanner—or key—onto each shaft and turning it, similar to winding a clock or wheellock pistol, in order to gradually flex and lock the individual fingers of the hand until the release was pressed. The mechanism could be hidden with a panel that had discreet holes for the spanners. Although the ratchet wheels, chains, and winding keys are reminiscent of clockwork, two experts in historical weapons have characterized 75 percent of the object's constructed parts, and especially the chains, as gunsmith technology.[75] Here the spring-powered wheel of the wheellock pistol, which used a short chain connected to a mainspring, is significant. A spanner turned the wheel until it locked under tension; pulling the trigger caused it to spin against a piece of iron pyrite, creating sparks to light priming powder.[76] It offered technological advantages over other firearms but was fragile and expensive to maintain, with some examples made up of more than fifty individual parts.[77] Wheellocks had become obsolete on the battlefield by the second half of the seventeenth century but remained popular in luxury handguns and rifles for elites long after.[78] The mechanical resemblance to this technology not only helps date the Braunschweig Hand, but also indicates a high level of sophistication and expense.

Locksmiths, clockmakers, and even gunsmiths possessed mechanical knowledge that could be used to make an artificial hand. However, different kinds of expertise were needed to craft the details of the hollow body that housed its mechanisms and the arm casing that connected it to a wearer. Let us turn our attention to these external components. Not only were they important to the successful operation of the prosthesis, but, as the Eisfeld Hand demonstrates, they could detract from or enhance its perceived quality, expense, and sophistication. The long arm casings of the Ruppin Hand and Braunschweig Hand, for example, display expert craftsmanship from armorers or fine metal

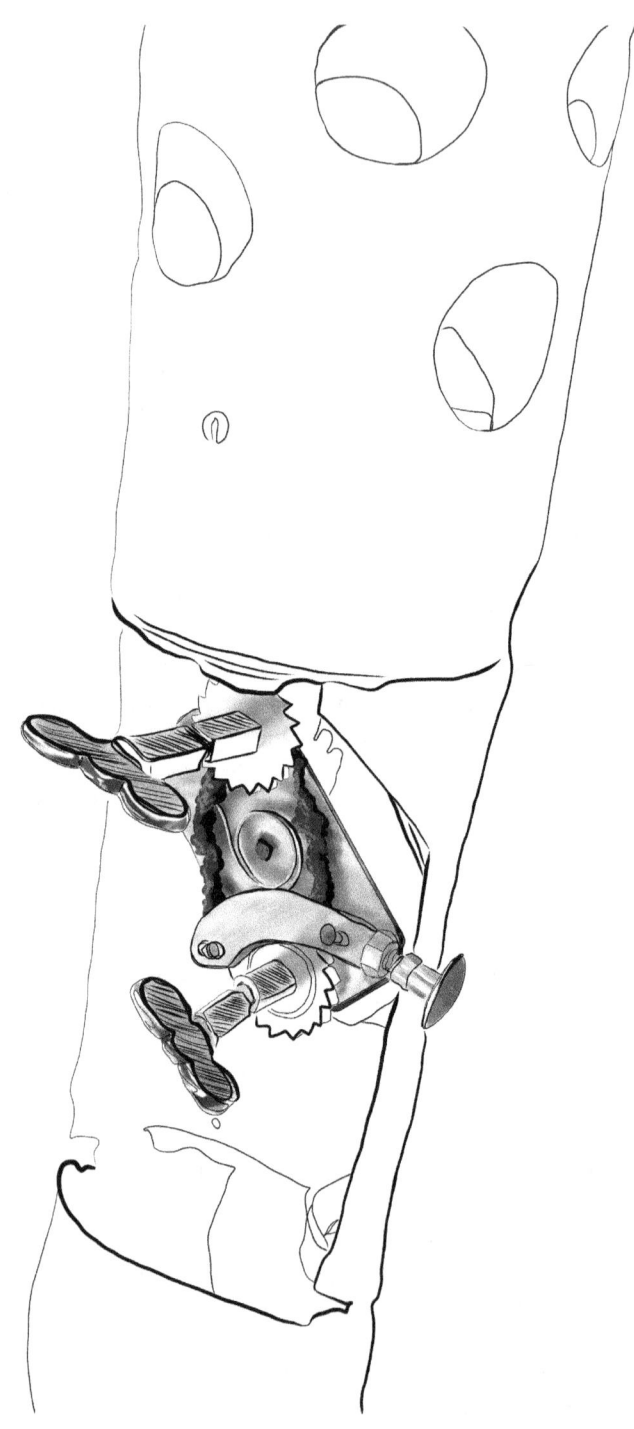

5.13 Wrist mechanisms of Braunschweig Hand with spanners placed on shafts.

smiths (figures 5.1, 5.12). The openwork lessens the objects' weights but does so through attractive and precise cutouts in the metal, one displaying narrow rectangles and the other circles.

A forearm casing of a right hand prosthesis in the possession of the Hessisches Landesmuseum Darmstadt draws attention to these components as separate pieces added to the wrists of mechanical hands (figures 5.14–5.15). Museum records purport that the Darmstadt Hand belonged to a Swedish officer during the Thirty Years' War and came into the possession of Hessian troops as a war trophy.[79] No extant records indicate the date or circumstances of the object's initial discovery, but its association with the Thirty Years' War may come from the location of the find near Arnsberg, where Swedish and Hessian troops skirmished several times.[80] After the occupation of Westphalia by Hessian-Darmstadt troops in the early nineteenth century, the prosthesis was sent from the Archiv der Landstände des Herzogtums Westfalen to Darmstadt, where Ludwig X of Hessen-Darmstadt, an avid collector of curiosities, had recently established a museum.[81] It has two blocks of curved fingers and an articulated thumb. The finger pairs can be pressed independently into three positions and released by a button on the top of the wrist. There are traces of paint in several places, as well as engraved wrinkles at the knuckles and the impression of fingernails. The openwork of the forearm casing features large rectangular and quadrantic cutouts. These are much larger than those of the Ruppin Hand or the Braunschweig Hand and significantly reduce the device's weight. Hinges and buckles allow the wearer to open and close the casing to put it on, wear it securely, and remove it. The bottom half of the casing is also shorter to facilitate easy movement of the elbow. The forearm's distal end is a decorative ring of half-circles that rest on top of the wrist like the cuff of a sleeve (figure 5.15). The visual effect highlights how the hand and the forearm are two separate pieces fused together to make a final product. This was skillfully accomplished. The half-circle pattern of the forearm "cuff" curls around a bolt, just visible at the bottom of the wrist in figure 5.15, where I postulate the proximal axis of the internal mechanisms is located. The fit of the forearm casing over the wrist is tailored exactly.

Just as the forms of natural hands vary, so too do those of artificial ones. It is a telling way in which the artifacts suggest an extension of bodily diversity into the material realm. The Darmstadt Hand, for instance, has two almost hemisphere-like bumps at the heel of the hand to imitate the curves of a palm (figure 5.15). The V-shape of the Ingolstadt Hand's palm uses the curve of the fixed thumb to create a more subtle effect (figure 5.7). Some hand casings are more flat and rectangular, including those of the Grüningen Hand and the Kassel Hand (figures 5.4, 6.4). This is also the case with the mechanically simpler of the two artificial hands purportedly worn by Götz von Berlichingen (figure 5.5).

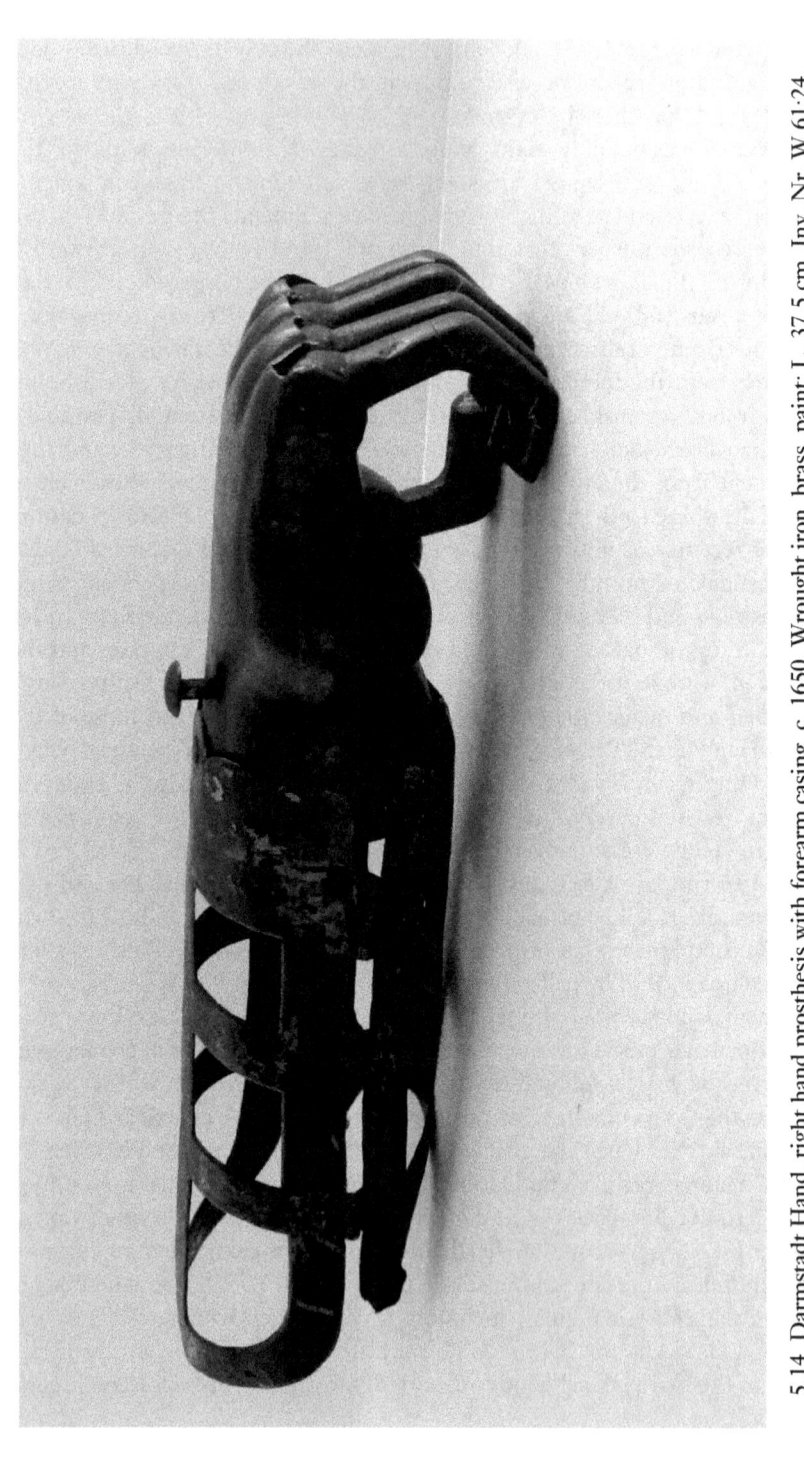

5.14 Darmstadt Hand, right hand prosthesis with forearm casing, c. 1650. Wrought iron, brass, paint; L. 37.5 cm. Inv. Nr. W 61:24. Hessisches Landesmuseum Darmstadt.

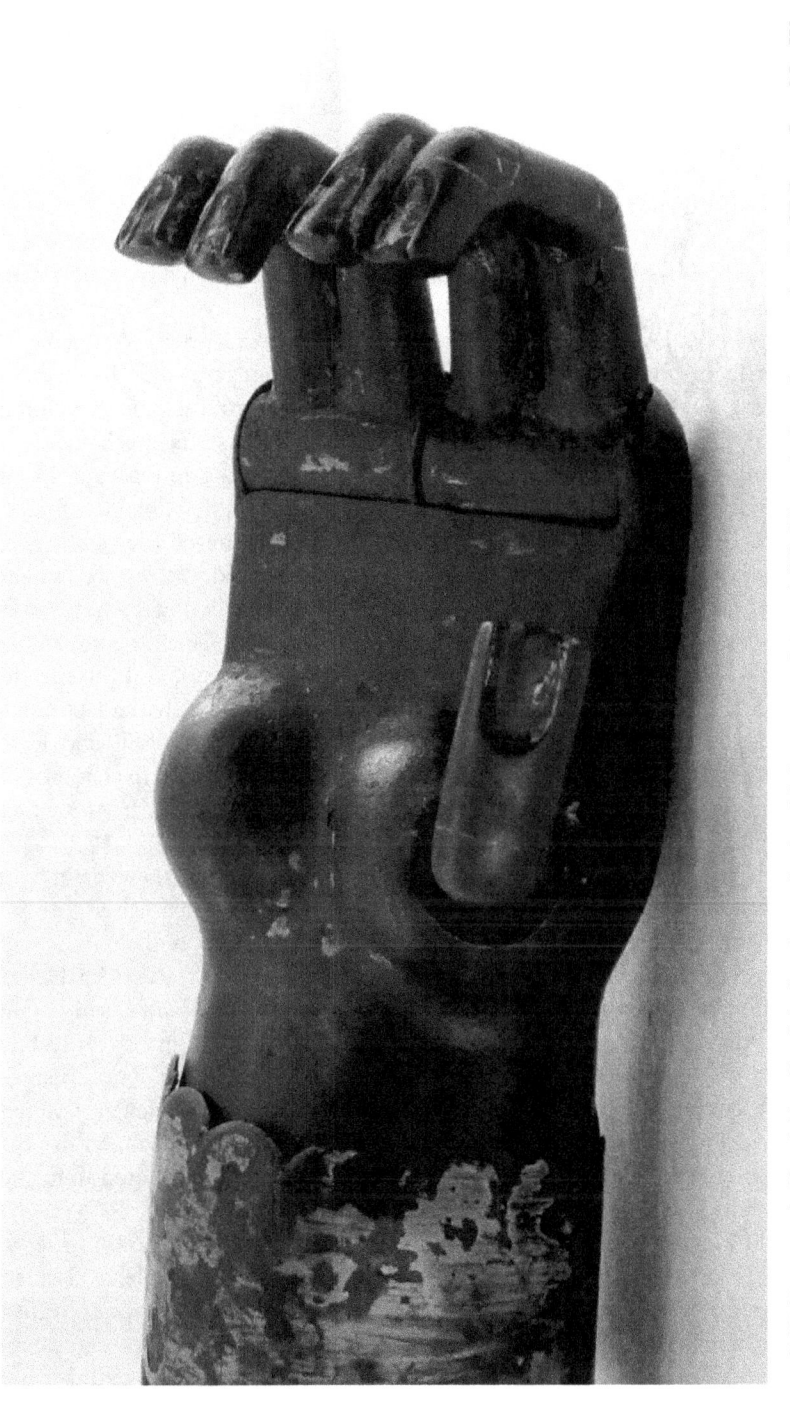

5.15 Darmstadt Hand (detail), right hand prosthesis with forearm casing, c. 1650. Wrought iron, brass, paint; L. 37.5 cm. Inv. Nr. W 61:24. Hessisches Landesmuseum Darmstadt.

The Ersthand (c. 1504–1510) also highlights differences in the shapes of fingers. Since the public debut of this right hand prosthesis in the late eighteenth century, its provenance has been described as a commission Götz made to a smith in Olnhausen.[82] Essentially, the inferred connection to Götz derived from geographic proximity. The artifact surfaced in Olnhausen, near the Berlichingen family seat of Jagsthausen in Baden-Württemberg, in 1793.[83] The owner, a smith, reported that it had been passed down for generations as a family heirloom. Observers quickly interpreted it as evidence of Götz's experience. Its appearance convinced them that he likely wore it with everyday apparel rather than with armor for battle.[84] Eventually it entered the private collection of the Berlichingen family, who preserve it today.[85] The artifact is made of iron, although the body and fingers could be made of a copper alloy.[86] Its surface is rough and exhibits heavy traces of flesh-colored paint. Engraved details depict wrinkles and fingernails. Its mechanisms—including two finger blocks, an articulated thumb, and a release button on the top of the wrist—are in fair condition and still operable. The little finger, which was broken off at its base when the hand first entered the public eye, was repaired c. 1980–1982.[87] As one scholar has remarked, the restored finger is probably smaller than the original. The differentiation in finger lengths may reflect modern rather than early modern aesthetics.[88] In several comparable artifacts—including the Kassel Hand, the Darmstadt Hand, and the Eisfeld Hand—the fingers have uniform, or nearly uniform, lengths and circumferences, except for the thumbs (figures 5.9–5.10, 5.15, 6.4). This may have simplified the manufacture of the parts for the artisan, pointing to elements of cost and production. It might also suggest design concerns, perhaps making an object more user-friendly.

Many objects have additional components attached to their hand and arm casings. A fragment of leather is still affixed to the proximal end of the Grüningen Hand's upper arm casing, and a leather strap remains wrapped around the Zweithand (figures 5.4, 5.6). The Ruppin Hand features buckles at the end of its forearm casing (figure 5.1). The Darmstadt Hand's arm casing also has hinges, buckles, and the remnants of a leather cord (figure 5.14). While blacksmiths and fine metal smiths could have formed the tubes of arm casings and the bodies of iron hands, other artisans had skillsets particularly suited to overseeing such composite products.[89] Armorers were accustomed to producing metal objects with textile components that had to be tailored to fit the human body.

A suit of armor required the talents of several different craft experts, especially if it was tailor-made or finely decorated. Early modern German cities were leading centers of armor production in Europe in the sixteenth century and into the seventeenth.[90] In centers such as Innsbruck, armorers were allowed to employ polishers, hammermen, locksmiths, and other specialized craftsmen in one workshop. By contrast, in places like Augsburg and Nuremberg, these individuals belonged to entirely separate shops working in conjunction with one another. When tailor-making a suit, the armorer obtained the client's dimensions by measuring, using clothing, or by creating a wax model of a limb. Thick plates of iron were cut with huge shears and roughly formed by hammermen. The armorer then fashioned the plates with hammers, anvil irons, stakes, and other tools. The component parts were smoothed, buffed, and embellished by a polisher and, in costly commissions, separate decorators or goldsmiths. The final stage of assembly involved locksmiths, who fitted straps, buckles, hinges, and other parts. Wealthy workshops could afford to employ locksmiths or to send pieces to a locksmith's shop, but smaller operations bought straps, buckles, hooks, hinges, and so forth from merchants to be assembled in-shop. The number of workshops involved in an armorer's order depended upon local regulations and the armorer's affluence. In Nuremberg, each master armorer was allowed two journeymen and four apprentices. To make a full suit of armor, some masters would have had to collaborate with others.[91]

Cooperation among multiple master artisans is evident in some artificial hands. Our discussion up to this point has emphasized metalworkers because most mechanical hands are primarily made of metal, with other materials attached. The Nuremberg Hand is the opposite: a wooden hand with iron pieces affixed to it. This object exhibits an integration of multiple crafts in vivid fashion, and thus provides a useful way to consider more broadly the context of the craft market, where the groups we have considered individually—locksmiths, armorers, and others—all plied their trades.

The Nuremberg Hand is a right, above-the-elbow arm prosthesis (figures 5.16–5.17). Its provenance and date of acquisition by the Germanisches Nationalmuseum are not known—its inventory card presents but a number and a single descriptive phrase. The hand is made entirely of unpainted wood, except for the iron nails that attach it to a leather sleeve, iron hooks embedded into the tips of three fingers, and the iron mechanism nailed into the palm. A recent examination of the hand's material has revealed that it is made of limewood or poplar.[92] It is superbly crafted to imitate human anatomy, with delicate fingernail, knuckle, and wrinkle details. The effect is strikingly lifelike. The wrist and each joint in the fingers are articulated, although three of the fingers are now missing. It is the work of a skilled woodworker, such as a joiner or even a sculptor—rival artisans in the craft market.[93] The sleeve nailed to the wooden wrist, which reaches a little above the elbow, signals the contribution of a leatherworker. There are two worn holes in the proximal end of the sleeve that could have been used to tie the leather to either the iron casing or the wearer's clothing.

A decorative armor-maker was certainly involved in fashioning the iron arm casing. The distal end of the casing fits around the wooden wrist and

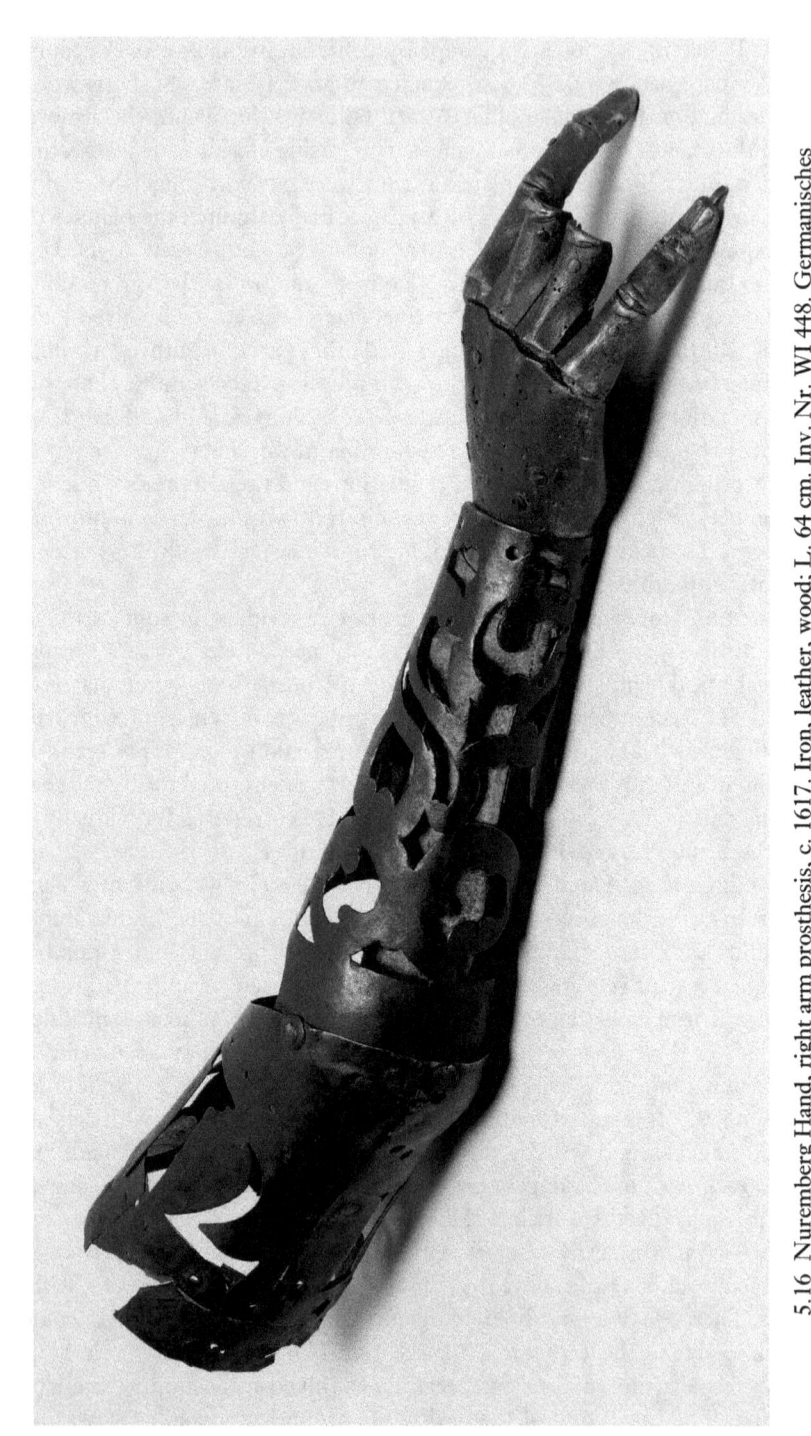

5.16 Nuremberg Hand, right arm prosthesis, c. 1617. Iron, leather, wood; L. 64 cm. Inv. Nr. WI 448. Germanisches Nationalmuseum (Nuremberg).

Mechanical hands 187

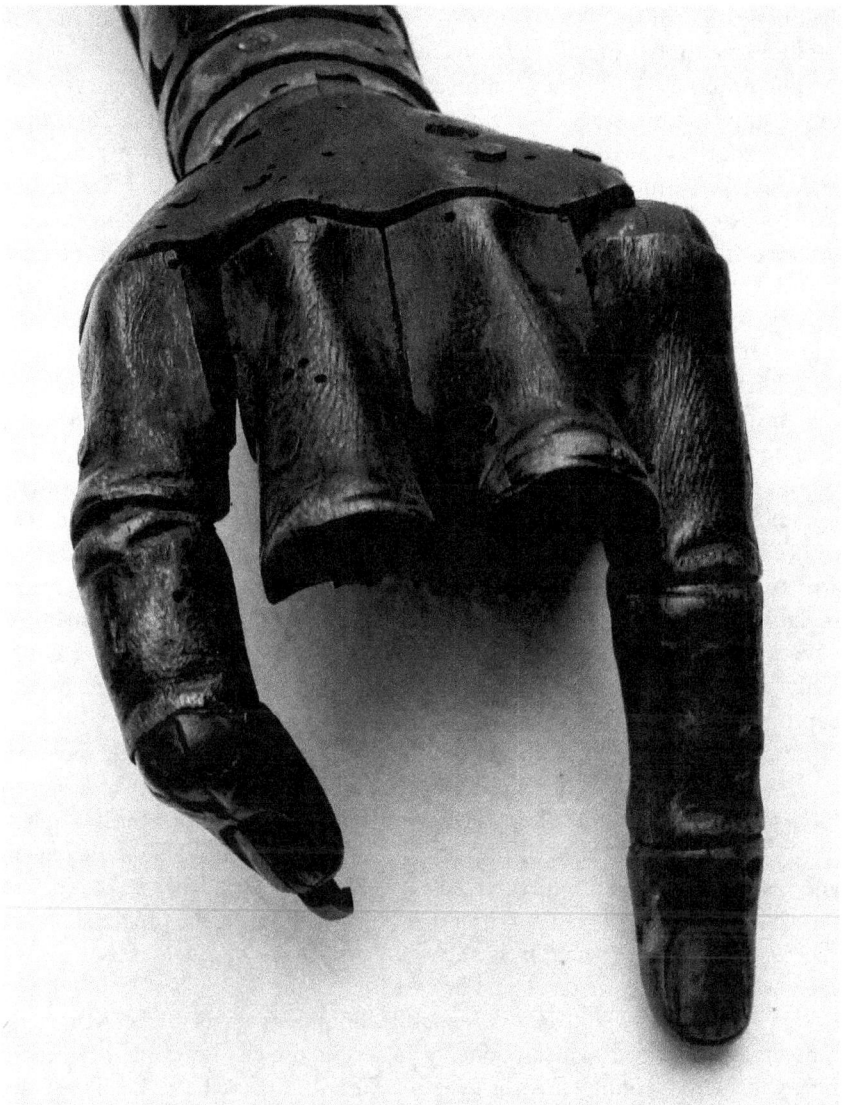

5.17 Fingers of Nuremberg Hand (detail), right arm prosthesis, c. 1617. Iron, leather, wood; L. 64 cm. Inv. Nr. WI 448. Germanisches Nationalmuseum (Nuremberg).

is kept in place only by its weight, rather than by nails. This means it could be removed from the hand and leather sleeve at the owner's discretion. There are perforations at the upper arm that could have been used to fasten the casing to the shoulder. There are also perforations near the wrist that could have been used to tie it to clothing if the wearer chose to conceal the arm beneath a shirt. The ornate pattern of the openwork served not only as costly decoration, but also to reduce weight.

The letters "AUG" and numbers "1," "6," "1," and "7" are carved out of the upper arm casing. A recent exhibition catalog states that AUG stands for the southwestern city of Augsburg, indicating its place of production, and mistakenly indicates that the numbers reference the year 1716.[94] Other experts associated with the museum believe AUG signifies a person's name, probably the object's owner, and that the numbers are intended to be read as 1617.[95] It is certainly possible that AUG indicates Augsburg. The hand may be made of limewood, which was widely used in southern Germany,[96] and while AUG may not have been a stamp for a particular workshop in Augsburg, the city was a major center of armor production. It is possible that indicating its place of production was part of a unique masterpiece, created by a journeyman for his guild's approval.[97] It seems clear that the numbers are intended to be read as 1617. Visually, the "1" and "6" are written above the letters AUG, with an embellished emphasis in between that draws the observer's eyes to begin reading at "1." In addition, the patternwork of the iron casing resembles other pieces of early seventeenth-century metalwork. The iron has also been blackened by a technique that involved covering the surface with oil and then heating it until it turned a dark color.[98] This was a corrosion inhibitor often used for armor at the turn of the century.[99]

The elbow joint and the iron mechanism in the wooden hand reveal the work of a locksmith. The articulated elbow uses a simple spring and pivot design to lock into three positions. The mechanism in the palm is a little more complex. Using the hooks embedded in the fingertips, the wearer could bend the fingers and insert the hooks into the three holes of the palm, where they would lock in place to create a circle. There is a release button located at the proximal end of the mechanism that, when pressed, would trigger the internal springs to free the hooks so that the fingers could be extended again.

The Nuremberg Hand displays expert techniques from distinct craft groups. The practices its material components suggest allow us to imagine the people involved in its production—the woodworker who carved the details of the knuckled hand, the leatherworker who provided a connective sleeve, the locksmith who fitted a gripping mechanism, and the armorer who formed the sheet iron, cut precise patterns, and burnished and blackened the surface of the arm casing. This prosthesis was an expensive and painstakingly executed piece that involved multiple master craftsmen.

This extraordinary example challenges us to ask a question every surviving artifact implicitly raises: How did it come to be? Few written sources indicate where one could go to commission a mechanical hand in early modern Europe. Götz von Berlichingen's autobiography never hints at how he obtained his.

In printed sources, Ambroise Paré referred to a Parisian locksmith in a chapter about artificial limbs.[100] Less precise is the heroicized posthumous account of Christian the Younger during the Thirty Years' War in the *Theatrum Europaeum*, which states only that the young duke commissioned an artful Dutch craftsman.[101] Other written sources give a clearer picture of workshops and artisans with skillsets amenable to the task. For example, there are isolated archival references to artisans producing prostheses. Ulrich Wagner, contracted to make an artificial hand in Fribourg in 1476, was a locksmith and clockmaker.[102] In 1541, an outstanding debt of four Gulden was owed to Philipp Ring, likely a Nuremberg leatherworker, involving an "iron hand."[103] The textual evidence does not contradict material culture and underscores the importance of locksmith techniques in the fabrication of mechanical hands. But artifacts tell us even more. They point to the contributions of craft groups that do not appear in written sources and display forms of artisanal collaboration at which the example of Philipp Ring can only hint. To understand how objects such as the Nuremberg Hand might have been made, we must turn to the craft market.

Locksmiths, armorers, and others belonged to the diverse range of artisans populating the early modern marketplace.[104] Many crafts shared a number of skills and tools, and it was possible to earn a living practicing multiple crafts.[105] However, particularly in German urban centers, there was usually a difference between who was *capable* of making a product or carrying out a task, and who was *allowed* to. Regulations that defined and enforced this distinction were local and could change according to shifts in the economy and the political hierarchy of a town or region.[106] To complicate matters further, craft trades (one's everyday occupation) did not always map seamlessly onto the organization of craft groups (one's guild).[107] Individual guilds could include a range of occupations, such as the smiths' guilds of Augsburg and Ulm, which both consisted of a wide variety of metalworkers.[108]

Increasing specialization was an important characteristic of craft trades in the early modern period. Municipal records in Nuremberg, for instance, registered an extensive list of distinct metalworking trades, distinguishing those who produced doorknobs from those who made curtain rods, scissors, or candelabras.[109] Against this backdrop, the flexibility of artisans to practice outside of one specialty was perhaps most importantly linked to the political status and interests of town guilds. Patricians could control market regulations, for example, as was the case in Frankfurt.[110] While some guilds sought to keep their crafts within a select pool of families, others accepted apprentices from a variety of backgrounds.[111] There could also be large disparities in wealth and resources both between trades and within a single trade.[112]

The fluidity of the craft market, increasingly recognized in recent scholarship, provided opportunities for artisans to fill custom orders.[113] Craftspeople who worked outside guilds contracted with customers independently—and often illegally. Craftspeople also used subcontracting, farming out a commission or part of a commission to others, either within or outside of the guild. While there are examples of regulations forbidding subcontracting, it was integral to the completion of a complex or high-quantity order. For instance, in Augsburg several shops were known to work together on individual orders. A well-off master furniture-maker might subcontract with smaller masters within his guild to make parts that would then be assembled in the contracting master's workshop. Guns and clocks were complex products that involved the work of several different craft processes. An early modern gun could pass through nine different workshops before the gunsmith presented the finished piece to the customer.[114]

Although craftwork became increasingly specialized through the early modern period, no craft trade specialized in artificial limbs. Moreover, the diversity of surviving prostheses suggests that no single group held a monopoly on their production. Sophisticated examples such as the Nuremberg Hand, which integrate expert-level workmanship from multiple craft groups, suggest cooperation among master artisans. The thick shroud of anonymity that hangs over these artifacts thins when we take this cooperation seriously and discuss mechanical hands as complex, custom orders.

Let us consider the Nuremberg Hand within this context (figures 5.16–5.17). Its most elaborate components are the wooden hand and iron arm casing. The level of skill evident in the metalwork suggests an urban rather than a rural production setting. Depending upon the city in which the object was made, the production of each component could have been highly specialized and under the regulation of several guilds. Also depending upon the city, a master craftsman could have had different levels of freedom to subcontract pieces of a special commission to other workshops or to collaborate with other masters. Perhaps a master joiner oversaw the commission and subcontracted to a locksmith, leatherworker, and armorer as needed. The creative mix of skills seen in this hand could also be the result of a journeyman using a workshop commission as an opportunity to create a masterpiece, for in such cases, stringent rules safeguarding specialized arts were sometimes lifted to allow the craftsman to showcase multiple abilities in one composite work. Another possibility could be a partnership between a master joiner and a master armorer, as families of different guilds often intermarried and worked closely together. Considering the wearer's role in its creation changes the kaleidoscope of options yet again. It is possible that its wearer had it made piecemeal, bringing it from one artisan to another to make additions and adjustments over time.

Formulating production narratives can help us think constructively about the puzzles different artifacts present. Let us return to the Eisfeld Hand and the mismatched quality of its craftsmanship (figures 5.9–5.10). It has sophisticated internal mechanisms paired with a shoddy wrist casing. Some deformity could be the result of corrosion, or a blemish exacerbated by decay. But the crooked line of perforations along the wrist, which in one area had to be redone after the craftsman punched two holes on the very edge of the metal, suggests either hurried or incompetent work, particularly when compared with the uniform perforations found at the wrist of the Ingolstadt Hand (figure 5.7). It seems odd that the level of care in this area would be so inferior to the main body and mechanisms of the artificial hand. These wrist perforations were functionally important: they helped fasten the prosthesis to its wearer.

When incorporated into a production narrative, several possibilities become apparent. The two parts could be the products of different workshops. For instance, the forearm casing of the Darmstadt Hand, with its precise fit on the main body of the hand and its clean openwork, likely resulted from the collaboration of multiple shops on a single order (figures 5.14–5.15). By contrast, the blemishes in the Eisfeld Hand's wrist casing make the prospect of two workshops coordinating one commission seem less probable. It is possible that the shops involved did not collaborate; perhaps after obtaining the mechanical hand from one artisan, the new owner took it to a blacksmith to have an inexpensive wrist casing added. The wearer could even have obtained additions and adjustments from yet another shop later. The small size and questionable quality of the Eisfeld Hand's wrist casing could also suggest its production fell into a gray area of the craft market—its producer could have been an expert in a different aspect of metalwork, or even a "false worker" who worked outside of guilds.[115] The entire object could have been made by one craftsman, or by one workshop whose expertise in mechanisms outstripped its competency with hammering, cutting, and perforating sheet metal. Thus, the Eisfeld Hand could conceivably have been made by one shop—perhaps a locksmith's—or artisans from multiple workshops.

Extant prostheses display such diversity in levels of skill and kinds of craft techniques that what might be plausible for one object's production narrative could be improbable for another. Artifacts must be examined individually. Yet systematically reading a prosthesis piece by piece does not pin down one production narrative for that object—it sketches out multiple possibilities. Scholars should embrace the utility of this unavoidable multiplicity, which affords a complex and surprising look at the effect of one individual's amputation on early modern communities. Artifacts show that the challenges of limb loss extended beyond an individual amputee and his or her family and into the shops of locksmiths, armorers, clockmakers, woodworkers, and any number of others.

Moreover, such an approach allows us to draw general conclusions about the production of mechanical limbs in early modern Germany. As Pamela Smith has said, "above all else, craft is productive knowledge and its products are records of practices as well as repositories of knowledge."[116] The diversity among surviving artifacts suggests these objects were made on an ad hoc basis, each a custom order. All take the recognizable form of a human hand and are passively operated. Yet no two artifacts execute any of this in exactly the same manner. The Nuremberg Hand, with claw-like fingertips designed to lock into a palm mechanism; the Braunschweig Hand, with its spanners to crank the mechanism like a clock; the Zweithand, with small leaf springs in every finger joint; and the Ingolstadt Hand, with its single external ratchet wheel—all of these are supplements for gripping and holding that imitate the movement and shape of a natural hand to different degrees. They display different ways of implementing a similar idea, tailored to the budgets and purposes of patrons as well as the skills and ingenuity of artisans. The nature of mechanical hand production was creative, adaptable, ad hoc, and collaborative.

Amputee-patrons—elusive and influential

Our analysis of material culture reveals that artisans from various craft groups created prosthetic hands on a case-by-case basis. These were custom orders. Just as we cannot definitively identify who wore them, we also cannot know whether their wearers personally commissioned them—or communicated their wishes through intermediaries—in every case. With this caveat in mind, I suggest that it is reasonable to assume their wearers were involved at some stage of their production, and that in many cases this was at the outset of the commission. This form of initiative and self-care in response to a radical bodily change fits well within the flexible vision of early modern "disability" described by Klaus-Peter Horn and Bianca Frohne. They argue that individuals and their families were expected to find solutions to challenging situations that mental and physical impairments could present. One was only viewed as "disabled"—a status Horn and Frohne carefully define as a perceived condition "justified and maintained by referring to a power that transcends any human effort to achieve 'ableness' and social adjustment"—in periods when accommodation was not possible.[117]

Multiple forms of textual evidence support the notion that the onus for procuring an artificial limb mostly fell on amputees and their families. Mareike Heide has gone so far as to describe prostheses as a "private affair" in early modern care.[118] Individuals who wore prostheses rarely appear in institutional records, including those of hospitals, alms and begging regulations, invalid houses, and other sources of public welfare. In exceptional cases when mentions of prosthesis-wearers surface, they involve false noses or wooden legs.[119] This suggests that owners of mechanical hands had the economic means and/or kin network that those who benefited from such sources of aid typically did not. As we have already seen, the surgical literature shows that most practitioners did not expect or seek a role in the process of obtaining a mechanical limb, with of course the exception of Paré.[120] The cultural narrative built around Christian the Younger in early modern chronicles reveals expectations that he himself commissioned a prosthesis from a craftsman.[121] Recent work in the Italian context has found a similar expectation expressed in a history of Venice. The author, Pietro Bembo (1470–1547), claimed that after suffering retaliatory amputations from a conquering force, three bombardiers told the Venetian Senate they would obtain iron hands.[122] Rare archival references to the fabrication of prostheses offer mixed possibilities: in one instance, a landgrave pays a gunmaker, locksmiths, and blacksmiths to create his artificial leg; in another, a town council pays a locksmith and clockmaker to produce an employee's iron hand.[123] Each piece of textual evidence offers an oblique view, some more revealing than others.

There is also the suggestive evidence of the artifacts themselves, and the craft practices involved in their production. Wrist openings, forearm or upper arm casings, leather sleeves, and other aspects of these objects required measurements to be fitted to the intended wearer, just as the components of a suit of armor or elaborate clothing. The irregular bump appearing around the wrist of the Ruppin Hand, an expansion made after the object was created, suggests that alterations were sometimes needed when the fit was not quite right (figure 5.1). The wearers of these objects must have been involved at some stage in order for artisans to determine the dimensions of their designs and the amount of material needed, which influenced the cost of the final product—something required to establish a contract for an order. While we must remain cautious, the written record, material culture, and the context of craft production strongly suggest wearers were involved in commissioning their prostheses. The initiative of an individual amputee was a key ingredient in the fabrication of a mechanical hand.

Considering these wearers as amputee-patrons emphasizes their role in driving material practices. "Patrons" signals many aspects of these individuals at once. It preserves the agency of both the amputee and the artisan, suggesting a form of partnership. Artisans' specialized knowledge and skills were needed to design and fabricate the internal mechanisms and external casings of iron hands. Yet those who wore them were more than consumers of a craft good. Amputees engaged in a form of "bodywork" by obtaining customized technologies that they used in different ways to adapt to a major bodily change.[124] Artisans applied their skills creatively to make such objects only at the behest of those who asked for them. "Patrons" highlights the active role amputees played in sponsoring and participating in material practices that experimented with new forms and materials for limbs, and consequently with the growing malleability of the body in early modern medicine.

"Patrons" also frames amputees who commissioned mechanical hands as customers. Their budgets ranged significantly, based on the technical sophistication and expense of materials apparent in surviving artifacts. One indicator of technical complexity is the extent of articulation in fingers, wrists, and elbows. Our pool of objects showcases a wide spectrum of movement. The simplest prostheses have fingers that move together in one block along a single axis at the base of the fingers, such as the Ingolstadt Hand (figure 5.7). More complex devices allow the fingers to lock into a greater variety of positions. The most basic of these have two finger blocks, as with the Ruppin Hand and the Eisfeld Hand (figures 5.1–5.2, 5.9): index and middle finger, and ring and little finger. The thumb can be rigid, as in the Grüningen Hand, or it can be moved separately, like the Darmstadt Hand (figures 5.4, 5.15). Artifacts with individual finger blocks have four rather than two wheels at their base so that each finger can move separately. The Kassel Hand, which also has a moveable thumb, is one example (figures 6.4–6.7). The most complex devices are articulated in every joint of each finger. Reconstructions of the Balbronn Hand not only flex each finger joint, but also have flexible wrists and elbows (figure 5.3). The Zweithand also has articulated finger joints and a flexible wrist (figures 5.6, 5.8). More articulation meant designing and fabricating more small parts—both mechanical gears and the external components of the hands, wrists, and even fingers that could house them—and a more time-intensive process fitting them together. The greater the variety of positions possible, the more sophisticated the internal mechanisms and the greater the cost.

Artifacts with internal mechanisms of comparable degrees of complexity could still represent a range of budgets. The mechanisms of the Eisfeld Hand resemble those of the Darmstadt Hand and the Ersthand (figures 5.5, 5.9–5.11, 5.14). All three use two finger blocks and a similar system of flat springs connected to a fixed rod at the wrist. They also share two levers located directly below a T-shaped release mechanism activated via an exterior button. In figure 5.11, the horizontal bar of the (upside-down) "T" is visible above the two levers located in the center of the image. Despite their comparable technology, the botched perforations of the Eisfeld Hand's wrist casing provide a sharp contrast to the Darmstadt Hand. Its forearm casing with openwork and precise half-circle patterns at the wrist indicates that it was a more elaborate and presumably more costly item. We can only speculate about the decision-making involved, but one amputee-patron spent far more than the other for a hand prosthesis with two-finger-block technology.

This is because fit and finish, as well as material quality, also contributed to cost. The individual components of composite orders added expense. For example, if the four Gulden owed to Philipp Ring in Nuremberg in 1541 were for leather or leatherwork to finish an iron hand, that component alone cost more than a quarter of a town surgeon's annual salary in nearby Munich, or four percent of a senior physician's.[125] When the different parts of an artificial hand came together, the final products could be enormously costly. The value of the Braunschweig Hand (figure 5.12) has been estimated to have equaled that of a large farm, including buildings, fields, and livestock.[126] This object, made of brass and other materials, not only includes circular openwork on the arm casing, but also incorporates a form of technology that increasingly became the preserve of elite consumers: the wheellock mechanism. The carved wood of the Nuremberg Hand (figure 5.17) is intricate enough to suggest the work of a master carver or the masterpiece of a joiner with the ambitions of a sculptor.[127] The Ingolstadt Hand (figure 5.7), by contrast, made entirely of painted iron and featuring a basic external locking mechanism, was simple enough to be affordable to a somewhat broader range of people—noble, patrician, wealthy merchant, military officer, and so on.

Careful analysis of these artifacts' materials, then, yields insights into the social status of their wearers. Both the Braunschweig Hand and the Balbronn Hand (figures 5.3, 5.12), two of the most technologically sophisticated prostheses in our source group, were found in church tombs, indicating that their wearers were individuals of high standing in their communities. Their prostheses represent the top of the market, but objects that were simpler to operate and less expensive were still unobtainable for most of the population. Indeed, the medievalist Simone Kahlow argues that it is difficult for scholars to distinguish between people of different social classes based on prosthetic artifacts in Europe *until* the appearance of iron hands at the turn of the sixteenth century.[128] Amputee-patrons were members of the upper circles of early modern society who commissioned artisans to make custom orders.

In the early modern craft market, commissions were conversations. A prospective customer presented a set of needs and wishes, and the artisan responded with proposals that fit the customer's budget and the artisan's skills (or access to others with skills). In some instances, such as tailors making clothing, artisans might carry out designs the customer made.[129] The technical complexity of mechanical hands suggests a customer's involvement in design could not be quite so complete, because of the specialized knowledge of mechanisms necessary. However, customers could still be involved in expressing what they wanted and could establish through a commission how the artisan would accomplish it. One example crops up in Geneva in 1587 with a contract made by the clockmaker Charles Cusin to produce an iron hand (*une main de fer*) for 20 *écus*.[130] It stipulated that the hand would have fingers that could be moved together or separately by winding crank handles (*les nilles*), reminiscent of the Braunschweig Hand's spanners (figures 5.12–5.13).[131] The customer wanted the ability to move the fingers separately—though the number of finger blocks is unclear—and Cusin's solution involved a mechanism the customer could wind at will. The resulting object did not approach the estimated value of the

Braunschweig Hand, but it was relatively expensive—the equivalent of over half a year's pay for a masonry day laborer in Geneva at the time.[132]

Prosthetic artifacts resulted from similar arrangements. The design and quality of materials and craftsmanship offer clues about what individual amputee-patrons *wanted* from these objects, and about how these objects *functioned* as works of embodied technology.[133] Early modern mechanical hands could not fully restore the use of amputated limbs. They did not erase the bodily change caused by amputations. Instead, each created a unique material lived experience—the way they fit and felt on the body, the routine patterns of movement their wearers developed to adjust fingers and activate release mechanisms, their appearance to wearers looking down at them in use, their appearance to others. Passively operated prostheses, they could serve different purposes.

Consider first the practical function of gripping and holding. This was, according to surgeons' definitions of a false restoration, the purpose of an artificial hand. An examination of material culture reveals a more complicated picture. Careful handling of the artifacts today shows that after centuries of corrosion, many are still capable of locking into positions that could facilitate carrying, lifting, or holding other objects. However, the more expensive and complex the artifact, the less user-friendly and efficient it was to operate. Stiff, slightly curved barrel fingers, which form a hook or O-shape when flexed, are faster and easier to move and adjust. The modest external spring of the Ingolstadt Hand, or the two-finger-block design of the Eisfeld Hand, made these simpler devices easier to use than more complex examples, like the Zweithand or the Braunschweig Hand (figures 5.6–5.7, 5.9, 5.12). Artifacts with fingers articulated in every joint offered a wide variety of positions, but that complexity also meant more complicated and time-consuming processes to arrange and adjust them. Moreover, the more intricate the internal mechanisms, the more delicate and prone to breaking. It is telling that the only instance in which Götz von Berlichingen refers directly to possessing an iron hand in his autobiography is when he mentioned a time it needed repairing.[134]

Elaborate arm casings could also make an object less user-friendly. The Kassel Hand and the Eisfeld Hand weigh just over a pound (figures 5.9, 6.4). The Grüningen Hand, with its wooden forearm, is about twice that (figure 5.4). By contrast, the Balbronn reconstruction weighs over three-and-a-half pounds and the Zweithand over three (figures 5.3, 5.6). The use of metal made these objects durable and incorporated mechanical designs that enabled moveable joints, but it also made them heavier to wear and lift, and more difficult to securely attach. In other words, an amputee-patron did not commission a more mechanically complex and elaborately artful prosthesis in order to grip or hold objects more efficiently or to wear it with greater ease and comfort. When discussing artificial limbs in today's parlance, it is common to distinguish between a "work arm," worn for everyday use, and a "Sunday arm," worn for special occasions.[135] Some early modern mechanical hands were probably worn more regularly than others, but all were forms of "Sunday arm." The artifacts in our pool reveal a spectrum rather than a binary. From the simplest to most sophisticated, they were all more complicated than required for everyday tasks.

This points us to more subjective functions. The most difficult of these to establish is what an object meant to the person who wore it. Consider the Balbronn Hand (figure 5.3). Did Hans van Mittelhausen express a wish to be buried wearing this iron arm? Was he concerned about how others would see his body after his death? Was the heavy metal device simply a clunky, impractical annoyance in need of constant repair, whose greatest value resided in the impression it made upon others? Or had it become, by the end, a familiar friend that formed an integral part of his own identity? Was it a mix of all of these? Even more intimate, and impossible to uncover, is the way early modern notions of an "ideal body" of two arms and two legs figured into Hans's understanding of the prosthesis. To what extent did he commission this object as a solution to social pressures to appear "normal" after the amputation of a limb? How much of the object's role as showpiece was meant to alter others' perceptions, and how much of it was meant to alter his self-perception?

Mechanical hands do offer evidence of the ways amputees sought to influence how others perceived them. Rare firsthand accounts[136] show that, for some, this undertaking could be well underway during post-operative convalescence. Mere weeks after the amputation of his left arm in 1622, Christian the Younger crafted perceptions of his injury from his sickbed in Breda. In a brief letter to his brother, Friedrich Ulrich of Braunschweig-Wolfenbüttel, he conveyed his gratitude for the "care and pity" his brother expressed for his "bruising."[137] "Praise be to God," he continued, that he could "occasionally walk and stand again."[138] He alluded to his future with confidence by assuring his brother that "even though the one arm is wanting, [I] hope to render good service to the Fatherland with the [other]."[139] In a few short sentences, he minimized the injury, conveyed he was not entirely bedridden, and asserted that he would be returning to the battlefield. Emphasizing his intention to fight with one arm echoes a strategy of self-fashioning found in Götz's autobiography. Götz concluded his description of his amputation and convalescence by declaring that he went on to war and feud "with one fist."[140] The remainder of the autobiography only mentions the missing hand in an aside.[141] Both examples suggest efforts to shape social perceptions. Götz, dictating to a scribe decades after the event, framed it as a triumph of his faith in God. Christian, writing to his brother in the midst of a difficult convalescence, appeared more immediately concerned with convincing his peers that his role and identity were unchanged by his injury.

Amputee-patrons drew from art and craft to influence others' perceptions after their stumps healed. They presented the likeness of a natural hand to the world around them. It was a likeness in form: each artifact includes a curved palm, four fingers, a thumb, and a wrist narrower than the main body of the hand. It could also be a likeness in color: multiple examples show signs of flesh-toned paint, including the Ingolstadt Hand and the Ersthand (figures 5.5, 5.7). The most visible portion of the devices—the base and length of the fingers—included other details modeled from nature. Every example from our pool has impressions of fingernails (figures 5.2, 5.15, 5.17). Many also display lines imitating wrinkled folds of skin at the knuckles. They were not designed to make owners appear to be wearing a cloth glove or steel gauntlet over a natural hand. They *were* the hand, and they were meant to appear that way. They could even be dressed like a natural hand: a contemporary who encountered Götz in 1512 noted that he "wore a glove on the iron hand."[142] Wrist or forearm casings, with perforations or straps to be secured to clothing or concealed beneath a sleeve, lacked the details of the artificial fingers. The Grüningen Hand, for instance, has a carefully painted hand, but an unadorned wooden forearm (figure 5.4). This suggests that in some cases these objects could allow the amputee-patron to appear inconspicuous to others at first glance.

The elaborate arm casings of the Nuremberg Hand and the Braunschweig Hand indicate that at other times the objects were intended to arrest the eye even at a distance (figures 5.12, 5.16). The weight of the metal casings for these above-the-elbow prostheses had to be carefully distributed. If they were attached only at the end of the upper arm casings, their centers of gravity would shift awkwardly with any attempt made to position their forearms parallel to the ground. The fragments of leather cords attached to artifacts only hint at methods early moderns might have developed to address this issue. Early twentieth-century designs used interconnected straps around the shoulder, torso, and leg to create a counterbalance for upper arm prostheses,[143] and it is possible early moderns employed combinations of straps beneath clothing for the same purpose. Placing the metal forearms into a form of sling, as if resting an injured arm, would have been another way to control the balance and weight of the device. Portraits of Christian the Younger made during his lifetime show him wearing his officer's sash as a sling with his left arm—which had been amputated above the elbow—seemingly intact, clad in armor, and resting in it.[144] While the simplicity of the arm casing of the Grüningen Hand suggests it was worn beneath clothing, the ornate openwork of the Nuremberg Hand and the Braunschweig Hand provided more options (figures 5.4, 5.12, 5.16). The leather sleeve fitted inside the arm casing of the Nuremberg Hand, for example, visually creates a solid surface through the metal openwork and conceals the length of the wearer's stump. The continuity of the piece suggests it was possible to wear it under clothing or in full view. With the casing under clothing, the lifelike wooden hand could have been inconspicuous until further examination led observers to admire its artistry (figure 5.17). If worn with portions of the casing visible, the striking black openwork irresistibly draws the eye, garnering immediate attention. Far from being subtle, ornate components suggest there could have been occasions when some amputee-patrons had no intention of blending in.

All mechanical hands were designed to impress observers upon closer inspection. Wearers could use them to perform demonstrations of technical virtuosity at the press of a button, the turn of a spanner, or the lift of an external lever. This was a simulation of movement achieved through custom mechanical designs. When the fingers are at rest, their bases sit parallel with the top of the hand. Flexion moves them, as natural fingers move, in the direction of the palm. The more complex its mechanisms, the more movement the object displayed. Articulating every joint of each finger did not offer a more efficient gripping or holding device than stiff-fingered prostheses. It imitated the anatomy of a human hand more closely. Surviving artifacts show that amputee-patrons valued this form of likeness and could obtain it at varying levels of expense and sophistication.

The more closely a prosthesis imitated nature, the more impressive it was. Most artifacts in our pool required a wearer to use a natural hand to press artificial fingers down into desired positions. The most artful examples move in ways that do not require this contact. The Braunschweig Hand's fingers, for example, would have curled at the turn of a spanner in the wrist, appearing to move of their own accord (figures 5.12–5.13). This was both reminiscent of an automaton—a mechanical marvel—and highly inefficient as an everyday aid for gripping and holding. The movements of the wooden Nuremberg Hand were less controlled than any of the iron hands—only three fingers could be locked in the mechanism located in its palm at one time (figures 5.16–5.17). But examining the artifact today reveals that this free movement of the wooden joints in each finger gives a more lifelike effect, allowing the fingers to settle in quite natural-looking positions when the hand is placed on different surfaces without requiring a wearer to passively adjust or lock them. The movement seems to flow from the object itself.

Mechanical hands took the forms they did in part because their wearers lived in a society that coveted ingenious and artful objects that blurred the boundaries of art and nature. This cultural trend appeared in its most enthusiastic form among the ruling classes. Princely connoisseurs assembled collections of cunning instruments and beautiful and rare objects to display in art cabinets (*die Kunstkammern*) and cabinets of curiosities (*die Wunderkammern*). They commissioned automata that carried goblets across tables, and chairs that played tricks on unwitting guests.[145] Instruments of navigation, timekeeping, and military technology were prized possessions.

The prestige associated with clever technical objects held multiple valences in early modern society. They were symbols of status and wealth that sparked conversation among guests, displayed learned interests, and even suggested the virtue of temperance. Engaging with mechanical objects in particular demonstrated a technical knowledge that was "tied not only to political authority but also to morality and wisdom."[146] When wondrous works were brought together into collections, they could convey political aims and tell dynastic stories.

It is hardly surprising that, within this context, a mechanical arm appeared in the *Kunstkammer* of Christian the Younger's descendants in Wolfenbüttel, displayed to visitors until the end of the eighteenth century as a family heirloom.[147] Neither the object nor images of it have survived. The Braunschweig Hand, dated to the seventeenth century, was found in a church tomb approximately ten miles from Wolfenbüttel (figure 5.12).[148] It is possible that the amputee-patron who commissioned the Braunschweig Hand wore and was buried with it, all while another mechanical limb was on display in the local ruler's art cabinet. The geographic proximity of these two objects—one that has survived, one that appears only in the written record—does not suggest a link between their wearers, but rather evokes a milieu that helps us to better understand the cultural meanings embodied in the prostheses. As one of the most elaborate artifacts in our source pool, the Braunschweig Hand gestures to a creative realm of artificial wonders imitating natural forms, made with cutting-edge technology. At the same time, it presents a tangible response to the loss of a limb, a prosthesis capable of holding other objects, a "false restoration" that facilitated an amputee's social adjustment after a traumatic injury. Less technically sophisticated objects show different combinations of practical function and more subjective functions, as well as different budgets. Some examples were more statement pieces than others—compare, for example, the ornate Nuremberg Hand with the simple Ingolstadt Hand (figures 5.7, 5.16). Yet all of the artifacts reveal in varying degrees an esteem for clever mechanical objects that can imitate the shape and movement of nature. They all suggest that amputee-patrons drew inspiration from a fashionable trend to manage the loss of a limb.

They did this against a backdrop of popular stereotypes that portrayed amputees and prostheses as symbols of poverty and misery. Visual and literary sources alike frequently depicted beggars with wooden legs and crutches, using these as stylized signs of weakness, helplessness, and need worthy of public aid or medical care.[149] In the wake of the Thirty Years' War, soldiers with missing limbs appeared in widely circulated broadsheets to evoke defeat, wretchedness, and the moral decay of the Holy Roman Empire.[150] How closely this symbolic imagery corresponded to everyday social experience has been rightly questioned. But it is apparent that amputee-patrons fashioned prostheses that inverted those negative stereotypes. Iron—an expensive, durable material—connoted strength, longevity, and wealth. Articulated fingers advertised self-sufficiency. They demonstrated functionality, even if this was more performative than practical in more elaborate examples. The mechanical workings of these objects also connected them to a cultural cache of intelligence, virtue, and competency. The likeness the prostheses presented operated on multiple levels, providing discretion (when desired) and embodying a form of cultural prestige. At first glance, the objects suggest wearers' desires to reestablish appearances or perceptions of bodily integrity that amputations altered. This undoubtedly played an important role in the process of obtaining artificial hands. But these objects also suggest *more*. Mechanical hands tapped into a nexus of positive cultural attributions by creatively harnessing art and craft.

In this way, amputee-patrons used objects not only to shape their social interactions, but also the meanings of bodily difference as early moderns perceived and/or experienced it.[151] The historian can only cautiously contemplate the significance each prosthetic artifact might have held for a wearer's identity, emotional well-being, ways of adopting new habits to perform everyday tasks, and configuring social relations. One thing we can know for certain: these objects symbolized a form of agency and control. Commissioning a mechanical hand—entering into dialogue with artisans—allowed an amputee-patron to stipulate the form, movement, and appearance of an artificial supplement. Katherine Ott has said that aesthetics "are illustrative of power."[152] While she was speaking of the limited power of the consumer apparent in the material culture of disability in modern America, her words resonate on multiple levels with the evidence of our early modern amputee-patrons. With no craft group specializing in artificial limbs, these individuals obtained objects uniquely designed to suit their needs, tastes, and budgets. The consumer *was* in control. Related to this was the socio-economic status of amputee-patrons: they were elites with the means to commission.

The artifacts suggest another form of power even more profound: the impact amputee-patrons had on the design of these devices, and how these devices in turn influenced early modern medical views. Recent scholars have posited a design model of disability in which design—defined as "processes of planning and making the material world"—has "played an active role in shaping the meaning of disability" in modern society.[153] Drawing on this notion in the early modern European context[154] highlights the role of amputee-patrons and artisans in expanding the malleability of the body. Each artifact represents an experiment. As a custom order, it was something new, to both the artisan and the amputee, which they created together. Surviving examples demonstrate that choices of materials, artful details, and forms of mechanisms made each prosthesis an exploration of desire, possibility, matter, and skill. These objects pushed far beyond the bounds of practical supplements. They were experiments in artificial intervention in the shape of the human body.

Allusions to these objects in surgical treatises, sources which give little attention to prostheses of any kind, suggest the efforts of a comparably small group of amputees had a significant impact on medical thinking. Surgeons referred to "iron hands" when discussing sites for upper limb amputations and reflected on them when formulating notions of false restorations of a limb. They said nothing of wooden hands, though these certainly existed, and only rarely referred to the use of leather. It is the *iron* hand that appears again and again. Obtaining an *iron* hand was the surgeon's recommended solution to replace an amputated one. The practices of amputee-patrons influenced how surgeons understood the benefits and utility of this prosthesis. Medical views of amputees' bodies were not simply dictated by early modern surgeons. The forces of influence undergirding medical notions of the "ideal" body—a body of certain harmonious proportions and symmetry—and how artificial materials could be used to achieve it were complex and multidirectional.

There are many layers of meaning in each prosthetic artifact, and I do not pretend to uncover them all here. Our investigation suggests that amputee-patrons drew inspiration from developing technology and cultural trends to commission artificial limbs that they found useful for navigating—in some combination—social interactions, the physical world of the everyday, and their own sense of identity. They embody the challenges many amputees managed after experiencing a seismic change to their bodies. Placing artificial limbs in the context of craft practices opens for scholars a crucial dimension of these objects—they were custom orders that required the talents of multiple artisans. The techniques and materials that comprise these anonymous objects can be tied, one by one, to physical spaces, economic activities, and social encounters.

Amputee-patrons are elusive historical actors. Yet their material practices were undoubtedly influential in the creation of the malleable body and, from the evidence of surgical literature, appear to have been highly effective in establishing and influencing early modern perceptions about the value and utility of their prosthetic devices. The loss of an upper limb created an opportunity unlike any other amputation. With his scalpel, the surgeon changed the body's form; with a mechanical hand, the amputee and the artisan changed it again.

Notes

1 E.g., Burhenne, *Prothesen*; Knoche, *Prothesen der unteren Extremität*; Putti, *Historic Artificial Limbs*. Short essays on individual objects also appear in local journals: e.g., Gosmann, "Die Arnsberger 'Eiserne Hand.'" A notable exception is Liebhard Löffler's *Der Ersatz*.

2 Kahlow, "Prothesen im Mittelalter"; Gagné, "Emotional Attachments"; Heide, "Arbeitsarm und Sonntagshand" and *Holzbein und Eisenhand*; Hausse, "The Locksmith, the Surgeon, and the Mechanical Hand."
3 Paré, *Les Oeuvres* (1579), 838–840, and *Wundt-Artzney* (1601), 951–952.
4 E.g., Purmann, *Wund-Artzney* (1692), 3:230; Jessen, *Wund-Artznei*, 208.
5 E.g., Knoche, *Prothesen der unteren Extremität*, 57–58.
6 E.g., Kahlow, "Archäologische Erkenntnisse zur Chirurgie und Prothetik," 346–347.
7 The artificial leg of Landgrave Friedrich II of Hesse-Homburg (1633–1708), which included a spring mechanism to articulate the foot, is one such exception: Heide, *Holzbein und Eisenhand*, 111–112, 115, 151–152.
8 *Preussische Staatszeitung*. Nr. 87. 24 March 1836; *Spenersche Zeitung*. Nr. 72. 25 March 1836. Unless otherwise noted, my descriptions in this chapter derive from examinations I conducted in 2012–2013. I am grateful to the museums and private owners who generously granted access to the artifacts, relevant institutional documentation, and insight from the professionals who oversee their preservation and care.
9 The roller on the buckles may suggest the object was made in the late sixteenth century: Dirk H. Breiding, conversation with author, Philadelphia Museum of Art, Philadelphia, 5 August 2014.
10 Breiding, "Techniques of Decoration." For a sixteenth-century example of openwork in decorative armor: Pyhrr and Godoy, *Heroic Armor*, 279, 283.
11 Hansjörg Albrecht, conversation with author, Museum Neuruppin, Neuruppin, Germany, 21 May 2013.
12 Forrer, "Die eiserne Hand," 103.
13 Société pour la conservation des monuments historiques d'Alsace, "Séance du 3 novembre 1856," 248–249.
14 Forrer, "Die eiserne Hand," 104–105; Löffler, "Neues von alten Händen," 79; Mechel, *Die eiserne Hand*, Tab. I–II.
15 Hornstein-Grüningen, *Erlebnisse*, 471.
16 Heide, *Holzbein und Eisenhand*, 122, 183.
17 On the importance of artifacts as objects that "actively shape and define disability" and mediate human relationships: Ott, "Disability Things."
18 On history of science: Dacome, *Malleable Anatomies*; Daston, *Biographies of Scientific Objects* and *Things that Talk*; Findlen, "Early Modern Things." On material culture and disability studies: Ulrich et al., *Tangible Things*, esp. p. 2; Mihm et al., *Artificial Parts, Practical Lives*; Ott, "Disability Things"; Gerritsen and Riello, "Introduction."
19 E.g., Siraisi, "Medicine, 1450–1620"; Rankin, *Panaceia's Daughters*; Cavallo, *Artisans of the Body*.
20 Fissell, "Introduction," 10–14; Horn and Frohne, "Fluidity"; Williamson and Guffey, *Making Disability Modern*.
21 Ott, "Disability Things."
22 Walz, "Die Armprothese," 55.
23 Frohne, "Performing Dis/ability?" 61. See also Heide, "Arbeitsarm und Sonntagshand," 119, and *Holzbein und Eisenhand*, 138.

24 E.g., Virdi, "Material Traces of Disability," 614.
25 Forrer, "Die eiserne Hand," 106.
26 Museé Historique, Strasbourg, inventory entry, Numéro 2750 a, b., 1 June 1953, Désignation de l'object: "Main de fer mécanique. ... Elle a servi sans doute au Junker Hans von Mittelhusen pour remplacer la main gauche et l'avant-bras estropiés peu dans les troubles de la Révolte des paysans en 1525." The entry cites Forrer's 1917 article under "Observations."
27 *Preussische Staatszeitung.* Nr. 87. 24 March 1836. Liebhard Löffler suggests the dating is related to an interest in linking the object to a knight who died in 1528 and notes that a sword and spurs were later salvaged from the area: *Der Ersatz*, 28.
28 Burhenne, *Prothesen*, 102–103; Wetz, "Zur Geschichte der Armprothetik," 154; Kahlow, "Prothesen im Mittelalter," 211.
29 Amirault, *La Vie de François, seigneur de La Noue*, 63.
30 Archives de l'Etat de Fribourg, Comptes des Trésoriers 148 b (2e semetre 1476), 64; Chapuis and Gélis, *Le monde des automates*, 2:309.
31 E.g., Lang, *Historischer Almanach* (1793) and *Historischer Almanach* (1794); Mechel, *Die eiserne Hand*.
32 Hornstein-Grüningen, *Erlebnisse*, 458: "Ritter Götz war durch Goethe plötzlich ein berühmter Mann und seine eiserne Hand eine unschätzbare Reliquie geworden," "'Hätte ich die Hand nie gesehen', schrieb Marquard, 'so sehr werde ich von allen Seiten um das Kleinod bestürmt'."
33 Ibid.
34 Putti, *Historic Artificial Limbs*, 2–3; Lang, *Historischer Almanach* (1793), 65–74.
35 Associations between Götz and iron hands are so well known in German culture that an iron hand appeared as the insignia of the 17th SS Panzergrenadier Division *Götz von Berlichingen* in World War II and today can be found on bottles of an "Iron Hand" (*Eiserne Hand*) series of wines, named for Götz, from a Württemberg-based winery: Cohn, "Götz von Berlichingen," 22; www.wzg-weine.de/unsere-weine/wuerttemberg-eiserne-hand (accessed 19 March 2021).
36 Forrer, "Die eiserne Hand," 103.
37 *Preussische Staatszeitung.* Nr. 87. 24 March 1836.
38 Hans-Christoph Freiherr von Hornstein, conversation with author, Riedlingen, Germany, 27 April 2013; Hornstein-Grüningen, *Erlebnisse*, 471.
39 www.sothebys.com/en/auctions/ecatalogue/2016/old-master-sculpture-l16231/lot.93.html# (accessed 29 March 2021).
40 E.g., Burhenne, *Prothesen*, 103, 105.
41 Mechel, *Die eiserne Hand*, Tab. I–II; Quasigroch, "Die Handprothesen," 26–27; Otte, "3D Computer-Aided Design Reconstructions."
42 Tobias Schönauer, conversation with author, Bayerisches Armeemuseum, Ingolstadt, Germany, 19 April 2013.
43 An exception is Liebhard Löffler's postulation that the wearer was a child on account of the object's size: *Der Ersatz*, 37; Quasigroch, "Die Handprothesen," 25. However, the Ingolstadt Hand—at 15 cm in length and nearly 10 cm broad—is not so small compared with other examples: the surviving hand fragment of the original Balbronn Hand is barely 16 cm in length.

44 Burhenne, *Prothesen*, 103: "vermutlich war das Halten der Zügel möglich."
45 "*Eisenhand* – um 1520 – Vermutlich verlor der Besitzer im Kampf die linke Hand und ersetzte sie durch diese Prothese." Bayerisches Armeemuseum online collection: Image 11 of 24, www.armeemuseum.de/de/fotogalerien/objekte.html (accessed 24 March 2016).
46 StdAM, KR 1551/52, 91r.
47 Hildanus, *Wund-Artzney*, 213: "haben doch ihr Mann/ und Freund/ auch die Krancke selbst begehrt/ daβ ihr der Arm abgenommen werde."
48 Ibid., 1192; Scultetus, *Wund-Artzneyisches Zeug-Hauβ* (1666), 2:182.
49 La Rocca, *European Armor*, 62; Topf, *Almain Armourer's Album*, 2–3, Plates IV, XVIII; Grancsay, "Hapsburg Locking Gauntlet."
50 Cf., Alexander, *Treasures Afoot*.
51 Ott, "Disability Things," 129.
52 Mechel, *Die eiserne Hand*.
53 See also Otte, "Christian von Mechel's Reconstructive Drawings."
54 Antje Scherner, conversation with author, Kassel, Germany, 23 April 2013.
55 At present the right block (index and middle fingers) only locks at the fourth increment, while the left locks in all positions.
56 Door, furniture, and casket locks: Pankofer, *Schlüssel und Schloss*, 60, 67; Welker, *Historische Schlüssel und Schlösser*, 14–16, 209–210, 264–266. Clocks: Maurice, *Die deutsche Räderuhr*, 1:81–126. Firearms: Hayward, *Art of the Gunmaker*, 1:263–277.
57 Landes, *Revolution in Time*, 208; Groiss, "Augsburg Clockmakers' Craft," 58.
58 Welker, *Historische Schlüssel und Schlösser*, 23.
59 Bedini, "Johann Wolfgang Gelb," 326–328, 331.
60 Maurice, *Die deutsche Räderuhr*, 1:137–146, 163–168; Mayr, *Automatic Machinery*, 6, 8–9.
61 Mayr, *Automatic Machinery*, 9; Keating, *Animating Empire*, 11; Landes, *Revolution in Time*, 212–215.
62 Farr, "Shop Floor," 42; Maurice and Mayr, *Clockwork Universe*, 173.
63 Bedini, "Johann Wolfgang Gelb," 323–326. For more on locksmiths: *AHRG*, 4:294–304; Welker, *Historische Schlüssel und Schlösser*; Eras, *Locks and Keys*.
64 Chapuis and Gélis, *Le monde des automates*, 1:191–230. On goldsmiths in Germany: *AHRG*, 5:6–10.
65 Keating, *Animating Empire*, 1–14, 91.
66 Maurice and Mayr, *Clockwork Universe*, 312–313, 317.
67 Ibid., 239, 274.
68 Bedini, "Role of Automata," 32.
69 Walz, "Die Armprothese," 55. The restorer received twelve fragments but determined one piece did not belong to the object: HAUM, copy of Olaf Wilde's "Restaurierungsbericht. Die künstliche Hand: HAUM Nr. Waf 11. Braunschweigisches Landesmuseum" (Braunschweig, 11 September 1997), 1, 4.
70 HAUM, copy of Wilde, "Restaurierungsbericht," 6.
71 For examples of the debate: Mayer, "Christian der Jüngere"; Walz, "Die Armprothese." Chapter 4 discusses Christian the Younger at length.
72 Gerchow, *Ebenbilder*, 260.

73 Löffler, "Die Braunschweiger Hand," 68–69.
74 Walz, "Die Armprothese," 59.
75 Löffler, "Die Braunschweiger Hand," 68.
76 Oakeshott, *European Weapons and Armour*, 38–39; Hayward, *Art of the Gunmaker*, 266–268; Karcheski, *Arms and Armor*, 100–103. For more on gunsmiths: *AHRG*, 4:305–309.
77 Karcheski, *Arms and Armor*, 100; Oakeshott, *European Weapons and Armour*, 39.
78 Battlefield use: Karcheski, *Arms and Armor*, 100–103. Luxury wheellock handguns: Pyhrr, *Firearms*.
79 While the object was on loan to the Sauerland-Museum (Arnsberg) during the spring of 2013, its display label stated: "Eiserne Hand eines schwedischen Offiziers im Dreißigjährige Krieg. Leihgabe des Hessischen Landesmuseum Darmstadt" (viewed 3 April 2013). This identification has carried over into sourcebooks and exhibition catalogs, with one going so far as to say the object functions like a piece of armor and need not necessarily be considered a prosthesis: Burhenne, *Prothesen*, 110–111.
80 The archive which originally held the object was dissolved and its records scattered, so we can only speculate about its discovery and what evidence may have existed to explain its designation as a war trophy. For an example: Gosmann, "Die Arnsberger 'Eiserne Hand,'" 27–28.
81 Walther, *Die Sammlungen*, 14; Burhenne, *Prothesen*, 111.
82 E.g., Lang, *Historischer Almanach* (1794); Mechel, *Die eiserne Hand*; Berlichingen-Rossach, *Geschichte*. Günther Quasigroch tackles these "fables," including one that claims Götz designed the prosthesis himself: "Die Handprothesen," 25.
83 Lang, *Historischer Almanach* (1794), 3.
84 Ibid., 4.
85 Berlichingen-Rossach, *Geschichte*, 475.
86 Quasigroch, "Die Handprothesen," 22.
87 Lang, *Historischer Almanach* (1794), 3, Plate 3; Quasigroch, "Die Handprothesen," 21. The finger appears broken in a photograph from a 1980 publication and restored in another from a 1982 publication; the latter mentions the restoration was recently completed: Löffler, "Götz von Berlichingen," 12; Quasigroch, "Die Handprothesen," 23.
88 Quasigroch, "Die Handprothesen," 22.
89 On blacksmiths in early modern Germany: *AHRG*, 4:234–263.
90 La Rocca, *European Armor*, 29–33.
91 Pfaffenbiehler, *Armourers*, 62, 65–66; Karcheski, *Arms and Armor*, 62, 64, 66–77.
92 Thomas Eser (Germanisches Nationalmuseum), email communication with author, 27 September 2014.
93 Baxandall, *Limewood Sculptors*, 112. Limewood carvings could be very lifelike; compare the Nuremburg Hand to the hands of Tilman Riemenschneider's statue of St. Matthew in Baxandall, *Limewood Sculptors*, 184, Fig. 116. For more on joiners: *AHRG*, 5:229–270.
94 Grossmann, *Mythos Burg*, 157. This is repeated in Heide, *Holzbein und Eisenhand*, 143–144.

95 Thomas Eser, conversation with author, Germanisches Nationalmuseum, Nuremberg, Germany, 7 May 2013.
96 On the artistic uses of limewood in early modern Germany: Baxandall, *Limewood Sculptors*.
97 Augsburg production and armorer stamps: Ffoulkes, *Armourer*, 13, 148; Karcheski, *Arms and Armor*, 62, 77; La Rocca, *European Armor*, 27, 146. Trial pieces made for guild approval: Pfaffenbiehler, *Armourers*, 26.
98 Conversation with Thomas Eser and museum staff, Germanisches Nationalmuseum, Nuremberg, Germany, 7 May 2013.
99 Metalworking techniques: Williams, *Knight and the Blast Furnace*; La Rocca, *European Armor*, 113. Locksmiths adapted the technique from armorers: Welker, *Historische Schlüssel und Schlösser*, 18.
100 Paré, *Les Oeuvres* (1579), 838.
101 Abelinus, *Theatrum Europaeum*, 668.
102 Chapuis and Gélis, *Le monde des automates*, 2:309.
103 Löffler, "Die Braunschweiger Hand," 68: "eyserin hanndt." The debt owed to Ring by the widow of another leatherworker could suggest coordination or sub-contracting between shops.
104 *AHRG*, 6 vols.
105 E.g., Ffoulkes, *Armourer*, 22, 44; Farr, *Artisans in Europe*, 98.
106 *AHRG*, 2:288–294.
107 Ibid., 1:99; Farr, *Artisans in Europe*, 98.
108 Groiss, "Augsburg Clockmakers' Craft," 58; Bedini, "Johann Wolfgang Gelb," 328.
109 Farr, "Shop Floor," 34; Strauss, *Nuremberg*, 134–136.
110 Soliday, *Community in Conflict*, 139.
111 Friedrichs, "Artisans and Urban Politics," 42; *AHRG*, 2:35–36.
112 Farr, *Artisans in Europe*, 119–127.
113 E.g., Farr, "Shop Floor," 27. The vision of artisans cooperating with others to fill orders appears in revisionist interpretations of guilds from the last two decades. These challenge traditional views characterizing them as forces of economic stagnation and instead outline a fluid craft economy in which trades came and went according to consumer demand. A summary of the debate: Soly, "Political Economy of European Craft Guilds," 45–46; Lis and Soly, "Subcontracting," 81; Epstein, "Craft Guilds in the Pre-modern Economy."
114 Farr, "Shop Floor," 39, 41, 47–49; Roper, *Holy Household*, 33. Subcontracting was also common among goldsmiths: Smith, "Sixteenth-Century Goldsmith's Workshop," 39.
115 Farr, "Shop Floor," 47.
116 Smith, "Making as Knowing," 20.
117 Horn and Frohne, "Fluidity," 40.
118 Heide, *Holzbein und Eisenhand*, 341.
119 Ibid., 112, 298; Heide, "'Kein rechte sonder ein gemachte Nasen.'"
120 Hausse, "The Locksmith, the Surgeon, and the Mechanical Hand"; Heide, *Holzbein und Eisenhand*, 123, 260.

121 Abelinus, *Theatrum Europaeum*, 668.
122 Gagné, "Emotional Attachments," 136.
123 Chapuis and Gélis, *Le monde des automates*, 2:309; Heide, *Holzbein und Eisenhand*, 111–112, 115.
124 On bodywork: Fissell, "Introduction," 10–14.
125 StdAM, KR 1541, 75v, 78r.
126 Löffler, "Die Braunschweiger Hand," 69.
127 Baxandall, *Limewood Sculptors*, 111–112.
128 Kahlow, "Prothesen im Mittelalter," 220.
129 O'Malley, "Little Gilded Shoes," 53; Baxandall, *Limewood Sculptors*, 102–103.
130 Babel, *Histoire corporative de l'horlogerie*, 49–50; Descaves, "Réponses."
131 Descaves, "Réponses."
132 A Genevan mason's daily wage was about 6 sols; 20 écus would have been the equivalent of at least 1200 sols. This estimate uses the following rates from 1542–1564: One écu was worth from four to seven Genevan florins and from forty-four to sixty sols. It also takes into account the heavy inflation Geneva experienced from the 1560s to 1600. Genevan masons' wages: Benedict, *Graphic History*, 172. Currency conversion rates: Valeri, "Religion, Discipline, and the Economy," 124. Inflation: Monter, *Studies in Genevan Government*, 26–27. Currency values: Braudel and Spooner, "Prices in Europe."
133 My approach is particularly influenced by Mihm et al., *Artificial Parts, Practical Lives*. See especially Ott, "Sum of Its Parts."
134 *MFH*, 118.
135 Burhenne, *Prothesen*, 102.
136 Medieval and early modern ego documents from individuals who survived amputation are scarce, and these give little attention to themes related to the injured body, recovery, or ways in which the loss of a limb impacted everyday experience: Heide, *Holzbein und Eisenhand*, 179; Frohne, "Performing Dis/ability?" 51–65.
137 NLA-WO-103, fol. 66r: "vorsorge unnd mitleidenn," "unser bekommener quetzuer."
138 Ibid.: "es Gott sei lob," "wiederumb hin und wieder gehe und stehe."
139 Ibid.: "Unnd ob zwarn der eine arm groes mangel erlitten, so verhoffe doch dem Vatterlandt noch mit dem ubrigen guitte diensten zu erweisen."
140 *MFH*, 77: "mit einer faust."
141 See Frohne's excellent textual analysis: "Performing Dis/ability?" 59–61.
142 Quasigroch, "Die Handprothesen," 21: "an der eysinen hand ein handschuch gehapt."
143 Burhenne, *Prothesen*, 107–108.
144 E.g., Mytens, *Christian, Duke of Brunswick and Lüneburg*, c. 1624, oil on canvas; Voerst, *CHRISTIANO D.G. POSTVLATO EP. HALBERSTADIENSI*, 1630–1645, engraving.
145 Maurice and Mayr, *Clockwork Universe*, 274; Koeppe, "Setting the Standard," 22.
146 Koeppe, "Setting the Standard," 19–21.

147 Lachmund, *De Ave Diomedea Dissertatio*, 11; [Sturm], *Des geöffneten Ritter-Platzes*, 142; Rehtmeyer, *Braunschweig-Lüneburgischen Chronica*, 1261; Brückmann, *Centuriae Tertiae Epistolarum Itinerariarum*, 974; Spehr, *Braunschweigischer Fürstensaal*, 291.
148 Walz, "Die Armprothese," 55.
149 Heide, *Holzbein und Eisenhand*, 278. Heide notes that institutional sources indicating recipients of public and private welfare do not support this early modern cultural stereotype and discusses other cultural meanings wooden legs could signify: Heide, 298, 279–281, 286. For a complex example in popular literature: Grimmelshausen, *Springinsfeld*.
150 E.g., Harms et al., *Deutsche Illustrierte Flugblätter*, 2:418–419, 486–487, 490–493.
151 Connected to this is the notion that social interactions play a fundamental role in defining the meaning of prostheses: Virdi, "Material Traces of Disability," 609.
152 Ott, "Disability Things," 27.
153 Guffey and Williamson, "Introduction," 1.
154 While the design model focuses on the industrialized world of the last two centuries, Nicole Belolan convincingly applies it to the improvised home creations and custom artisanal orders of the eighteenth century: "Material Culture of Gout."

6

Prosthetic technology on the move

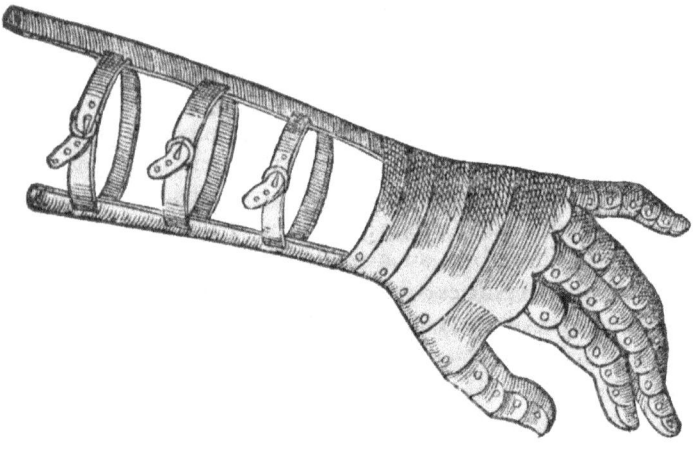

In 1575, Ambroise Paré published an image displaying the internal mechanisms of an iron hand. It was one of four illustrations of mechanical limbs—two hands, an arm, and one leg—that appeared in his book of artificial body parts within his monumental surgical treatise, *Les Oeuvres*.[1] He provided readers with woodcuts of artificial limbs that could, as he wrote in the chapter preface, "perform voluntary motions following nature as closely as art can."[2] The designs were precious, and only "obtained by heartfelt supplications from someone named *le petit Lorrain*—a locksmith living in Paris, an *homme de bon esprit*."[3] In his entreaties to the locksmith, Paré insisted on acquiring more than just images. He carefully recorded "the names and explanation of each part pictured, made in the proper terms and words of the artisan."[4] Image and text together formed a report of the surgeon's persistent consultations with the petit Lorrain. As Paré explained to readers, he gathered information from one locksmith "so that every locksmith or clockmaker may well understand, and make similar artificial arms or legs."[5] The mechanical limbs in Paré's *Oeuvres* were not fanciful designs, but rather echoes of three-dimensional objects already worn by amputees in the early modern period, and which survive in museums and private collections today. With its publication, Paré's *Oeuvres* reveals a moment in which ongoing practices of technical crafts, including those of the locksmith and clockmaker, appeared in the literature of another kind of craft: surgery.

Though a French practitioner, Paré was an influential voice in the surgical discourse that developed and circulated in the Holy Roman Empire through vernacular works. The 1601 and 1635 translations of his *Oeuvres*, entitled *Wund-Artzney*, presented the mechanical hand image directly to German surgeons and barber-surgeons in their own language. But the chapter in which it appeared had changed. The discussion in the preface was similar but not the same as the original French. And the image's explanatory text with the "proper terms and words of the artisan" was gone. The movement of prosthetic technology into German surgical treatises was not straightforward, nor was what it conveyed to German readers clear-cut. As the work of a vernacular surgeon, Paré's *Wund-Artzney* presents a perspective both localized (a German translation for German-speaking readers) and connected to a wider medical world. It is with that wider medical world—the original context of the mechanical hand woodcut's creation in France—that we must begin to follow the image's dissemination and meaning in the Holy Roman Empire. Exploring this movement is a culminating point in the second half of our story of the malleable body. We have seen surgeons discuss artificial limbs as false restorations, and the role of amputees and artisans in developing mechanical hands as artful objects that performed a myriad of functions for their wearers. Equipped with an understanding of mechanical hand production and the influence of amputee-patrons, we turn now to Ambroise Paré's famous woodcut ready to reinterpret its long-held significance in the history of medicine.

This chapter revolves around one sixteenth-century surgeon's attempt to capture and preserve a device designed by a master locksmith. Using evidence from extant artifacts and early modern surgical texts, it analyzes the widely circulated images of mechanical limbs from Paré's *Oeuvres* and their transmission into German print. In particular, it focuses on the best known of the designs—a woodcut of the internal mechanisms of an iron hand—to explore the technical knowledge that the image contains and the ways in which this knowledge may have been conveyed to early modern viewers over several editions and translations. At different points in the dissemination of *Les Oeuvres*, mistakes in the publication reveal a fundamental misunderstanding of the way the technology depicted in the woodcut worked. Yet the image probably retained its practical purpose when shown, as Paré directed, not to surgeons or learned physicians, but to the trained eye of the artisan.

Artisans were a crucial audience for the mechanical limb woodcuts appearing in *Les Oeuvres*. To consider their perspective, I utilize evidence of extant artifacts to contextualize Paré's publication within the flexible nature of prosthesis production. In particular, a side-by-side comparison of Paré's mechanical hand woodcut with the interior of the sixteenth-century Kassel Hand (figures 6.4–6.5) anchors Paré's printed image in craft practices. The creative environment of artificial limb design and construction allows us to consider the woodcut's potential usefulness to different viewers, offering new insight into its transmission. Paré's image provided a broad suggestion of mechanical relationships meant to be in dialogue with the skills and inclinations of the individual craftsman rather than a recipe for exact replication. The mechanical hand woodcut thus presents a form of technical knowledge transfer that was endlessly adaptable to the experiences of artisans from different craft groups.

This chapter opens a new set of investigative possibilities for Paré's writings. Paré looms large in the history of medicine for his innovations as a surgical practitioner, including his treatment of gunshot wounds and his rediscovery of the ligation of blood vessels.[6] Recent studies have analyzed Paré as an author, from the organizing framework of his treatises to the role of translation in transforming editions of his works.[7] This chapter focuses on mechanical limbs and examines an influential part of Paré's work through the lens of material culture, then explores the movement of craft knowledge through print. Paré's book of artificial body parts serves as the chief textual source available to historians for the study of early modern artificial limbs. Yet the author's relationship to the mechanical limb designs in his treatise has often been misconstrued. While scholars such as Reed Benhamou have accurately noted the contributions of the locksmith—the petit Lorrain—to Paré's text, a common mischaracterization of Paré as the inventor of these designs persists, particularly in medical literature and popular textbooks.[8] Restoring the role of the locksmith in Paré's *Oeuvres* not only clarifies Paré's role in the development of prosthetic technology, but also introduces a craft workshop context that is crucial to examining the function of the mechanical hand woodcut as it was disseminated across Europe in translated editions.

This investigation engages in particular with two bodies of scholarship involving practical knowledge and knowledge-making: one that focuses on craft, and another that explores early modern print. Over the last two decades, scholars have given increasing attention to craft knowledge and practices, as well as their relationship to textual knowledge traditions. Historians such as Chandra Mukerji and Pamela Smith have examined craft knowledge as a set of practices preserved through collective memory, and as a way of knowing nature derived from hands-on experience with natural materials.[9] Scholars have also emphasized the social practices essential to learning, knowing, and doing in the early modern workshop.[10] Recent work has considered these elements—hands-on activity and social relationships—as essential to structures of practical knowledge, which underwent continuous reorganization.[11] This chapter considers how master craftsmen familiar with various spring-driven mechanisms could bring their knowledge to bear when viewing the prosthetic hand design in *Les Oeuvres*. Master craftsmen constituted a distinct audience for Paré's chapter on artificial limbs. The potential utility of the woodcut design for this audience should be understood within the adaptable and collaborative processes of making and doing in a workshop.

This chapter also draws from a range of scholarship that examines the role of print in accumulating, appropriating, and communicating traditions of oral or unwritten knowledge, whether local and indigenous (specific to a place or population), or tacit and technical (hands-on practices passed on verbally and/or learned through observation and experience). Its approach engages with work on early modern technological literature, which purportedly aimed to transmit hands-on practices through text and image. Pamela O. Long has described technological books as "trading zones" in which substantive exchanges of knowledge took place between artisans and learned men.[12] Eric H. Ash's study of technical treatises argues for the rise of "expert mediators," who used printed works to claim an abstract theoretical understanding of technical processes that elevated them above—and at the expense of—traditional craft practitioners.[13] I suggest that Ambroise Paré, as an author who included a locksmith's designs in his medical text, was a kind of intermediary, moving information from one context to another. However, the transmission of Paré's *Oeuvres* into the German vernacular shows that despite its appearance in printed surgical treatises, prosthetic technology remained the domain of early modern artisans.

Text and artifact: mechanical limbs in *Les Oeuvres*

The intricate visual presentation of mechanical limbs in Ambroise Paré's *Oeuvres* was an extraordinary exception to the norms of surgical literature. Paré, who began his medical career as an obscure barber-surgeon, was a renowned author and surgeon to four French kings.[14] After the success of his treatise on gunshot wounds in 1545, he published extensively on surgical operations, anatomy, birth defects, putrefaction, and pestilential diseases, among other topics. In 1575, he compiled his previous publications along with new material into a massive volume entitled *Les Oeuvres de M. Ambroise Paré, conseiller et premier chirurgien du roi* (Paris, 1575). He dedicated Book XXII of his *Oeuvres* to artificial parts for the correction of defects in the body and included chapters on noses, ears, eyes, hands, arms, and legs.[15] The book is remarkable for its attention to objects over reconstructive surgery, its inclusion of mechanical limbs, and its numerous woodcuts, which overshadow the written text and give the treatise the feel of a pattern book. *Les Oeuvres* became a common reference point for prostheses in surgical literature within the Holy Roman Empire and across Europe.[16] It went through multiple editions in France, in both the vernacular and Latin, within two decades.[17] The collected works appeared in German and Dutch print shops fairly early.[18] In the 1603 edition of his *Gründlicher Bericht*, the surgeon Fabry von Hilden informed readers that he saw no need to explain wooden legs and iron hands because Paré's detailed work was available to all diligent German surgeons in their own language.[19]

Artificial arms, hands, and legs are the subject of Chapter XII, which provides images of upper and lower limb prostheses accompanied by explanatory text.[20] The chapter consists of less than four pages and six woodcuts. The preface informs readers that Paré made several entreaties to a Parisian locksmith, known as the petit Lorrain, in order to obtain the designs displayed in the woodcuts. The author explained that he was careful to preserve the terminology used by his consultant so that any locksmith or clockmaker (*Serrurier ou horologeur*) could understand the designs.[21] The explanatory text, then, attempted to transmit the words of the petit Lorrain directly to the reader. The devices portrayed in the woodcuts had the dual function of copying both the motion and appearance of a patient's missing limb. According to the chapter preface, the artificial limbs "serve not only for the movement of lost parts, but also for their beauty and adornment."[22] They were intended as metal imitations of the natural body.

Paré made no secret of the petit Lorrain's involvement in Chapter XII: the author's prefatory text to the images explicitly cites the locksmith as the source of the designs. His account suggests that the artisan was reluctant to share his craft with the surgeon. Indeed, an English translation from 1634 interpreted Paré's description of his supplications as financial offers, and told readers that Paré paid the locksmith a substantial sum.[23] The desire to protect trade secrets within individual workshops fit well within traditions of early modern craft knowledge, which was usually passed down orally during years of apprenticeship.[24] Paré's preface highlights the role of the petit Lorrain because the locksmith's extensive involvement was unique to Chapter XII, setting it apart from the other chapters in Book XXII. Paré reproduced the locksmith's words without adding glosses of his own. Chapter XII, accordingly, exposes the reader of Paré's surgical treatise to artisans, craft practices, the rituals of knowledge exchange, and an entire world of prosthesis production occurring outside of the surgeon's practice.

Chapter XII has three woodcuts of upper limb prostheses.[25] The first (figure 6.1) displays the internal mechanisms of an iron hand.[26] The hand is articulated in four fingers, with a rigid thumb and wrist.[27] The individual components in the image are numbered from one to nine and are briefly described in text positioned to the right of and directly beneath the woodcut. The numbered descriptions make up what Paré referred to as the exact terminology of the Parisian locksmith. Three terms are of especial interest for the vocabulary of Paré's consultant: *gaschettes* (components 3 and 5), *estoqueaux* (component 4), and *les lames des doigts* (component 9). *Gaschette*, probably an early spelling of *gâchette*, could refer to part of a lock or a lever-like piece in a gunlock connected with the trigger mechanism. In both contexts, the *gaschette* holds other pieces

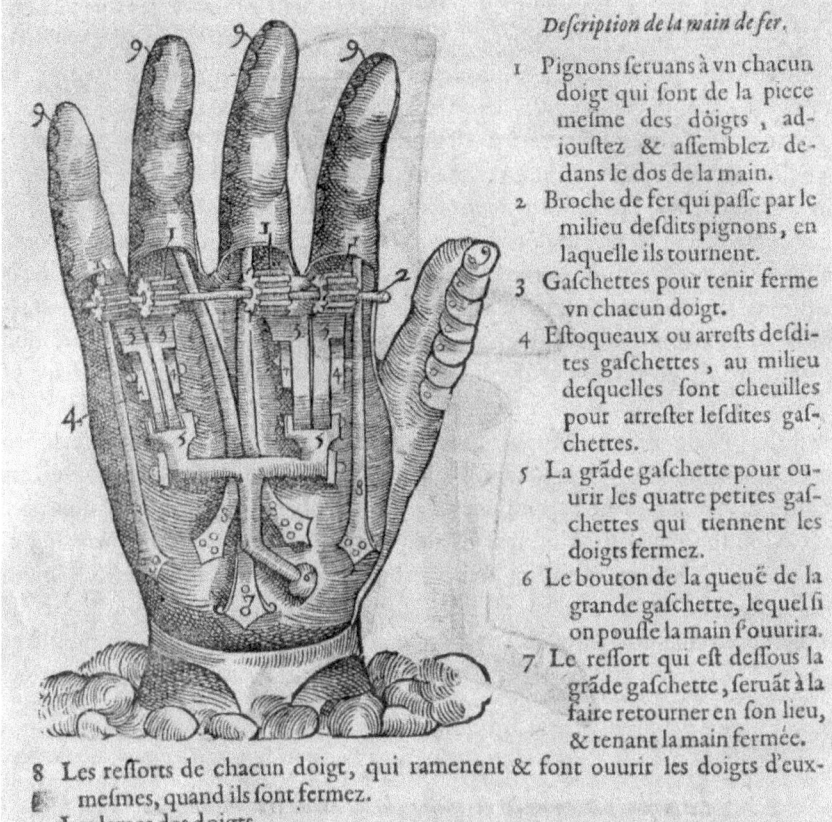

Description de la main de fer.

1 Pignons feruans à vn chacun doigt qui font de la piece mefme des doigts, adiouftez & affemblez dedans le dos de la main.
2 Broche de fer qui paffe par le milieu defdits pignons, en laquelle ils tournent.
3 Gafchettes pour tenir ferme vn chacun doigt.
4 Eftoqueaux ou arrefts defdites gafchettes, au milieu defquelles font cheuilles pour arrefter lefdites gafchettes.
5 La grãde gafchette pour ouurir les quatre petites gafchettes qui tiennent les doigts fermez.
6 Le bouton de la queuē de la grande gafchette, lequel fi on poufle la main f'ouurira.
7 Le reffort qui eft deffous la grãde gafchette, feruãt à la faire retourner en fon lieu, & tenant la main fermée.
8 Les refforts de chacun doigt, qui ramenent & font ouurir les doigts d'eux-mefmes, quand ils font fermez.
9 Les lames des doigts.

6.1 Mechanical hand in Ambroise Paré, *Les Oeuvres* (Paris, 1614), 902 (detail).

in place until acted upon.[28] The woodcut features four small *gaschettes*, "to hold each finger fast," and one large *gaschette* connected to the external release button, "to open the four little *gaschettes*."[29] *Estoqueaux* is a period spelling of the plural of *étoquiau*, which refers to a stopper, catch, or "click" within horology, or a stay pin within locksmithing. In both professions, this part prevents another part from moving or rotating beyond a certain point.[30] In the woodcut, the *estoqueaux* are stoppers of the *gaschettes*, and have pins or bolts (*chevilles*) in their centers for this purpose.[31] While *lame* generally means a narrow metal strip, in this context it is certainly the more precise armorer's term that refers to "narrow strips of steel riveted together horizontally."[32] These were used in those parts of plate armor which required greater mobility, such as portions of the solleret or sabaton (protective covering for the foot), taces (plates at the bottom of the cuirass, or breastplate), or gauntlets.[33] Paré's woodcut shows this technology of riveted, overlapping plates applied to the fingers of a prosthesis to enable flexion. The terms Paré recorded suggest the range of craft groups that would have been familiar with the language and mechanical principles the woodcut attempts to convey: locksmiths, gunsmiths, clockmakers, and armorers.

The next woodcut (figure 6.2) demonstrates how to fit the iron hand on a patient's forearm using three straps with buckles. Although the components of this image are not labeled, the *lames des doigts* listed in the text accompanying the first woodcut can be understood as overlapping plates that begin at the base of the wrist and continue to the base of the fingers, where the pattern continues with smaller *lames* on each individual finger. A third woodcut (figure 6.3) illustrates a left arm prosthesis that includes an articulated elbow joint in addition to the articulated fingers of the hand. The proximal end of the arm displays a series of cords threaded through perforations at the edge of the metal. The cords in this illustration support the assumption that similar perforations seen in extant artifacts were intended to help secure prostheses to their wearers (figure 5.7).[34] The arm's components, also numbered from one to nine, are labeled in the accompanying text located below the image. The mainspring in the elbow mechanism is a spiral torsion spring similar to the mainspring found in watches and spring-driven clocks. According to Paré's text, it must be made of tempered steel and three feet or more in length.[35] When describing the curve

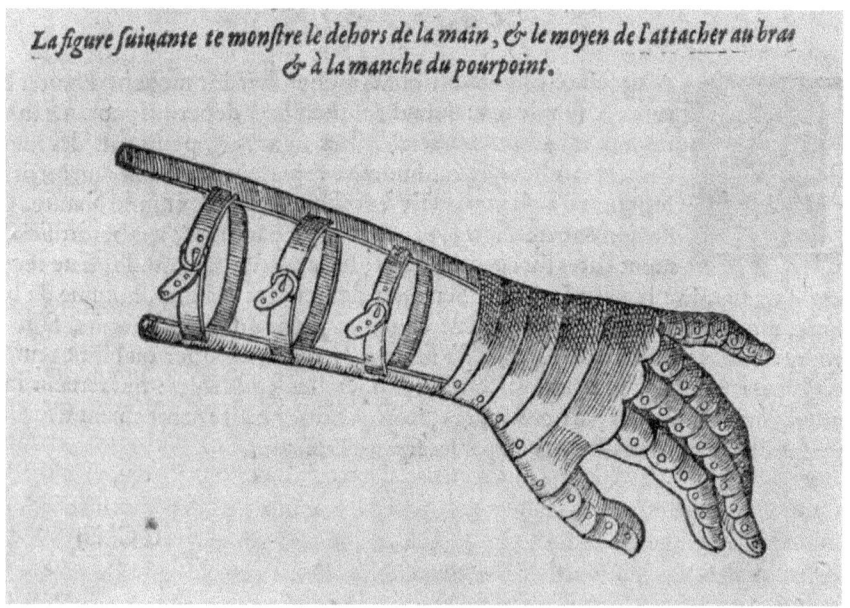

6.2 Artificial hand with strap fastenings in Ambroise Paré, *Les Oeuvres* (Paris, 1614), 902 (detail).

Prosthetic technology on the move 217

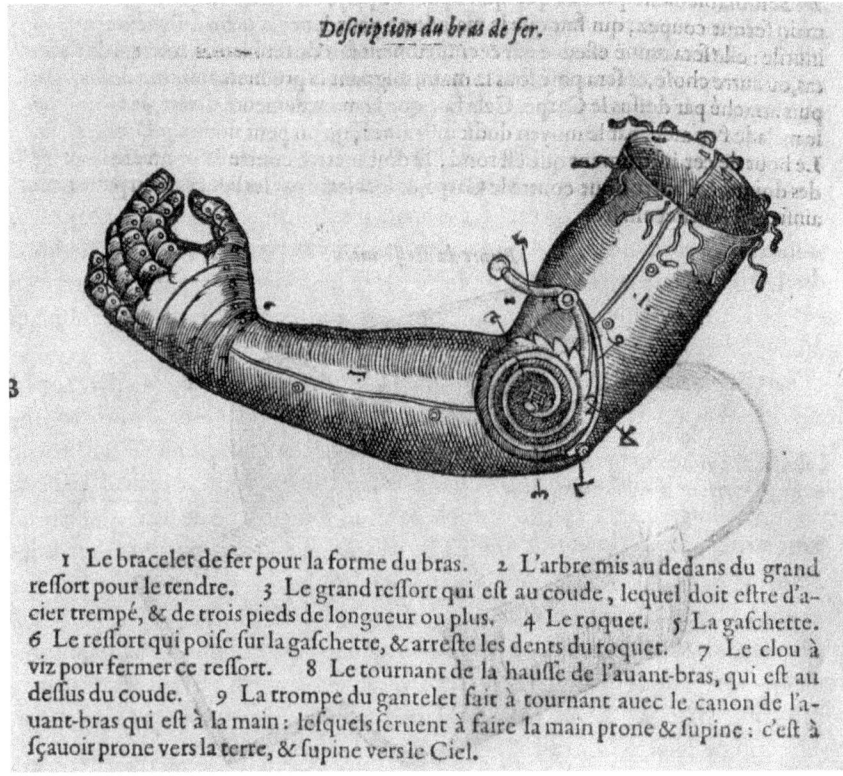

6.3 Artificial arm in Ambroise Paré, *Les Oeuvres* (Paris, 1614), 903 (detail).

of the wrist, Paré's consultant referred to the gauntlet (*gantelet*), the base of which should be placed at an angle with the forearm. The woodcuts display technical elements relevant to the practices of multiple craft groups.

Extant artifacts and knowledge of craft production shed much-needed light on the ways in which these designs related to actual practices of making artificial hands.[36] As our analysis of artifacts in Chapter 5 revealed, no single craft group had a monopoly on their production. The variety of crafts represented in the technical terms of Paré's text supports this evidence. Paré's reliance on the locksmith to provide the designs for Chapter XII also mirrors the need for an artisan's specialized technical knowledge to devise the precise mechanical layouts of these objects as custom orders. Moreover, the expensive materials and cutting-edge technology evoked in the woodcuts and their explanatory text underline that these were objects only the surgeon's wealthy patients could afford. We can see reflected in Chapter XII, then, the resourcefulness, flexibility, technical sophistication, and luxury characteristic of mechanical limb production in the early modern period.

Evidence from material culture provides a general setting in which to place Chapter XII of Paré's book. Comparing the mechanical hand woodcut systematically to an early modern artifact anchors the petit Lorrain's designs more firmly in workshop production. The internal mechanisms of the iron hand in *Les Oeuvres* are strikingly similar to those of the sixteenth-century Kassel Hand, a right hand prosthesis in the collections of the Staatliche Museen Kassel (figure 6.4).[37] The precise date of the artifact's creation has not been fixed; it could predate Paré's original 1575 publication by seventy years, or it could be directly contemporary to it. As we have seen, its four functioning fingers can be locked individually in seven different positions, and released by pulling a switch located on the wrist beneath the palm.

The basic principle of flexion and extension through toothed wheels, pawls, and release switches is shared by most extant hand prostheses. However, the designs of the Y-shaped lever acting on four mounted pawls are extraordinarily similar in the Kassel Hand and Paré's woodcut. In both the woodcut and the artifact, the fingers are attached at their bases to four toothed wheels that sit on a common axis (figures 6.1, 6.5–6.6). The wearer operates the mechanisms from the outside by using his or her other hand to push the fingers downward into the desired position. As each wheel turns, it moves against a pawl, or what Paré's text labels a *petite gaschette*, a flat pivoted lever which catches on the teeth and prevents the wheel from rolling. The four pawls are mounted on bases, which Paré's consultant termed *estoqueaux*, that hold the pawls. In Paré's woodcut these bases have stopping pins, which keep the pawls from pivoting too far in one direction. The Kassel Hand has two pairs of flat springs bolted between the mounted pawls. These serve the same purpose by applying downward pressure to the proximal end of each pawl. Both artifact and woodcut have a large Y-shaped lever connected to the external release button. Paré's consultant referred to this as *la grande gaschette*, or the main lever, which acts on the four pawls in order to release the toothed wheels and open the fingers. In the Kassel Hand, this Y-shaped main lever consists of two parts: a vertical shaft that extends from the release trigger on the exterior of the wrist through the interior of the hand's shell; and a solid triangular plate with a wedge-like thickness that stretches horizontally from the vertical shaft of the main lever to just beneath the proximal ends of the pawls. The release trigger, once pressed, acts on the vertical shaft of the main lever, which pushes the solid triangular plate forward. The wedge-like body of the plate moves beneath the ends of all four pawls at once and forces them upward, creating a controlled seesaw motion of the pawls that removes pressure from the toothed wheels and allows the fingers to move freely again.

Yet though artifact and woodcut share comparable internal layouts, they ultimately present different versions of a mechanical hand. The Kassel Hand has a solid sheet-metal exterior and barrel fingers that flex only at their base (figure 6.4). The woodcut displays a prosthesis with an exterior made up almost

Prosthetic technology on the move 219

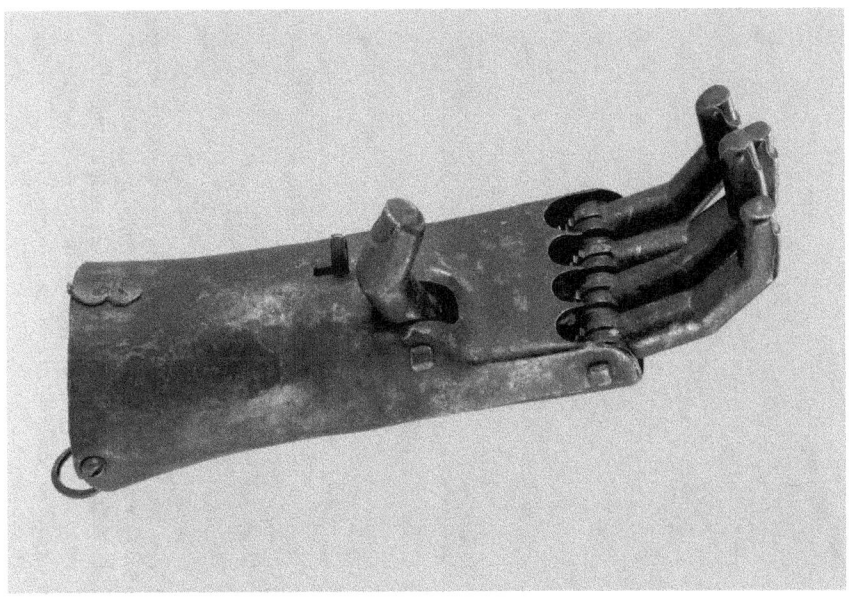

6.4 Kassel Hand, right hand prosthesis, sixteenth century. Wrought iron, L. 23.5 cm. Inv. Nr. KP B XIV.32. Museumslandschaft Hessen Kassel.

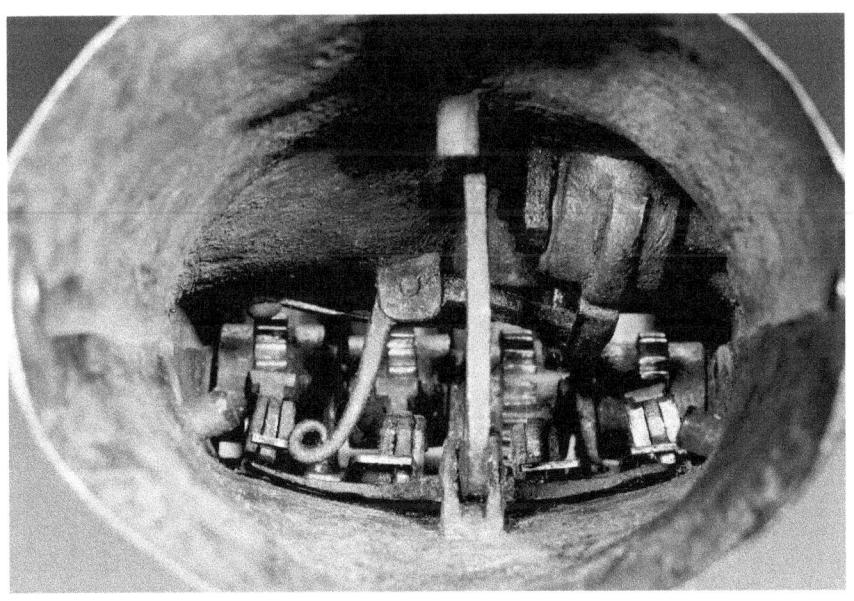

6.5 Internal mechanisms of Kassel Hand, right hand prosthesis, sixteenth century. Wrought iron, L. 23.5 cm. Inv. Nr. KP B XIV.32. Museumslandschaft Hessen Kassel.

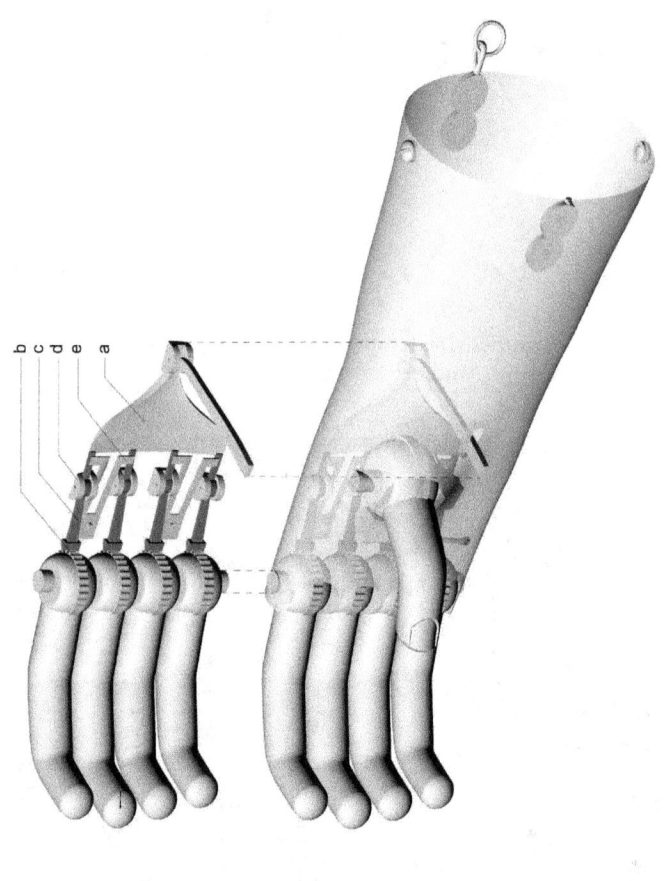

6.6 Diagram of Kassel Hand mechanisms: four fingers currently functioning. a. Y-shaped main lever consisting of two parts: a vertical shaft that extends from the release trigger on the exterior of the wrist through the interior of the hand's shell; and a solid triangular plate of wedge-like thickness that stretches horizontally to just beneath the proximal ends of the pawls. b. Toothed wheel (one of four) that rotates forward and backward to flex or extend the corresponding finger. c. Pawl (one of four) that catches in the grooves of the toothed wheel. d. Base on which the pawl is mounted (one of four) that allows the pawl to pivot. e. Flat spring pair (one of two) that prevents the pawls from pivoting too far in one direction by applying downward force.

entirely of riveted metal strips, similar to a gauntlet in a suit of armor. The Kassel Hand, with its articulated thumb (figure 6.7), is also technically more complex. These differences in construction would not only have made a visual difference, but could also have resulted in different weights, forms of movement, and cleaning or preservative regimens. The creation of the two hands would also have called for different materials and required different kinds of skills. The presence of strong similarities alongside startling differences that we see in the Kassel Hand and Paré's woodcut is characteristic of the diversity found among surviving artifacts of mechanical hands and arms.

A side-by-side comparison between Paré's woodcut and the Kassel Hand demonstrates that the printed image reflected existing early modern trends in prosthetic limb technology. The petit Lorrain's design aligns with the mechanisms of extant artifacts. The importance of this connection between print and artifact for our understanding of Paré's chapter on artificial limbs cannot be overstated. As previous studies have shown, illustrations of instruments in surgical treatises could convey fantasy theories or serve simply decorative functions with little practical meaning.[38] The Kassel Hand shows that Paré's woodcut was not simply a curious image: the design represented a viable way to create a moving hand prosthesis. The Kassel Hand also provides an example of how the petit Lorrain's design might appear in motion, and even offers insight into the relative ease or difficulty of operating an object with a similar mechanical layout.

As a workable model, the woodcut's ability to convey the petit Lorrain's designs to readers outside of France holds significance for the study of technical knowledge transmission, and for our broader understanding of relationships among knowledge, text, and image in the early modern period. The artifact comparison stirs a new set of questions about the woodcut's function in early modern surgical treatises. It provides a compelling workshop context with which to consider whether or not the transmission of the petit Lorrain's designs could feasibly have been achieved. The role of craft production in the initial creation of the image allows us to consider its purpose in Paré's surgical treatise from the perspective of an artisan—such as a locksmith or clockmaker. Put simply, if the mechanical hand design in Chapter XII came from one artisan's workshop, what might have happened when a reader brought the printed image into another?

Craft knowledge in motion

In several early modern crafts, making or copying drawn designs was a core practice, vital to creating objects.[39] Drawings passed down from master to apprentice in the workshop could be exact patterns to replicate precisely. Very few survive in manuscript form. Published models were often decorative

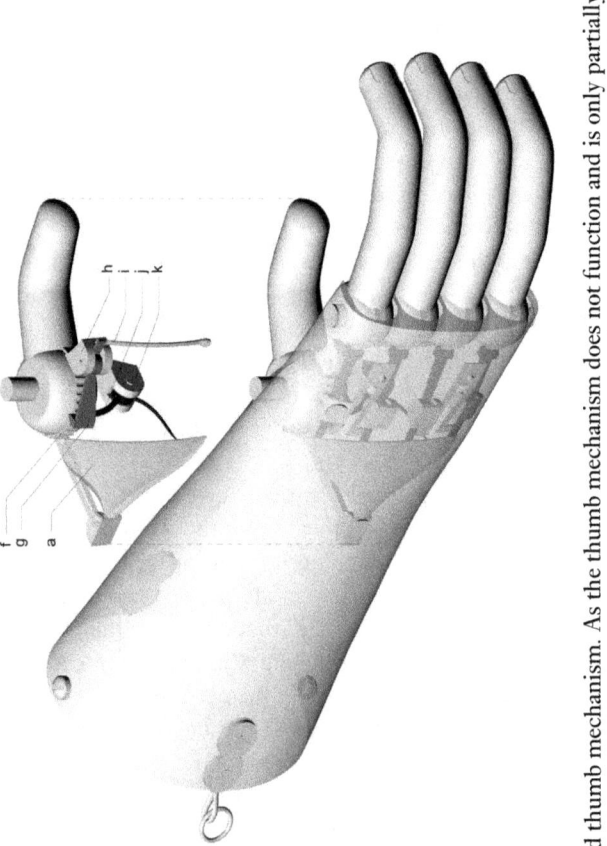

6.7 Diagram of Kassel Hand thumb mechanism. As the thumb mechanism does not function and is only partially visible, this speculative explanation is based on what is observable and an analysis of the other fingers. f. Toothed wheel that rotates forward and backward to flex or extend the thumb. g. Pawl, in the form of a curved tab, that catches in the grooves of the toothed wheel. h. Base on which the pawl is mounted that allows it to pivot. i. Curved flat spring that prevents the pawl from pivoting too far in one direction. j. Curled thumb lever that, when activated, presses on the pawl to release the toothed wheel. k. Mount for curled lever which allows it to pivot. a. Y-shaped main lever consisting of two parts: a vertical shaft that extends from the release trigger on the wrist's exterior through the interior of the hand's shell; and a solid triangular plate of wedge-like thickness that stretches horizontally to just beneath the curly end of the thumb lever. This configuration would suggest that when the thumb functioned, activating Y-shaped main lever (a) pushed the triangular plate forward beneath thumb lever (j) and caused it to pivot, applying pressure on pawl (g) to release toothed wheel (f).

patterns rather than working diagrams.[40] The images of prosthetic limbs that appear in Paré's *Oeuvres* represent a distinctive compromise: neither standard surgical knowledge nor standard craft practice. The petit Lorrain was reluctant to share his design of the mechanical layout of an iron hand, and the resulting woodcut does not offer such intimate, even secret, detail. It is a schematic model offering a set of ideas for the artisan posed with the challenge of making a mechanical limb.

According to the preface to Chapter XII, Paré attempted to document the petit Lorrain's method of making mechanical limbs so that he could commission them from other artisans in the future. By publishing the locksmith's designs, the surgeon was recording and disseminating craft knowledge rather than producing it himself. Extant artifacts that predate *Les Oeuvres* by several decades make this abundantly clear.[41] His efforts to codify this craft knowledge in written form fit within a broad early modern trend to transmit hands-on practices into print in diverse forms, including theoretical treatises on technical professions, practical manuals, and books of secrets.[42] Paré's endeavor to obtain designs from a craftsman focused exclusively on the production of mechanical limbs. In contrast to the other kinds of prostheses in Book XXII, such as leather ears and painted eyes, these devices were beyond the surgeon's ability to design or construct. All Paré needed was to know how to commission them. The language other authors used shows that they shared this perspective. When referring to Paré's instructions on artificial legs and hands, Fabry von Hilden uses the phrase "wie man ... anfertigen lassen ... soll" ("how one is to have made" or "how one should have made").[43] Fabry's language clarifies that Paré's chapter teaches diligent surgeons how to *have prostheses made*, rather than how to *make prostheses*.

Paré's intention to commission prostheses using the designs in Chapter XII raises questions that extend beyond text and image, and into the relationship between written and tacit knowledge—the oral information passed down from master to apprentice, the unspoken tricks learned from years of experience, the materials or techniques kept secret to protect business.[44] The way in which Paré attempted to codify and share prosthesis designs reveals how he thought about craft knowledge and its ability to travel. He believed the combination of word and image would give him and others the power to communicate with artisans. Paré's work was primarily written for medical practitioners—particularly surgeons and barber-surgeons who could not read Latin. By using the locksmith's words in a surgical text, Paré was furnishing surgeons with a vocabulary that would facilitate dialogue with the artisans he advised his readers to consult, transforming the surgeon into a mediator between patients and artisans. For surgeons, including Paré himself, the mechanical hand woodcut and its explanatory text served as an early modern way to black box—that is, to bypass the technical details of—prosthetic limb technology.[45] The surgeon did not need to know how or why the mechanisms of the design worked—or even be able to identify the mechanisms themselves. In theory, the surgeon only needed to show the image to the artisan and read the accompanying text aloud in order to commission an artificial hand.

It would be easy to dismiss Paré as an optimist. For the most part, the translation of *Les Oeuvres* out of the French vernacular removed the local detail of Chapter XII. This is particularly evident in the Latin and German translations published in Frankfurt in the quarter century following the success of the first French edition. Paré's chapter on artificial limbs changed in two crucial ways as it traveled to the Holy Roman Empire. First, due to choices made by the translators in rendering Paré's words, the details the author provided about which artisans could be consulted to make prostheses disappeared from the preface. In the German translation by Peter Uffenbach, Paré's reasoning for obtaining the petit Lorrain's designs was "so that afterwards in case of necessity I could have others made accordingly."[46] The only artisan who appears is the petit Lorrain, whom the German translation refers to as a "blacksmith" (*einem Schmiedt*) experienced in these matters rather than as a locksmith.[47] The Latin edition similarly calls the petit Lorrain a "most ingenious smith" (*ingeniosissimo fabro ferrario*).[48] Paré's original explanation about obtaining the vocabulary and images so that any locksmith or clockmaker could understand is absent from both the Latin and German editions.

The second major change—and by far the more significant—was the omission of explanatory text for the mechanical limbs, which left the illustrations even barer and more decontextualized. The images themselves were preserved in detail, including the numbering of individual components. The technical terms that corresponded with the numbers were initially dropped in the first Latin translation of *Les Oeuvres*, supervised by Jacques Guillemeau (1550–1613), a pupil of Paré, and published in Paris in 1582.[49] Chapter XII of the Latin translation published by a German print shop in Frankfurt a little more than a decade later is nearly identical to it.[50] In its treatment of the explanatory text, the German translation issued by the same print shop followed the example of its Latin predecessor.[51] The Holy Roman Empire was not the only place in which the petit Lorrain's technical terms disappeared. The English translation of 1634 also printed the mechanical limb woodcuts without the corresponding text.[52] Paré's original preface indicated that the woodcuts should be shown to an artisan, who could understand the designs by seeing the image and reading the accompanying text. Yet in the vast majority of translated editions, half of Paré's intended formula for communicating this craft knowledge was missing from the page.

At first glance, Chapter XII's transformation in Latin, German, and English editions might appear to be simply the stripping away of local detail. However, the editions issued from Dutch print shops suggest a more complicated and contingent course of textual transmission. Historians of science have examined knowledge-making processes in which local knowledge is rendered universal.[53] From this perspective, if the petit Lorrain's technical terms were too specific to have universal application, then their omission could be understood as an attempt to make Chapter XII legible to a wider European audience. After all, the mechanical hand, arm, and leg designs are the only three woodcuts in all of Book XXII accompanied by technical jargon—and they were the only ones whose explanatory text seemed to experience difficulty traveling. The accompanying text of the other images uses general description, such as a wooden leg prosthesis whose components are identified simply as a cushion on which to rest the patient's stump, and buckles with which to secure the leg.[54] Yet Dutch editions reveal that the petit Lorrain's vernacular, technical terminology was not too local to travel, even if it did not in most cases. The preface to the first Dutch translation, published in Dordrecht in 1592, retains Paré's allusion to the petit Lorrain as a locksmith (*Slotmaker*), and repeats his intention to present a design understandable to every locksmith and clockmaker (*elck Horologimaker ende Slotmaker*). The Dutch translation also includes explanatory text on all three woodcuts of mechanical devices.[55] A translation of French technical jargon into another vernacular language, and even into Latin, was possible.[56] How, then, can we account for the inclusion and exclusion of the explanatory text in the changing forms of Chapter XII when Paré considered it so important to provide the petit Lorrain's terminology in his original edition?

In large part, the forms that translated editions of Chapter XII took outside of France were contingent upon which version of Paré's work the print shop used as a model: the French vernacular (Paris, 1585), the Latin (Paris, 1582), or a combination of both. On its very title page, the Dutch translation announces that it is based on the so-called fourth French edition, published in Paris in 1585.[57] In imitation of this edition, the book of artificial body parts appears as Book XXIII rather than Book XXII, and it retains the explanatory text of Chapter XII in its entirety. By contrast, the Latin edition published in Frankfurt in 1594 is a self-proclaimed reprint of Jacques Guillemeau's Latin translation of 1582. Following Guillemeau's edition, the book of prostheses remains Book XXII, and Chapter XII drops the explanatory text from the mechanical limbs. The first German translation does the same.[58] Rather than follow one model, the first English translation is a hybrid, "translated out of Latin and compared with the French."[59] The translator, Thomas Johnson (d. 1644), used Guillemeau's Latin edition for the bulk of the treatise. Accordingly, Chapter XII omits the explanatory text for the mechanical limb woodcuts. However, after the manner of the vernacular French edition, the book of prostheses appears as Book XXIII. The choices made in these early editions of Paré issued by Dutch, German, and English print shops influenced the way Chapter XII continued to be printed in these different areas of Europe.

The omission of explanatory text for the mechanical hand woodcut in most translated editions of Chapter XII, then, largely hinged on the decision to drop the petit Lorrain's technical jargon in the first Latin translation of 1582. Isabelle Pantin's work on early modern translation describes this edition as "almost a new version" of *Les Oeuvres*, its translation out of the vernacular signaling a change in the role and envisioned reception of the treatise.[60] The alterations to Chapter XII in Guillemeau's edition—which consequently disrupted Paré's formula of text and image to communicate with artisans—point to the significance of multiple audiences for Paré's work. The intended audience for the first Latin translation transformed the function of the explanatory text. The mechanical designs in Chapter XII were part of a vernacular craft, and rendering the text into Latin would not have helped most craftsmen to better understand the images. It is possible that Guillemeau opted to omit the petit Lorrain's terminology rather than offer a translation because it would have been unintelligible to both Latinate and vernacular audiences: learned readers would not understand the mechanisms; craftsmen would not understand Latin.

The interests of Latinate audiences could change over time. Nearly a century after the publication of Guillemeau's edition, an engraved copy of Paré's woodcut image appeared in Jan Baptist van Lamzweerde's *Appendix* (Leiden, 1693) with a Latin translation of the technical jargon. By that time, learned readers were interested in and familiar with technical descriptions of scientific apparatus and its uses from authors such as Robert Hooke, Isaac Newton, and Antoni van Leeuwenhoek. In Lamzweerde's publication, the explanatory text for the petit Lorrain's mechanical hand was directed at the educated and curious medical reader, not a master locksmith looking at encoded instructions.

Paré had a particular vernacular viewership in mind for the petit Lorrain's designs. His stated intention for the mechanical limb woodcuts and their explanatory text was for readers to show them to craftsmen. Artisans from craft groups that worked with spring-driven mechanisms were a crucial audience for Chapter XII—a necessary audience, if the designs were to be used to commission prostheses. In order to explore the mechanical hand woodcut's capacity to communicate the technical information of the petit Lorrain's design, it is essential to consider the various forms of the chapter from the perspective of a master craftsman. As we will see, with and without explanatory text, and even with and without printed errors, the petit Lorrain's schematic diagram for the internal mechanisms of an iron hand could have had practical uses for the artisan.

Many historians have been skeptical of the printing press's impact on the transfer of craft techniques. Stephan Epstein, for instance, has stated that "published, 'disembodied' technical knowledge did not disseminate well."[61] Manuals contained either too little or too much of the information needed for a task, and often omitted practitioners' tricks. Apprenticeship was essential for the transfer of technical knowledge because most craft knowledge was tacit, learned as one was socialized into a craft, and it took many years of practice to acquire and hone such skills.[62] The distinction to be made when discussing Paré's woodcuts, however, is that there was no craft group that specialized in mechanical prostheses or underwent apprenticeship to become prosthesis-makers. Chapter XII addressed artisans from different craft groups who were applying their skills in creative ways to carry out the custom orders of amputee-patrons. Even when the explanatory text was present in an edition, it simply conveyed sets of relationships between the components, using specialized terms for each component, rather than offering explanations of how the components were made or how they worked. Epstein argued that the nature of craft learning limited the utility of print to communicate technical knowledge. Yet years of practical experience would have made Paré's woodcut legible to artisans familiar with spring-driven mechanisms. To make sense of the petit Lorrain's design, a master craftsman needed some prior understanding of the mechanical relationships the image presented.

The picture did not have to convey precise instructions to be useful.[63] It rendered the petit Lorrain's specific production process abstract and the particular objects that he made general.[64] Viewing it evoked knowledge of mechanical relationships. For a talented artisan in one of the craft groups that worked with mechanisms (locksmiths, gunsmiths, clockmakers, and so forth), the image could call to mind specialized knowledge required to achieve flexion and extension in an artificial hand. Whereas a general viewer might see an interesting puzzle, an experienced artisan viewing the woodcut could use his knowledge of mechanisms to supply meaningful connections between components, making sense of the device as a whole by intuiting patterns of mechanical principles represented on the page. The details involved in bringing those relationships into being once they were suggested were up to the individual craftsman. Craft knowledge, as Pamela Smith argues, required constant experimentation, investigation, and adaptation to changing conditions.[65] Paré's woodcut evoked mechanical possibilities. The schematic diagram was one way to spark the imagination of a craftsman who had never made a mechanical limb—a taking-off point rather than a recipe to be copied with precision. The result would not be a duplication of the objects crafted in the petit Lorrain's workshop, but rather a distinctive adaptation of the ideas presented in the petit Lorrain's design.

The presence of numbers within the woodcut image underlines its potential to communicate technical knowledge across various editions and translations of Paré's *Oeuvres*. Copies of the original woodcut that appeared in translated editions always included numbers, despite the omission of the explanatory text with which the numbers were intended to correspond (figure 6.8). The consistent inclusion of numbers could suggest that translators, artists, editors,

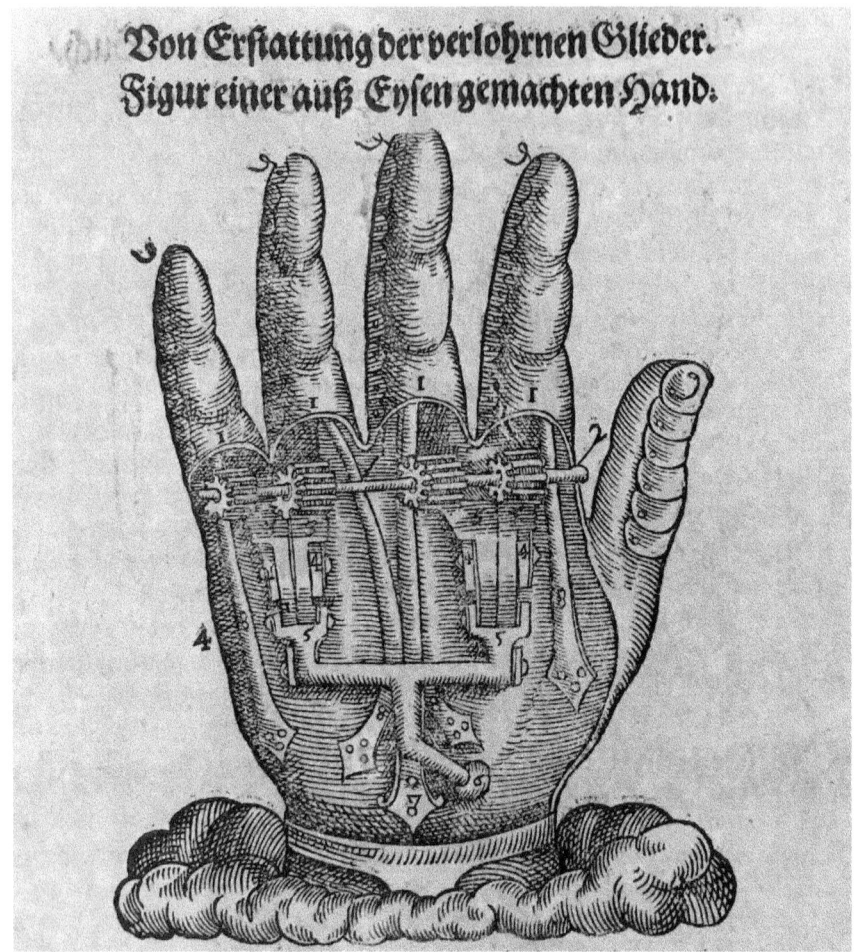

6.8 Mechanical hand in Ambroise Paré, *Wund-Artzney* (Frankfurt am Main, 1635), 749 (detail).

and printers intended to preserve the practical dimension of the image for readers who chose to follow Paré's example and consult with craftsmen. After all, the numbers on their own would have guided the knowledgeable viewer's eyes through the image in a way that signaled implicit relationships between individual components. The numbers tell a story (figure 6.9). Ones point to the wheels at the base of the fingers. Below, a two directs the eyes to the axis on which the wheels sit. Threes mark short levers that touch the wheels; fours identify the bases on which the short levers are mounted. Two fives draw the eyes from the ends of a Y-shaped lever, situated just below the fours, to a shaft that leads to a round button marked with the number six. In a nearly straight

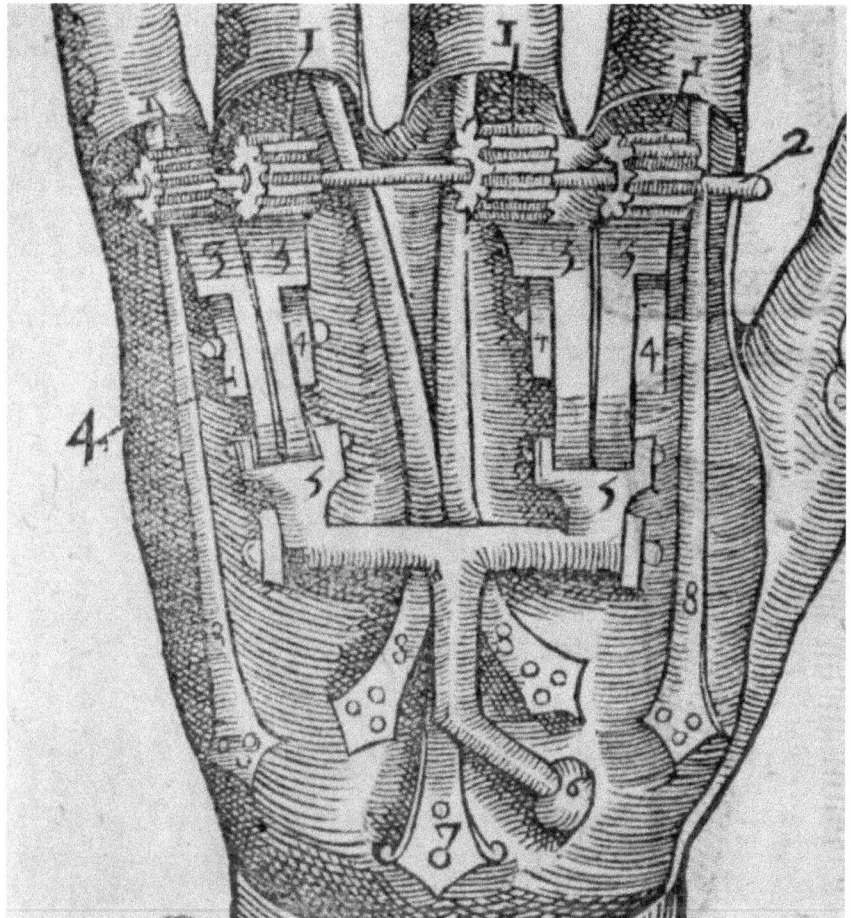

6.9 Artificial hand mechanisms in Ambroise Paré, *Les Oeuvres* (Paris, 1614), 902 (detail).

line down the page, numbers one through six have walked us through the lock and release mechanism of the hand in a logical order, putting each component in a coherent relationship with the numbers that come before and after it.

The remaining numbers then draw the viewer's attention back up the page: from the release button, the viewer's eyes move to seven, the base of the mainspring. Close above are eights that fan out in a V-shape along four springs, and guide the eyes upward through each of the four fingers. At the tip of each finger is a nine, indicating the looped pattern that textures the exterior of the hand (figure 6.1). From seven to nine, the order of the components emphasizes that the fingers are fully articulated. The numbers seven and eight indicate springs running through each finger, while nine draws attention to overlapping plates

230   *The malleable body*

recognizable to metalworkers as a technique used to enable flexibility. The numbers help viewers make necessary connections as their eyes move around the page.

Still, a problem remains. One telling error recurs in the dissemination of the woodcut, an error that shows that translators, editors, artists, and printers did not understand—or at least fully understand—the way the components worked. In the French edition, the explanatory text clearly states there are four little *gaschettes*, or pawls mounted on bases; but in many versions of the woodcut, at least one of the four is mislabeled (table 6.1). The confusion may trace back to the lines of the artists and cutters who worked on the original woodblock for the first edition of *Les Oeuvres*, which appeared in 1575. A line of shading runs through the top of the threes within the little *gaschettes*. The resultant pooling of ink along this line in prints obfuscates the top half of the number carved into each *gaschette*, creating the impression of a five in two of the four components. The 1579 edition displays the same problem—at

Table 6.1 Les petites gaschettes

	Year	Location	Language	gaschette	gaschette	gaschette	gaschette
1	1575	Paris	French	3	3	3	3
2	1579	Paris	French	3	3	3	3
3	1582	Paris	Latin	3	3	3	3
4	1585	Paris	French	3	3	3	3
5	1592	Dordrecht	Dutch	3	3	3?	3
6	1594	Frankfurt am Main	Latin	3	3	?	5
7	1601	Frankfurt am Main	German	3	3	?	?
8	1612	Frankfurt am Main	Latin	3	3	5?	5
9	1614	Paris	French	3	3	3	3
10	1634	London	English	4	3 (inverted)	3 (inverted)	3 (inverted)
11	1635	Frankfurt am Main	German	3	3	5	5?
12	1636	Amsterdam	Dutch	3	3	3	3
13	1649	London	English	4	3 (inverted)	3 (inverted)	3 (inverted)
14	1693	Leiden	Latin	3	3	3	3

Notes: This table lists the numbering of the four *petites gaschettes* within images of the mechanical hand design from a sampling of printed works. The component numbers appear as they do on the page, from left to right.

Sources: 1) Paré, *Les Oeuvres* (1575), 724; 2) Paré, *Les Oeuvres* (1579), 839; 3) Paré, *Opera Ambrosii Parei* (1582), 668; 4) Paré, *Les Oeuvres* (1585), 916; 5) Paré, *De chirurgie* (1592), 841; 6) Paré, *Opera Chirurgica* (1594), 656; 7) Paré, *Wund-Artzney* (1601), 724; 8) Paré, *Opera Chirurgica* (1612), 493; 9) Paré, *Les Oeuvres* (1614), 902; 10) Paré, *Workes* (1634), 881; 11) Paré, *Wund-Artzney* (1635), 748; 12) Paré, *De chirurgie* (1636), 701; 13) Paré, *Workes* (1649), 586; 14) Lamzweerde, *Appendix*, Tab. 8.

first glance it appears that one of the small *gaschettes* is labeled five instead of three. The ambiguity in the first two vernacular editions is less apparent in the first Latin translation (Paris, 1582), which printed the image from the same block but clearly numbers the little *gaschettes* as threes. But the Latin translation printed in Frankfurt in 1594, although a self-proclaimed reproduction of Guillemeau's 1582 edition, did not accurately copy the numbering of the parts in the image. Instead, only two of the four small *gaschettes* are clearly numbered correctly. The mistake was repeated in the German translation issued from the same shop a few years later. In fact, the version of the mechanical hand image—with its numbering error—that circulated in the Holy Roman Empire was consistent across several Latin and German translations because the shop printing them reused the same woodblock (figure 6.8).[66] Bafflingly, the first English translations, published in 1634 and 1649, erroneously number one of the little *gaschettes* as four. For about a century, ordinary readers were not expected to understand the woodcut, and the mislabeled *gaschette* suggests that many involved in printing it—not to mention those reading it—did not.

It is impossible to know with absolute certainty whether or not a mislabeled *gaschette* would confound an artisan looking at the woodcut. However, an approach that considers the years of experience and specialized training characteristic of workshop practices provides one way to divine what an early modern craftsman's response might have been. As no more than half of the small *gaschettes* were mislabeled in any given edition (see table 6.1), the sequential chain of numbers in the lock and release mechanism always remained intact for at least two fingers, usually three, of the mechanical hand (the thumb was not articulated). A craftsman only needed to notice the pattern—the implied relationship between components—once for the woodcut to prompt his particular knowledge of mechanisms as described above. A recalibration of what scholars expect the woodcut to successfully convey is crucial here. We must not envision the woodcut as a blueprint to be copied precisely. Even if, for instance, a master locksmith looking at the 1635 German edition (figure 6.8) did not assume that the mislabeled *gaschette* in the index finger was a printer's error, and instead believed that he did not fully understand how that particular part of the hand operated, he could shrug his shoulders and then turn to creating the prosthesis he envisioned. His vision probably would spring from the mechanical principles recalled after looking at the woodcut—the principles he detected in the chain of components in the ring finger and the little finger, whose small *gaschettes* are clearly and correctly labeled, and whose operations he could fully understand. One mislabeled *gaschette* was probably not serious enough to destroy the logical relationships between components for the metalworker's eye, or disrupt the woodcut's ability to inspire the artisan.

The woodcut of the petit Lorrain's mechanical hand served multiple purposes in Paré's book of prostheses: it was interesting for readers to look at, its complexity and the story of its acquisition contributed to an impressive image of the author as an avid learner and possessor of information, and it could be used as a base model to present to a craftsman when commissioning a prosthesis. All of these functions remained intact in the German translations; the woodcut was not simply reduced to a curious illustration when it appeared without explanatory text. This of course does not mean that German surgeons were actually lugging Paré's hefty tome around the marketplace to negotiate commissions for artificial limbs in the shops of locksmiths and clockmakers. In fact, there is no indication that they became involved in procuring mechanical hands for patients. But with the petit Lorrain's design, they could have. The woodcut presents a schematic diagram that was largely inaccessible to ordinary readers—with or without the accompanying text. Yet for the trained eye of the artisan, the image contained useful suggestions of mechanical relationships for the design of an artificial limb. Indeed, a French locksmith treatise of 1627, entitled *La fidelle ouverture de l'art de serrurier*, includes a chapter on mechanical limbs that demonstrates just this. The chapter begins by acknowledging Paré's treatise, and then presents a modified version of the petit Lorrain's mechanical hand that features two pairs of moveable fingers.[67] The design is distinctly different from the petit Lorrain's, yet the corresponding images clearly play on those appearing in Paré's *Oeuvres*. The author, Mathurin Jousse (1575–1645), a master locksmith who published treatises on architecture and carpentry among other technical subjects, offers an example of an artisan who was not only exposed to Paré's chapter on artificial limbs, but also displayed a creative response to the petit Lorrain's mechanical layout. The flexible nature of mechanical limb production in early modern Europe created opportunities for master craftsmen to apply their specialized skills to create prostheses. In this context, the technical information conveyed by the mechanical hand woodcut in Paré's *Oeuvres* had the potential for boundless adaptation, its utility to artisans contained not in the possibility for exact replication, but rather in its capacity to spark the imaginations of artisans from diverse craft groups.

The surgeon as intermediary

The image of the internal mechanisms of an iron hand appearing in Ambroise Paré's *Oeuvres* contains layers of meaning that were accessible in different ways and in varying degrees to those who created it, published it, and viewed it for over a century. The woodcut displayed the design of a Parisian locksmith who rendered an intricate workshop practice into a broad schematic representation that communicated information while safeguarding his precise process of production. Paré, surgeon and author, obtained an image and text he could use to commission prostheses for future patients, and that he could circulate through print to share with other medical practitioners. The majority of surgeons and general viewers of the image, which appeared in multiple editions of Paré's *Oeuvres* in various languages in various lands through the late sixteenth and seventeenth centuries, likely gazed on it with curiosity, without understanding the technical knowledge contained in it; some may have even brought the image to artisans in order to facilitate the commissioning of an artificial limb. Master craftsmen of different craft groups, by contrast, could have grasped the main mechanical relationships appearing in the image by applying their specialized knowledge, and were capable of considering the petit Lorrain's suggestions in their own designs. Thus, the mechanical hand woodcut reveals a complex story about the creation, control, and transmission of technical knowledge in early modern Europe. Exploring this story offers insights into issues far broader than the history of Paré's surgical writings.

One area of insight involves the communication of technical knowledge. This study of the mechanical limb woodcuts in Paré's *Oeuvres* provides a vision of technical knowledge transfer that was purposely adaptable to the skills of multiple craft groups. Master craftsmen constituted a distinct audience for Paré's chapter on artificial limbs. Their years of experience predisposed them to recognize mechanical relationships within the petit Lorrain's design for a prosthetic hand, and the adaptable character of workshop environments and the nature of mechanical limb production made the design potentially useful for them. Rather than a formula to be replicated exactly, the petit Lorrain's designs presented a jumping-off point for artisans tasked with creating an artificial limb. This utility points to a form of technical knowledge transmission through print that was versatile and flexible.

This analysis of the potential utility of Paré's woodcut is made possible only by examining the evidence of material culture. Extant artifacts of prostheses reveal that creativity and improvisation characterized mechanical limb production in the sixteenth and seventeenth centuries. A comparison between the mechanical layout of the petit Lorrain's prosthetic hand design and the internal mechanisms of the sixteenth-century Kassel Hand particularly grounds Paré's woodcut in ongoing practices of creating prosthetic technology in this period. Within the context of craft workshops and the evidence of artifacts, assessing the fluidity of the mechanical hand woodcut in its legibility to multiple craft groups is a more accurate way to measure the potential success of transferring knowledge than its ability for duplication. The case of mechanical limbs raises the question not only of what other kinds of early modern technology might be studied from a similar perspective, but also of what other ways we might use material culture to reassess well-known printed sources.

A second area of insight relates to the history of prosthetic technology and surgery. The transmission of Paré's *Oeuvres* supports the conclusion that mechanical limbs remained squarely in the domain of artisans in the early modern period. Paré's publication did not challenge or significantly alter artisans' control over the design and production of mechanical limbs. Indeed, scholarship on early twentieth-century prosthetic technology suggests that artificial limb design remained an artisanal undertaking for centuries.[68] Prosthetic technology, then, developed along a remarkably different arc than did other examples of early modern collaborations between authors of printed texts and practitioners of technical crafts, including navigation and architecture. An examination of Paré's text provides some explanation for this development. Paré did not attempt to master the information needed to fabricate a limb, or even claim to comprehend the petit Lorrain's design in his publication. His treatise made no effort to render the images and technical jargon of the explanatory text legible to a general audience. In consequence, surgeons reading Paré's *Oeuvres* did not understand the design, and could not contribute alterations to the design or suggest additional devices of their own. Master craftsmen, by contrast, were capable of both.

The mechanical hand woodcut of *Les Oeuvres*, which circulated throughout Europe in multiple editions and translations for over a century, began with a conversation between Ambroise Paré and a Parisian locksmith. What can we make of the relationship between Paré and the petit Lorrain? The interaction Paré described in his chapter preface falls short of a true "trading zone": there was no reciprocal exchange of skills and knowledge, only the surgeon entreating the artisan for copies and explanations of his designs.[69] To some extent, Chapter XII reveals Paré's ambitions to become a "facilitator of knowledge."[70] In his attempt to provide general readers schematic designs to show to an artisan, the woodcuts and explanatory text in his chapter on artificial limbs demonstrate his efforts to acquire knowledge that could be used to mediate, as Eric H. Ash has written, "between a body of specialized skills and information on the one hand and the patron who required and paid for it on the other."[71] The vital link between Paré's professional aspirations and the petit Lorrain's designs was, of course, the amputee-patron. If artisans remained in control of prosthetic technology, amputee-patrons remained in control of its commissioning and the collaborative role this entailed.

Notes

1 Paré, *Les Oeuvres* (1575), 724–725. My references and quotations from the French are drawn from the second edition: Paré, *Les Oeuvres* (1579).
2 Paré, *Les Oeuvres* (1579), 838: "representent les mouvements volontaires, de tant pres qu'il est possible à l'art ensuivre nature."

3 Ibid.: "i'ay par grande priere recouvert d'un nommé le petit Lorrain, Serrurier demeurant à Paris, homme de bon esprit."
4 Ibid.: "les noms & explication de chacune partie desdits pourtraicts, faite en propres termes & mots de l'artisan."
5 Ibid.: "à fin que chacun Serrurier ou horologeur les puisse bien entendre, & faire bras ou iambes artificielles semblables."
6 On gunpowder: DeVries, "Military Surgical Practice," 131–146; Lindemann, *Medicine and Society*, 132.
7 E.g., Berriot-Salvadore and Mironneau, *Ambroise Paré*. Paré has also been studied for his book on monsters and prodigies: Huet, "Monstrous Medicine."
8 On Benhamou's analysis: "Artificial Limb in Preindustrial France," 836–837. Mischaracterizations: Engstrom and Van de Ven, *Physiotherapy*, 1; Rang and Thompson, "History of Amputations and Prostheses," 5; Thurston, "Paré and Prosthetics," 1117; Krebs, *Groundbreaking Scientific Experiments*, 224; Wetz, "Zur Geschichte der Armprothetik," 156.
9 Mukerji, *Impossible Engineering*, 225; Smith, *Body of the Artisan*.
10 Smith, "Sixteenth-Century Goldsmith's Workshop," 34, 38; Epstein, "Property Rights," 383.
11 Valleriani, "Epistemology of Practical Knowledge," 2–3.
12 Long, *Artisan/Practitioners*, 125.
13 Ash, *Power, Knowledge, and Expertise*, 16–17.
14 For a classic biography: Malgaigne, *Surgery and Ambroise Paré*. For a more recent example: Poirier, *Ambroise Paré*.
15 This chapter refers to Paré's book of artificial body parts as Book XXII unless indicating a specific edition or translation of *Les Oeuvres* in which it appears as Book XXIII.
16 E.g., Jessen, *Wund-Artznei*, 206–208.
17 Earliest French-language editions: Paré, *Les Oeuvres* (1575); Paré, *Les Oeuvres* (1579); Paré, *Les Oeuvres* (1585); Paré, *Les Oeuvres* (1598). First Latin translation: Paré, *Opera Ambrosii Parei* (1582).
18 German and Latin translations printed in Frankfurt am Main: Paré, *Opera Chirurgica* (1594); Paré, *Wundt-Artzney* (1601); Paré, *Opera Chirurgica* (1612); Paré, *Wund-Artzney* (1635). Dutch editions: Paré, *De chirurgie* (1592); Paré, *De chirurgie* (1604).
19 Hildanus, *Gründlicher Bericht*, 140.
20 Although the chapter originally appeared as Chapter XI in the first edition (Paris, 1575), I refer to it by its common sequencing label as Chapter XII. It first appeared as Chapter XII in the second edition (Paris, 1579), and remained so in subsequent editions in French, as well as in Latin, Dutch, German, and English translations.
21 Paré, *Les Oeuvres* (1579), 838.
22 Ibid.: "servent non seulement à l'action des parties couppees: mais aussi à la beauté & ornement d'icelles."
23 Paré, *Workes*, 880.
24 Long, *Artisan/Practitioners*, 4.

25 A fourth woodcut of a leather hand was added by the 1585 French-language edition published in Paris, but it did not appear in German editions: Paré, *Les Oeuvres* (1585), 917.
26 The figures from Chapter XII of the French edition appearing in this chapter are taken from the 1614 Paris printing, in which all components are numbered correctly and clearly.
27 See Karpinski, *Studien über künstliche Glieder*, 34.
28 Diderot and Félice, *Encyclopédie*, 21:12–13.
29 Paré, *Les Oeuvres* (1579), 889. "3 Gaschettes pour tenir ferme un chacun doigt," "5 La grande gaschette pour ouvrir les quatre petites gaschettes, qui tiennent les doigts fermez."
30 Diderot and Félice, *Encyclopédie*, 17:433.
31 Paré, *Les Oeuvres* (1579), 839. "4 Estoqueaux ou arrests desdites gaschettes, au milieu desquelles sont chevilles pour arrester lesdites gaschettes."
32 Ffoulkes, *Armourer*, 162.
33 Ibid., 166; La Rocca, *European Armor*, 36.
34 See Chapter 5.
35 Paré, *Les Oeuvres* (1579), 840. A spring (6) above the *gaschette* (5) catches in the teeth of the *rocquet* (4), and is held firm by a nail-screw (7). In the middle of the spiral mainspring is a shaft (*l'arbre*) that continues into a cavity for the extension of the arm (2).
36 On the production and functions of mechanical hands, see Chapter 5.
37 See Chapter 5.
38 E.g., Savage-Smith, "Exchange of Medical and Surgical Ideas."
39 E.g., Groiss, "Augsburg Clockmakers' Craft," 78; O'Malley, "Little Gilded Shoes," 54.
40 A rare example appears in Maurice, "Jost Bürgi," 88.
41 See Chapter 5.
42 E.g., Long, "Power, Patronage, and the Authorship of *Ars*"; Eamon, *Science and the Secrets of Nature*; Harkness, *Jewel House*, 211–241; Smith, "Codification of Vernacular Theories."
43 Hildanus, *Gründlicher Bericht*, 140.
44 On tacit knowledge: Long, *Openness, Secrecy, Authorship*.
45 For the concept of black boxing in sixteenth-century technical manuals: Ash, *Power, Knowledge, and Expertise*, 150.
46 Paré, *Wund-Artzney* (1635), 748: "damit ich nachmals im Fall der Noht/ etwan andere darnach könte machen lassen."
47 Ibid.
48 Paré, *Opera Chirurgica* (1594), 656.
49 Paré, *Opera Ambrosii Parei*, 668–669.
50 Paré, *Opera Chirurgica* (1594), 657–658.
51 Paré, *Wundt-Artzney* (1601), 951–952.
52 Paré, *Workes*, 881–882.
53 E.g., Chambers and Gillespie, "Locality in the History of Science"; Turnbull, "Traveling Knowledge."
54 Paré, *Les Oeuvres* (1579), 841.
55 Paré, *De chirurgie* (1592), 840–842.

56 For the Latin translation: Lamzweerde, *Appendix*, 17–22.
57 Janet Doe clarifies there was no third French edition—the so-called fourth edition of 1585 came directly after the second edition of 1579: *Bibliography*, 121.
58 Paré, *Wundt-Artzney* (1601), 951–952.
59 Paré, *Workes* (1634), title page.
60 Pantin, "Role of Translations," 167. See also Pantin, "La traduction latine des Oeuvres d'Ambroise Paré."
61 Epstein, "Property Rights," 383.
62 Ibid. Epstein consistently argues ten years is the amount of time it takes to become an expert. For more on apprenticeship: Epstein, "Craft Guilds, Apprenticeship, and Technological Change."
63 Compare this with Wolfgang Lefèvre's discussion of machines: "Limits of Pictures," 81–82.
64 On codified practical knowledge as a conceptual knowledge structure characterized by increased abstraction: Valleriani, "Epistemology of Practical Knowledge," 5.
65 Smith, "Sixteenth-Century Goldsmith's Workshop," 44.
66 Doe, *Bibliography*, 188.
67 Jousse, *La fidelle ouverture de l'art de serrurier*, 122–124. For a discussion of Jousse and the later development of locksmith literature in Germany: Welker, *Historische Schlüssel und Schlösser*, 9, 19–20.
68 E.g., Linker, *War's Waste*.
69 See Long, *Artisan/Practitioners*, 95.
70 Eric H. Ash has applied this concept, originally discussed in a different context by Lisa Jardine and Anthony Grafton, to the role of Thomas Digges in the reconstruction of the Dover Harbor in the 1580s: Ash, "'A Perfect and an Absolute Work'"; Jardine and Grafton, "'Studied for Action.'"
71 Ash, "'A Perfect and an Absolute Work,'" 267.

Epilogue

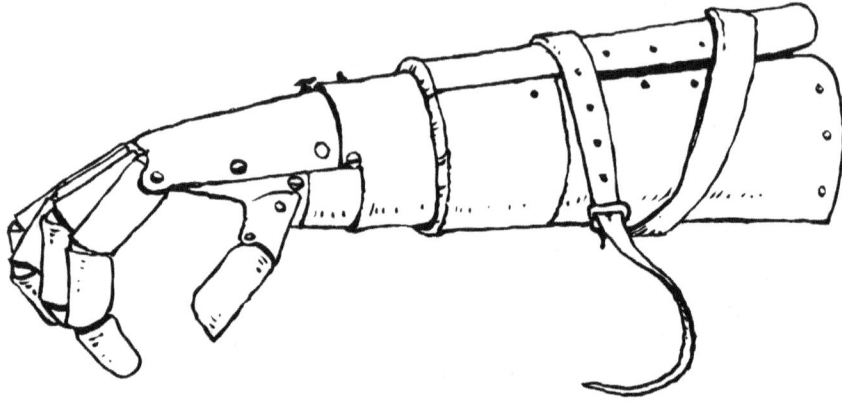

Elana Duffy chose to remove her right foot and part of her leg in late summer 2019. In an essay she wrote for *The New York Times* a year later, she reflected on her decision and the events that followed. She had been a soldier in the U.S. Army in Iraq in 2005 when she sustained a combination of complicated head and leg injuries. They led to fourteen years of "nearly constant, and sometimes excruciating, pain." With a right ankle that rolled when she put weight on it and an impaired sense of balance, she discovered that even stepping off a curb became dangerous. The original injuries repeatedly caused new ones, compounding the damage. Her doctor, a limb reconstruction and replacement surgeon, suggested osseointegration within a list of potential treatments. It is a form of amputation in which the surgeon inserts a titanium rod into the bone that extends beyond the stump and ends in a "node" to which one can attach devices for different activities. For Duffy, this meant attachments suited for "walking, kayaking, diving and climbing." Her doctor acknowledged that it was "a drastic option" not because the procedure was still relatively new or involved directly connecting human bone with an artificial implant, but because it was the only one involving amputation. "The risk of the operation going wrong was low," she writes, "but was I really willing to cut off a part of my leg?" With her decision to move forward, she became one of the first individuals in the United States to undergo osseointegration for a lower leg injury.[1]

The account of her months-long recovery paints a complex picture, a combination of liberating ("I felt more free than I had in years") and difficult ("there are still hard days"). She tells readers the overall improvement in her quality of life was undeniable: "I am living mostly pain-free, and I was finally able to get back on a rock wall." An avid climber, she describes changing old techniques to use her new climbing foot. In this activity and in others, using her prosthesis appears as an ongoing series of developments, choices, and adjustments. Duffy writes that she was "still working on stairs," while running was a future goal. She also reports anticipated new attachments: a swimming foot and a running foot. "I'm happier with Peggy (the name I've given the new leg)," she writes, "than I'd been with my natural foot in many years." "Giving up my leg," she concludes, "meant getting back the rest of my life."[2]

A veritable chasm seemingly separates this twenty-first-century example from the one with which this book began: Götz von Berlichingen's autobiographical account of the loss of his hand in 1504. Duffy's surgeon turns to amputation not as a final resort—a life-saving measure—but instead presents it as one of several treatment options. Rather than a private enterprise of amputees and the technical domain of artisans, her prosthetic limb is fully medicalized: her surgeon inserted a metal rod that became a permanent part of her stump. After the procedure, Duffy describes herself as "bionic."[3] Her prosthesis is immutable yet ever changing, a base to attach a growing number of devices, some yet to be conceived of and created, for every manner of activity. It encompasses many forms of an artificial foot all at once. Her modern account suggests a form of surgical and prosthetic interventionism beyond the wildest dreams of early modern surgeons. Moreover, the clarity of Duffy's voice in it has no parallel in sixteenth- and seventeenth-century sources. Her first-person account illuminates one person's direct experience with the force of a blazing sun. In comparison, we have been working by meager candlelight to recover something of early modern communities facing the cold fire, patients experiencing phantom pain, and amputee-patrons commissioning iron hands.

To be sure, there are some familiar resonances: the patient deliberates with her social circle before deciding on an amputation procedure, and her continuing activities to obtain and adjust prosthetic feet tailored to her various needs and interests would be familiar enough to amputee-patrons with mechanical hands. Even the concept of removing a portion of a lower leg to enhance one's quality of life was not unknown in early modern surgical literature. Defending the utility of short lower leg stumps, Ambroise Paré described a patient who had his long lower leg stump amputated "five fingers under the knee" so that he could move about more quickly.[4] Still, that patient's decision shortened an existing stump; his choice was not the same as the one Duffy made four centuries later.

A modern procedure like osseointegration reflects broader assumptions about surgical and artificial intervention characteristic of biomedicine today. The human body is composed of replaceable parts—not only arms and legs, but also hearts and lungs. It is something humans can change and mold. We take for granted that medical professionals can and should perform invasive procedures that alter the size, shape, texture, and movement of limbs—natural and artificial—to preserve or improve a patient's quality of life. Testing the boundaries of this understanding outside of medicine (and sometimes the law) are body modification practices that integrate living tissue with artificial parts. Implanting powerful magnets in the tips of fingers, for instance, amplifies sensory experience with novel zaps to the nerves when touching everyday objects. These are not medical procedures, yet they reflect a shared and unspoken belief about human ability to alter the physical body to enhance one's encounter with the world. Our early modern story is about how embodied practices in the sixteenth and seventeenth centuries created the first stirrings of this belief within Western medicine.

In the early modern period, intervention in the body was an arena explored in surgical techniques and textual debate, in the material practices amputee-patrons sponsored and the resulting objects artisans made. Early moderns did not invent amputation or prosthetic limbs, but they did develop new techniques and technologies that existed alongside inherited ones. With hands-on practices and technical treatises, they investigated and interrogated these subjects more deeply and systematically than their predecessors. In short, they created a multiplicity of practices *and* ideas surrounding the body, amputation, and artificial limbs. The nascent but growing perception of the body as something that human hands could alter came from increasing numbers of examples of alterations. I have called this transformation the rise of the malleable body not because it resulted in a "modern" vision of intervention, like Athena springing fully formed from Zeus's head. There was no direct or inevitable line of progression from early modern to contemporary practices, and the distance between Western medicine in the sixteenth century and modern biomedicine is vast. Yet we need the story of early modern actors—amputees like Götz von Berlichingen and surgeons like Fabry von Hilden—to make sense of a modern story like Elana Duffy's. This book argues that over the course of the early modern period, surgical and artisanal experimentation and discussion expanded the number and degree of interventions one could obtain and consequently influenced expectations about what was possible. This newfound malleability of the body was less discovered than created, an unstable but powerfully alluring perception shaped by scalpels, forged in furnaces, and articulated through text and object.

This book set out not only to explore the nature of this transformation, but also to examine how it occurred. During our investigation of the body taken apart and put back together, we have seen the contributions of many actors. Recording their thoughts and experiences, surgeons described the human body as sacred raw material in one breath and compared handling it to making a snowball in another. They learned about the body through physical techniques and discussions surrounding them. Their treatises could at times portray bodies in generalized ways, but practitioners operated on individuals. Patients held more power in the early modern medical marketplace than today, and surgeons' treatises reveal different ways they exerted influence on surgical practice. Amputations took place with their consent, and practitioners adapted their methods when pressed, whether hiding cautery irons from view or undertaking a technique recommended by a rival consultant.[5] Amputees whose stumps healed adapted to new challenges in ways that could inform and contribute to surgeons' discussions. This book has focused on elite amputee-patrons because they drove material practices that developed a new prosthetic technology—mechanical hands. These not only represented a new frontier in the making of artificial limbs to serve aesthetic and practical purposes, but they also came to hold a particularly powerful symbolic function in the conceptualization and discussion of amputees in surgical literature. Other members of early modern communities also played important roles. Surgeons consulted patients' families, friends, and even pastors to decide whether to perform amputations. Amputees also brought artisans from different craft workshops—locksmiths, blacksmiths, clockmakers, and so on—into explorations of the body by commissioning custom artificial limbs. They applied their specialized skills in novel ways to craft devices that met the requirements of their patrons.

The malleable body arose from embodied forms of knowledge-making. Among surgeons, these manifested in multiple ways. We find a surgical epistemology in amputation techniques characterized by intersecting questions—worked through again and again in operations and reflective writing—of physical matter, the human, and the surgeon's role. Amputation remained an extreme measure throughout the early modern period; yet its goals also developed into something more complex and variegated than in earlier centuries. Working with bodies transformed surgeons' understandings over four generations or so about what it was they were doing when they cut off a limb. They were no longer simply saving a life. They were enhancing the future movement of the body, they were defending its material integrity, or they were doing some combination of both. Surgeons continued to make meaning through their encounters with bodies after the operation. Discussions of false imaginations (what we have called early modern "phantom limbs") and false restorations (artificial body parts) show complex relationships between direct experience from surgical activities and the conceptual frameworks found in a growing corpus of surgical literature.

Mechanical hands offer another view of embodied knowledge-making, this time outside of the surgeon's practice. Artisans and amputees participated in the creation of these objects in different ways. Amputee-patrons articulated their wants and needs, expressing ideas about the appearance and movement of their bodies, and how they envisioned the effect a mechanical device would have on them. Artisans applied their skills, technical knowledge, and creativity to design an object to meet the patron's criteria. Each artificial hand was a custom order, an artisanal experiment. The earliest surgical literature about artificial limbs was based on these ongoing activities, not the other way around. Once the objects were crafted, amputee-patrons wore them, operated them, and took them to other workshops for modifications or repairs. Together, the material efforts of amputee-patrons and artisans expanded prosthetic options and their meanings, from the discreet hand to the showpiece arm. Allusions to iron hands in surgical literature point to the multidirectional influence of practices and ideas surrounding the body. Amputee-patrons convinced surgeons that iron hands were useful and artful; surgeons situated the objects in a conceptual framework that presented them to readers as the ideal "solution" to the loss of a limb. The knowledge to produce this technology became valuable enough for one surgeon to attempt to codify and disseminate, but in practice it appears to have remained the domain of artisans.

This book began with the firsthand account of the most widely known amputee-patron of the sixteenth century—the knight Götz von Berlichingen. His figure looms large in German culture, Goethe's dramatic portrayal coloring so much of our present perception of early modern prosthetic limbs. His autobiography was the natural starting place for a story about amputation and prostheses in early modern Germany. As we reach the end of my telling, I suggest we think about how this story might look from other scholarly perspectives. A social perspective might consider the relationship between attitudes toward risky surgical operations and other developments, such as increased competition and increased medicalization of urban society. A broader geographical perspective would test the cultural particularities of the malleable body. With its large-scale centers of print and skilled artisanal production, its fascination with the *Wunderkammer*, and its experience with sustained warfare, early modern Germany was perhaps an ideal environment for a gradual transformation of the body. Examining vernacular print in other regions would reveal more about the relationship between university-educated and master–apprentice-trained authors and their contributions to a textual discourse available to barber-surgeons. An expanded study of surviving artifacts from early modern Europe, particularly a comparison of internal mechanisms and estimated dates of production, would also paint a much larger picture. A compilation of data might even allow us to identify and reconstruct the movement of prosthetic technology in much the same way as surgical treatises reveal the movement of amputation techniques. Reed Benhamou once stated that our technical knowledge of early modern artificial limbs is, apart from the woodcuts of Ambroise Paré, anecdotal.[6] This book shows that it does not have to be.

The malleable body signified an early modern perception—an idea—that gradually arose out of practices. It was a perception of possibility and capacity for change. So, too, the work of writing about this historical transformation has led this book's author to develop a perception of the possibilities lying dormant in a fledgling academic subfield. A cultural history of medicine, technology, and the body was bound to poke about in odd and seemingly unconnected places because of the questions that animate it and the different disciplines that inspire it. Early modern European surgery is particularly suited for such an endeavor because it touches on so many threads of academic discourse at once—learned and vernacular medicine, Renaissance anatomy, artisanal/craft knowledge, practical knowledge-making, material culture, print culture and the history of the book, technology, the history of the body, and disability history. The latter has conventionally existed in opposition to the history of medicine, though scholars like Beth Linker have made cogent cases in recent years for the advantages of working across both fields.[7] This book shows that we can learn more about early modern surgeons, medical knowledge, and knowledge-making by considering the agency and contributions of actors who experienced mental or physical difference, as well as considering ideas about the body advanced by historians of disability. In fact, including these changes the stories that historians of medicine have told: mechanical hands, so long considered the invention of one surgeon, become the collaborative creations of amputees and artisans, whose material efforts influenced surgeons' treatises. The development of surgical literature about this subject makes little sense without the activities of amputee-patrons and artisans.

In what other ways would an inclusive approach enhance our understanding of premodern medicine and the body? Early modern surgery is a growing field, poised to draw from the most innovative methods of new and more established areas of study alike without becoming institutionally entrenched in them. Let its future scholars take full advantage of the intellectual possibilities. Let its future chart new realms.

Notes

1 Elana Duffy, "I Got Blown Up in Iraq. Years Later, Amputating My Leg Set Me Free," *The New York Times*, 10 September 2020.
2 Ibid.
3 Ibid.

4 Paré, *Wund-Artzney* (1635), 421: "fünff Finger unter dem Knie."
5 E.g., Solingen, *Hand-Griffe*, 376; Hildanus, *Wund-Artzney*, 304.
6 Benhamou, "Artificial Limb in Preindustrial France," 837.
7 Kudlick, "Social History of Medicine and Disability History"; Linker, "On the Borderland of Medical and Disability History."

Bibliography

Full references for manuscript sources, artifacts, and periodicals are in the notes and captions.

Manuscript and artifact collections

Archives de l'Etat de Fribourg
Bayerisches Armeemuseum, Ingolstadt
Deutsches Historisches Museum, Berlin
Germanisches Nationalmuseum Nürnberg
Herzog Anton Ulrich-Museum, Braunschweig
Hessisches Landesmuseum Darmstadt
Museé Historique, Strasbourg
Museum Eisfeld
Museum Neuruppin
Museumslandschaft Hessen Kassel
Niedersächsisches Landesarchiv Wolfenbüttel
Schlossmuseum Götzenburg, Jagsthausen
Stadtarchiv Augsburg
Stadtarchiv München
Stadtarchiv Ulm

Artworks

Bruegel the Elder, Pieter. *The Beggars*. 1568. Oil on wood, 18.5 × 21.5 cm. RF 730, The Louvre, Paris.

Mytens, Daniel. *Christian, Duke of Brunswick and Lüneburg (1599–1626)*. C. 1624. Oil on canvas, 220.6 × 140.0 cm. RCIN 405885, Royal Collection Trust, United Kingdom.

Voerst, Robert van. *CHRISTIANO D.G. POSTVLATO EP. HALBERSTADIENSI*. 1630–1645. Engraving with etching, 25.4 cm × 18.8 cm (sheet of paper). RCIN 610172, Royal Collection Trust, United Kingdom.

Printed works

Abelinus, Johann Philipp. *Theatrum Europaeum* [...]. Frankfurt, 1662.
Agricola, Johann. *Chirurgia parva oder kleine Wund-Artzney* [...]. Nuremberg, 1643.
Alberti, Leon Battista. *De re aedificatoria*. Florence, 1485.
Albucasis. *On Surgery and Instruments: A Definitive Edition of the Arabic Text of Albucasis, with English Translation*. Edited and translated by M. S. Spink and G. L. Lewis. London: Wellcome Institute, 1973.
Alexander, Kimberly S. *Treasures Afoot: Shoe Stories from the Georgian Era*. Baltimore: Johns Hopkins University Press, 2018.
Ames, Edward, and Nathan Rosenberg. "Changing Technological Leadership and Industrial Growth." *The Economic Journal* 73:289 (1963): 13–31.
Amirault, Moyse. *La Vie de François, seigneur de La Noue* [...]. Leiden, 1661.
Arcaeus, Franciscus. *Fraxinalensis, der Artzney Doctoris und Wund-Artzts / Zwey Chirurgische Bücher* [...]. Nuremberg, 1674.
Arrizabalaga, Jon, John Henderson, and Roger French. *The Great Pox: The French Disease in Renaissance Europe*. New Haven: Yale University Press, 1997.
Ash, Eric H. "'A Perfect and an Absolute Work': Expertise, Authority, and the Rebuilding of Dover Harbor, 1579–1583." *Technology and Culture* 41:2 (2000): 239–268.
———. *Power, Knowledge, and Expertise in Elizabethan England*. Baltimore: Johns Hopkins University Press, 2004.
Babel, Anthony. *Histoire corporative de l'horlogerie, de l'orfèverie et des industries annexes*. Geneva: A. Jullien, 1916.
Barbette, Paul. *Chirurgische und Medicinische Wercke* [...]. Hamburg, 1677.
———. *Chirurgische und anatomische Schrifften* [...]. Frankfurt am Main, 1694.
Baudaert, Willem. *Memorien* [...] *beginnende met het jaer 1620. Ende eyndigende in Nov. d. jaers 1624*. Vol. 2. Arnhem, 1625.
Baumann, Reinhard. *Landsknechte: Ihre Geschichte und Kultur vom späten Mittelalter bis zum Dreißigjährigen Krieg*. Munich: C. H. Beck, 1994.
Baumgartner, R. "Fußprothese aus einem frühmittelalterlichen Grab aus Bondaduz-Kanton Graubünden/Schweiz." *Helvetia archaeologica* 13 (1982): 155–162.
Baxandall, Michael. *The Limewood Sculptors of Renaissance Germany, 1475–1525: Images and Circumstances*. New Haven: Yale University Press, 1980.
Bearden, Elizabeth B. *Monstrous Kinds: Body, Space, and Narrative in Renaissance Representations of Disability*. Ann Arbor: University of Michigan Press, 2019.
Bedini, Silvio A. "Johann Wolfgang Gelb of Ulm: 17th Century Lock and Instrument Maker." *Physis* 3:2 (1961): 322–333.
———. "The Role of Automata in the History of Technology." *Technology and Culture* 5:1 (1964): 24–42.
Belolan, Nicole. "The Material Culture of Gout in Early America." In Williamson and Guffey, *Making Disability Modern*, 19–42.
Benedict, Philip. *Graphic History: The Wars, Massacres and Troubles of Tortorel and Perrissin*. Geneva: Droz, 2007.

Benhamou, Reed. "The Artificial Limb in Preindustrial France." *Technology and Culture* 35:4 (1994): 835–845.
Berlichingen, Götz von. *Mein Fehd und Handlungen*. Edited by Helgard Ulmschneider. Sigmaringen: Thorbecke, 1981.
Berlichingen-Rossach, Friedrich Wolfgang Götz von. *Geschichte des Ritters Götz von Berlichingen mit der eisernen Hand und seiner Familie*. Leipzig: Brockhaus, 1861.
Bernstein, Frances L. "Rehabilitation Staged: How Soviet Doctors 'Cured' Disability in the Second World War." In Burch and Rembis, *Disability Histories*, 218–236.
Berriot-Salvadore, Évelyne, and Paul Mironneau, eds. *Ambroise Paré (1510–1590): pratique et écriture de la science à la Renaissance: actes du Colloque de Pau, 6–7 mai 1999*. Paris: H. Champion, 2003.
Bertolini Meli, Domenico. "'Ex Museolo Nostro Machaonico': Collecting, Publishing, and Visualization in Fabricius Hildanus." *Journal of the History of Medicine and Allied Sciences* 72:1 (2017): 98–116.
Bertolini Meli, Domenico, and Cynthia Klestinec. "Renaissance Surgery Between Learning and Craft." *Journal of the History of Medicine and Allied Sciences* 72:1 (2016): 1–5.
Blankaart, Steven. [...] *Chirurgische Abhandlung Der so genennten Frantzosen* [...]. Leipzig, 1699.
Bok, Marten Jan. "Christian von Braunschweig in den Niederlanden." In *Der Krieg als Person: Herzog Christian d. J. von Braunschweig-Lüneburg im Bildnis von Paulus Moreelse. Ausstellung im Herzog Anton Ulrich-Museum Braunschweig, 16. März bis 14. Mai 2000*, edited by Jochen Luckhardt and Nils Büttner, 15–39. Braunschweig: Herzog Anton Ulrich-Museum, 2000.
Bontekoe, Cornelis. *Newes Gebäw der Chirurgie* [...]. Hannover, 1687.
Borgognoni, Teodorico dei. *The Surgery of Theodoric: ca. A.D. 1267*. 2 vols. Translated by Eldridge Campbell and James Colton. New York: Appleton-Century-Crofts, Inc., 1960.
Botallo, Leonardo. *Opera omnia medica & chirurgica*. Annotated by Johannes van Horne. Leiden, 1660.
———. *Zwey Chirurgische Bücher* [...]. Nuremberg, 1676.
Brachelius, Johann Adolph. *Kriegs- und Friedens Historia* [...] *Von Anno 1618. biß ins Jahr 1652* [...]. Cologne, 1657.
Braudel, F. P., and F. Spooner. "Prices in Europe from 1450 to 1750." In *The Cambridge Economic History of Europe*. Vol. 4. Edited by E. E. Rich and C. H. Wilson, 374–486. Cambridge: Cambridge University Press, 2008.
Bredekamp, Horst. *Lure of Antiquity and the Cult of the Machine: The Kunstkammer and the Evolution of Nature, Art and Technology*. Princeton: Markus Wiener Publishers, 1995.
Breiding, Dirk H. "Techniques of Decoration on Arms and Armor." In *Heilbrunn Timeline of Art History*. New York: The Metropolitan Museum of Art, 2000–. www.metmuseum.org/toah/hd/dect/hd_dect.htm (October 2003) (accessed 24 March 2016).
Brockliss, Laurence, and Colin Jones. *The Medical World of Early Modern France*. Oxford: Oxford University Press, 1997.

Brückmann, Franz Ernst. [...] *Centuriae Tertiae Epistolarum Itinerariarum LXXV*. Braunschweig: Schroeder, 1756.
Brugis, Thomas. *Vade Mecum Chirurgicum Oder Reise-Gefehrte* [...]. Hamburg, 1684.
Brunschwig, Hieronymus. *Dis ist das buch der Cirurgia* [...]. Augsburg, 1497.
Burch, Susan, and Michael Rembis, eds. *Disability Histories*. Chicago: University of Illinois Press, 2014.
Burhenne, Verena, ed. *Prothesen von Kopf bis Fuß: Katalog zur gleichnamigen Wanderausstellung des Westfälischen Museumsamtes, Landschaftsverband Westfalen-Lippe*. Münster: Landschaftsverband Westfalen-Lippe, 2003.
Burres, Lorenz. *Ein new Wund Arzney Büchlein* [...]. Frankfurt am Main, 1549.
Bynum, W. F., and Roy Porter, eds. *Companion Encyclopedia of the History of Medicine*. 2 vols. New York: Routledge, 1994.
Cabré, Montserrat. "From a Master to a Laywoman: A Feminine Manual of Self-Help." *Dynamis* 20 (2000): 371–393.
Carrera, E. "Anger and the Mind–Body Connection in Medieval and Early Modern Medicine." In *Emotions and Health, 1200–1700*, edited by E. Carrera, 95–146. Leiden: Brill, 2013.
Cavallo, Sandra. *Artisans of the Body in Early Modern Italy: Identities, Families and Masculinities*. Manchester: Manchester University Press, 2010.
Celsus, Aulus Cornelius. *De Medicina*. 3 vols. Translated by W. G. Spencer. Cambridge, MA: Harvard University Press, 1935–1938.
Chamberland, Celeste. "Honor, Brotherhood, and the Corporate Ethos of London's Barber-Surgeons' Company, 1570–1640." *Journal of the History of Medicine and Allied Sciences* 64 (2009): 300–332.
Chambers, David Wade, and Richard Gillespie. "Locality in the History of Science: Colonial Science, Technoscience, and Indigenous Knowledge." In *Nature and Empire: Science and the Colonial Enterprise*, edited by Roy MacLeod, 221–240. Chicago: University of Chicago Press, 2001.
Chapuis, Alfred, and Edouard Gélis. *Le monde des automates: étude historique et technique*. 2 vols. Paris, 1928; reprinted Geneva: Slatkine, 1984.
Chauliac, Guy de. *The Cyrurgie of Guy de Chauliac*. Edited by Margaret S. Ogden. London: Oxford University Press, 1971.
Christian II, Prince of Anhalt-Bernburg. *Tagebuch Christians des Jüngeren, Fürst zu Anhalt: niedergeschrieben in seiner Haft zu Wien* [...] *nach dem Ms. der Herzogl. Bibl. zu Cöthen*. Edited by G. Krause. Leipzig: Dyk, 1858.
Clark, Stuart. *Vanities of the Eye: Vision in Early Modern European Culture*. New York: Oxford University Press, 2007.
Cock, Emily. *Rhinoplasty and the Nose in Early Modern British Medicine and Culture*. Manchester: Manchester University Press, 2019.
Cohn, Henry J. "Götz von Berlichingen and the Art of Military Autobiography." In *War, Literature, and the Arts in Sixteenth-Century Europe*, edited by J. R. Mulryne and Margaret Shewring, 22–40. Basingstoke: Macmillan, 1989.
Conrad, Lawrence I., Michael Neve, Vivian Nutton, Roy Porter, and Andrew Wear. *The Western Medical Tradition, 800 BC to AD 1800*. Cambridge: Cambridge University Press, 1995.

Crawford, Cassandra. *Phantom Limb: Amputation, Embodiment, and Prosthetic Technology*. New York: New York University Press, 2014.
Dacome, Lucia. *Malleable Anatomies: Models, Makers, and Material Culture in Eighteenth- Century Italy*. Oxford: Oxford University Press, 2017.
Daston, Lorraine, ed. *Biographies of Scientific Objects*. Chicago: University of Chicago Press, 2000.
———, ed. *Things that Talk: Object Lessons from Art and Science*. New York: Zone Books, 2004.
———. "The History of Science and the History of Knowledge." *KNOW: A Journal on the Formation of Knowledge* 1:1 (2017): 131–154.
Davids, Karel. "Shifts of Technological Leadership in Early Modern Europe." In *A Miracle Mirrored: The Dutch Republic in European Perspective*, edited by J. Lucassen and K. Davids, 338–366. Cambridge: Cambridge University Press, 1995.
De Moulin, Daniel. "Paul Barbette, M.D.: A Seventeenth-Century Amsterdam Author of Best-Selling Textbooks." *Bulletin of the History of Medicine* 59:4 (1985): 506–514.
———. *A History of Surgery: With Emphasis on the Netherlands*. Dordrecht: Martinus Nijhoff Publishers, 1988.
Della Croce, Giovanni Andrea. *Officina aurea [...] Wund-Artzney [...]*. Frankfurt, 1607.
DeMaitre, Luke. *Medieval Medicine: The Art of Healing, from Head to Toe*. Santa Barbara: Praeger, 2013.
Descartes, René. *The Philosophical Writings of Descartes*. 3 vols. Translated by John Cottingham, Robert Stoothoff, and Dugald Murdoch. Cambridge: Cambridge University Press, 1984–1991.
Descaves, Lucien. "Correspondance medico-littéraire: Réponses." *La Chronique Médicale: revue mensuelle de médecine historique, littéraire & anecdotique* 31 (March 1924): 88.
Devisse, Jean, and Michel Mollat. *From the Early Christian Era to the "Age of Discovery": Africans in the Christian Ordinance of the World*. Translated by William Granger Ryan. Vol. 2, Pt. 2 of *The Image of the Black in Western Art*, edited by David Bindman and Henry Louis Gates, Jr. London: The Belknap Press, 2010.
DeVries, Kelly. "Military Surgical Practice and Gunpowder Weaponry." *Canadian Bulletin of Medical History* 7:2 (1990): 131–146.
———. "Sites of Military Science and Technology." In *Early Modern Science*, edited by Katherine Park and Lorraine Daston, 306–319. Vol. 3 of *The Cambridge History of Science*. Cambridge: Cambridge University Press, 2006.
DeVries, Kelly, and Robert Douglas Smith. *Medieval Military Technology*. 2nd ed. Tonawanda: University of Toronto Press, 2012.
Diab, Mohammad. *Lexicon of Orthopaedic Etymology*. Amsterdam: Harwood Academic Publishers, 1999.
Diderot, Denis, and Fortuné Barthélemy de Félice, eds. *Encyclopédie ou dictionnaire raisonné des connoissances humaines*. Vol. 17. Yverdon, 1772.
———, eds. *Encyclopédie ou dictionnaire raisonné des connoissances humaines*. Vol. 21. Yverdon, 1773.
Dietz, Johann. *Meister Johann Dietz, des grossen Kurfürsten Feldscher und königlicher Hofbarbier*. Ebenhausen bei München: W. Langewiesche-Brandt, 1915.

DiMeo, Michelle, and Sara Pennell. *Reading and Writing Recipe Books, 1550–1800*. Manchester: Manchester University Press, 2013.
Doe, Janet. *A Bibliography, 1545–1940, of the Works of Ambroise Paré, 1510–1590: premier chirurgien & conseiller du roi*. Amsterdam: G. Th. Van Heusden, 1976.
Dormandy, Thomas. *The Worst of Evils: The Fight Against Pain*. New Haven: Yale University Press, 2006.
Duden, Barbara. *The Woman Beneath the Skin: A Doctor's Patients in Eighteenth-Century Germany*. Translated by Thomas Dunlap. Cambridge: Harvard University Press, 1991.
Dürer, Albrecht. *Opera Alberti Dureri* [...]. Arnhem, 1604.
Eamon, William. *Science and the Secrets of Nature: Books of Secrets in Medieval and Early Modern Culture*. Princeton: Princeton University Press, 1994.
Ecker-Offenhäußer, Ute. "Joseph Schmid. Handwerkschirurg und Schriftsteller in Augsburg im 17. Jahrhundert." *Medizin, Gesellschaft, und Geschichte: Jahrbuch des Instituts für Geschichte der Medizin der Robert Bosch Stiftung* 15 (1996): 117–139.
———. "*wie man sich in Sterbensläuffen nach eines jeden Beutel praeservieren und verwahren soll* – Volkssprachlich-medizinischer Buchdruck in Augsburg im 17. Jahrhundert." In *Augsburger Buchdruck und Verlagswesen. Von den Anfängen bis zur Gegenwart*, edited by Helmut Gier and Johannes Janota, 947–962. Wiesbaden: Harrassowitz Verlag, 1997.
Engstrom, Barbara, and Catherine Van de Ven. *Physiotherapy for Amputees: The Roehampton Approach*. Edinburgh: Churchill Livingstone, 1993.
Epstein, Stephan R. "Craft Guilds, Apprenticeship, and Technological Change in Preindustrial Europe." *The Journal of Economy History* 58:3 (1998): 684–713.
———. "Property Rights to Technological Knowledge in Premodern Europe, 1300–1800." *The American Economic Review* 94:2 (2004): 382–387.
———. "Craft Guilds in the Pre-modern Economy: A Discussion." *Economic History Review* 61:1 (2008): 155–174.
Eras, Vincent J. M. *Locks and Keys throughout the Ages*. Amsterdam: H. H. Fronczek, 1957.
Eyler, Joshua R., ed. *Disability in the Middle Ages: Reconsiderations and Reverberations*. Farnham: Ashgate, 2010.
Fabricius ab Aquapendente, Hieronymus. *Pentateuchos Chirurgicum* [...]. Frankfurt am Main, 1592.
———. *Wund-Artznei* [...]. Nuremberg, 1673.
Farr, James R. "On the Shop Floor: Guilds, Artisans, and the European Market Economy, 1350–1750." *Journal of Early Modern History* 1:1 (1997): 24–54.
———. *Artisans in Europe, 1300–1914*. Cambridge: Cambridge University Press, 2000.
Ferragud, Carmel. "Wounds, Amputations, and Expert Procedures in the City of Valencia in the Early Fifteenth Century." In Tracy and DeVries, *Wounds and Wound Repair*, 233–251.
Ferri, Alfonso. *De Sclopetorum sive archibusorum vulneribus libri tres* [...]. In *Thesaurus chirurgiae*, edited by Peter Uffenbach. Frankfurt, 1610.
Ffoulkes, Charles John. *The Armourer and His Craft, from the XIth to the XVIth Century*. New York: B. Blom, 1967.

Ficarra, Bernard J. *Essays on Historical Medicine*. New York: Froben Press, Inc., 1948.

Findlen, Paula. "Early Modern Things: Objects in Motion, 1500–1800." In *Early Modern Things: Objects and Their Histories, 1500–1800*, edited by Paula Findlen, 3–27. New York: Routledge, 2013.

Finger, Stanley, and Meredith P. Hustwit. "Five Early Accounts of Phantom Limb in Context: Paré, Descartes, Lemos, Bell, and Mitchell." *Neurosurgery* 52:3 (2003): 675–685.

Fissell, Mary. "Introduction: Women, Health, and Healing in Early Modern Europe." *Bulletin of the History of Medicine* 82:1 (2008): 1–17.

Forrer, Robert. "Die eiserne Hand von Balbronn (Elsaſs)." *Zeitschrift für historische Waffenkunde* 7:4 (1917): 102–107.

Fracchia, Carmen. "Spanish Depictions of the Miracle of the Black Leg." In Zimmerman, *One Leg in the Grave Revisited*, 79–91.

French, Roger. *Dissection and Vivisection in the European Renaissance*. Aldershot: Ashgate, 1999.

Friedrichs, Christopher R. "Artisans and Urban Politics in Seventeenth-Century Germany." In *The Artisan and the European Town, 1500–1900*, edited by Geoffrey Crossick, 41–55. Brookfield: Ashgate, 1997.

Frohne, Bianca. *Leben mit "kranckhait." Der gebrechliche Körper in der häuslichen Überlieferung des 15. und 16. Jahrhunderts. Überlegungen zu einer Disability History der Vormoderne*. Affalterbach: Didymos-Verlag, 2014.

———. "Performing Dis/ability? Constructions of 'Infirmity' in Late Medieval and Early Modern Life Writing." In Krötzl et al., *Infirmity*, 51–65.

———. "The Cultural Model." In Nolte et al., *Dis/ability History*, 61–63.

Furttenbach, Joseph. *Architectura Recreationis* [...]. Augsburg, 1640.

Gadebusch Bondio, Mariacarla. *Medizinische Ästhetik. Kosmetik und plastische Chirurgie zwischen Antike und früher Neuzeit*. Munich: W. Fink, 2005.

———. "Anatomie der Hand und anatomisches Handwerk vor und nach Andreas Vesal." In *Die Hand. Elemente einer Medizin- und Kulturgeschichte*, edited by Mariacarla Gadebusch Bondio, 79–116. Berlin: Lit, 2010.

———. "On the Function, Utility, and Fragility of the Nose: Early Modern Patients and Their Surgeons." *Nuncius* 32 (2017): 25–51.

Gagné, John. "Emotional Attachments: Iron Hands, their Makers, and their Wearers, 1450–1600." In *Feeling Things: Objects and Emotions through History*, edited by Stephanie Downes, Sally Holloway, and Sarah Randles, 133–153. Oxford: Oxford University Press, 2018.

Galen. *De sanitate tuenda libri sex*. Cologne, 1526.

———. *Opera omnia*. Vol. 18, edited by Karl Gottlob Kühn. Leipzig, 1829.

Garrison, Fielding H. *Notes on the History of Military Medicine*. Hildesheim; New York, 1970.

Gehema, Janus Abraham à. *Wolversehener Feld-Medicus* [...]. Hamburg, 1684.

———. *Der krancke Soldat* [...]. Stettin, 1690.

———. *Der Qualificirte Leib-Medicus*. Stettin, 1690.

———. *Zwantzig sonderbahre Chirurgische Observationes* [...]. Frankfurt am Main, 1690.

———. "Wie die Wunden der Soldaten ins gemein zu tractiren und zu curiren [...]." In *Chirurgische Schriften*, by Johann von Muralt. Basel, 1691.
Gelfand, Toby. *Professionalizing Modern Medicine: Paris Surgeons and Medical Science and Institutions in the 18th Century*. Westport: Greenwood Press, 1980.
Gelman, Georgius. *Chirurgiae tripartita flora. Das ist: Dreyfache Chyrurgische Blumen* [...]. Frankfurt, 1680.
Gerchow, Jan, ed. *Ebenbilder: Kopien von Körpern—Modelle des Menschen*. Ostfildern-Ruit: Hatje Cantz, 2002.
Gerritsen, Anne, and Giorgio Riello. "Introduction: Writing Material Culture History." In *Writing Material Culture History*, edited by Anne Gerritsen and Giorgio Riello, 1–14. London: Bloomsbury Academic, 2015.
Gersdorff, Hans von. *Feldbuch der Wundarznei*. Strasbourg, 1517.
Gosmann, Michael. "Die Arnsberger 'Eiserne Hand'—Ein Relikt aus dem Dreißigjährigen Krieg." *Heimatblätter. Zeitschrift des Arnsberger Heimatbundes* 22 (2001): 27–32.
Gottfried, Johann Ludwig. *Johann Ludwig Gottfrieds Fortgesetzte Historische Chronick* [...]. Vol. 2. Frankfurt am Main, 1745.
Gowland, Angus. "Melancholy, Imagination, and Dreaming in Renaissance Learning." In Haskell, *Diseases of the Imagination*, 53–102.
Grafton, Anthony. "Philological and Artisanal Knowledge Making in Renaissance Natural History: A Study in Cultures of Knowledge." *History of Humanities* 3:1 (2018): 39–55.
Grancsay, Stephen V. "A Hapsburg Locking Gauntlet." *The Metropolitan Museum of Art Bulletin* 32:8 (1937): 188–191.
Greflinger, Georg. *Der Deutschen Dreyßig-Jähriger Krieg*. Munich: Fink, 1983.
Greiff, Sebastian. *Apologia und Refutation* [...]. Frankfurt, 1589.
———. *Vom Cometen Anno 1596* [...]. Erfurt, 1596.
———. *Wundartzeney* [...]. Schleusingen, 1622.
———. *Wolbewärte Wundarzney* [...]. Schleusingen, 1630.
Grimmelshausen, Hans Jakob Christoffel von. *Der seltzame Springinsfeld* [...]. Paphlagonia, 1670.
Grob, Alexa, and Hans Joachim Winckelmann. "Das Collegium Medicum zu Ulm." *Sudhoffs Archiv* 98:1 (2014): 109–123.
Groebner, Valentin. *Defaced: The Visual Culture of Violence in the Late Middle Ages*. Translated by Pamela Selwyn. New York: Zone Books, 2004.
Groiss, Eva. "The Augsburg Clockmakers' Craft." In Maurice and Mayr, *Clockwork Universe*, 57–86.
Grooss, K. S. *Cornelis Solingen: A Seventeenth-Century Surgeon and his Instruments*. Leiden: Museum Boerhaave, 1990.
Grossmann, G. Ulrich, ed. *Mythos Burg: eine Ausstellung des Germanischen Nationalmuseums Nürnberg, 8. Juli bis 7. November*. Dresden: Sandstein Verlag, 2010.
Guffey, Elizabeth, and Bess Williamson. "Introduction: Rethinking Design History through Disability, Rethinking Disability through Design." In Williamson and Guffey, *Making Disability Modern*, 1–13.

Gunnoe Jr., Charles D. "Paracelsus's Biography among His Detractors." In Scholz Williams and Gunnoe Jr., *Paracelsian Moments*, 3–18.

Gurlt, Ernst Julius. *Geschichte der Chirurgie und ihrer Ausübung: Volkschirurgie, Altertum, Mittelalter, Renaissance*. 3 vols. Berlin: Hirschwald, 1898.

Hale, J. R. *War and Society in Renaissance Europe, 1450–1620*. New York: St. Martin's Press, 1985.

Harkness, Deborah. *The Jewel House: Elizabethan London and the Scientific Revolution*. New Haven: Yale University Press, 2007.

Harms, Wolfgang, Michael Schilling, and Andreas Wang, eds. *Deutsche Illustrierte Flugblätter des 16. und 17. Jahrhunderts. Die Sammlung der Herzog August Bibliothek in Wolfenbüttel: kommentierte Ausgabe*. 3 vols. Munich: Kraus International Publications, 1980–1989.

Harrington, Joel. *The Faithful Executioner: Life and Death, Honor and Shame in the Turbulent Sixteenth Century*. New York: Farrar, Straus and Giroux, 2013.

Hasegawa, Guy R. *Mending Broken Soldiers: The Union and Confederate Programs to Supply Artificial Limbs*. Carbondale: Southern Illinois University Press, 2012.

Haskell, Yasmin, ed. *Diseases of the Imagination and Imaginary Disease in the Early Modern Period*. Turnhout: Brepols, 2011.

———. "Introduction: When is a Disease Not a Disease? Seeming and Suffering in Early Modern Europe." In Haskell, *Diseases of the Imagination*, 1–17.

Hauri, Dieter. *Die Steinschneider: Eine Kulturgeschichte menschlichen Leidens und ärztlicher Kunst*. Berlin: Springer, 2013.

Hausse, Heidi. "Bones of Contention: The Decision to Amputate in Early Modern Germany." *The Sixteenth Century Journal* 47:2 (2016): 327–350.

———. "The Locksmith, the Surgeon, and the Mechanical Hand: Communicating Technical Knowledge in Early Modern Europe." *Technology and Culture* 60:1 (2019): 34–64.

Hayward, John F. *The Art of the Gunmaker*. 2 vols. London: St. Martin's Press, 1962.

Heide, Mareike. "'Kein rechte sonder ein gemachte Nasen'—Prothesenträger_innen in Frühneuzeitlichen Versorgungssystemen?" In Nolte et al., *Dis/ability History*, 374–377.

———. *Holzbein und Eisenhand: Prothesen in der Frühen Neuzeit*. New York: Campus Verlag, 2019.

———. "Arbeitsarm und Sonntagshand – Handprothesen in der Frühen Neuzeit." In Jütte and Schmitz-Esser, *Handgebrauch*, 111–134.

Herls, Cornelis. *Examen Chirurgiae oder der Wund-Artzney [...]*. Nuremberg, 1692.

Herrlinger, Robert. "Die Anatomie des Jost Amman: und die Illustration zu Feyerabends Paracelsus-Ausgabe von 1565." *Sudhoffs Archiv für Geschichte der Medizin und der Naturwissenschaften* 37:1 (1953): 23–38.

Hildanus, Wilhelm Fabricius. *De Gangraena et Sphacelo, Das ist: Von dem Heissen und Kalten brandt [...]*. Cologne, 1593.

———. *Gründlicher Bericht vom heissen und kalten Brand*. Edited by Erich Hintzsche. Basel, 1603; reprinted Bern: Huber, 1965.

———. *De combustionibus [...]*. Basel, 1607.

———. *New Feldt-Artzney-Buch [...]*. Basel, 1613.

———. *Lithotomia Vesicae, Das ist: Gründtlicher Bericht von dem Blaterstein* [...]. Basel, 1626.

———. *Lithotomia Vesicae: That is, An accurate description of the Stone in the Bladder* [...]. London, 1640.

———. *Wund-Artzney* [...]. Frankfurt am Main, 1652.

———. *Opera observationum et curationum medico-chirurgicarum*. Frankfurt, 1682.

Hintzsche, Erich. *Guilelmus Fabricius Hildanus: 1560–1634*. Hilden: Lindopharm Rönsberg, 1973.

Hintzsche, Erich. Introduction to Hildanus, *Gründlicher Bericht*, 7–22.

Hirsch, August, ed. *Biographisches Lexikon der hervorragenden Ärzte aller Zeiten und Völker*. 5 vols. 3rd ed. Munich: Urban & Schwarzenberg, 1962.

Horn, Klaus-Peter, and Bianca Frohne. "On the Fluidity of 'Disability' in Medieval and Early Modern Societies: Opportunities and Strategies in a New Field of Research." *The Imperfect Historian: Disability Histories in Europe*, edited by Sebastian Barsch, Anne Klein, and Pieter Verstraete, 17–40. Frankfurt am Main: Peter Lang, 2013.

Hornstein-Grüningen, Edward von. *Die von Hornstein und von Hertenstein Erlebnisse aus 700 Jahren; ein Beitrag zur schwäbischen Volks- und Adelskunde*. Konstanz: Pressverein, 1911.

Huet, Marie-Hélène. "Monstrous Medicine." In *Monstrous Bodies/Political Monstrosities in Early Modern Europe*, edited by Laura Lunger Knoppers and Joan B. Landes, 127–147. Ithaca: Cornell University Press, 2004.

Issickemer, Jakob. *Das buchlein der zuflucht zu Maria der muter gottes in alten Oding* [...]. Nuremberg, 1497.

Jardine, Lisa, and Anthony Grafton. "'Studied for Action': How Gabriel Harvey Read His Livy." *Past and Present* 129 (1990): 30–78.

Jessen, Johannes Jessenius von. *Anweisung zur Wund-Artznei* [...]. Nuremberg, 1674.

Joël, Franz. *Chirurgia oder Wund-Artzney* [...]. Nuremberg, 1680.

Joubert, Laurent. *Traitté des arcbusades* [...]. Lyon, 1581.

Jousse, Mathurin. *La fidelle ouverture de l'art de serrurier* [...]. La Fleche, 1627.

Jütte, Robert. "A Seventeenth-Century German Barber-Surgeon and His Patients." *Medical History* 33:2 (1989): 184–198.

———. *Ärzte, Heiler und Patienten: Medizinischer Alltag in der frühen Neuzeit*. Munich: Artemis & Winkler, 1991.

Jütte, Robert, and Romedio Schmitz-Esser, eds. *Handgebrauch: Geschichten von der Hand aus dem Mittelalter und der Frühen Neuzeit*. Paderborn: Wilhelm Fink, 2019.

Kahlow, Simone. "Prothesen im Mittelalter—ein Überblick aus archäologischer Sicht." In *Homo Debilis. Behinderte—Kranke—Versehrte in der Gesellschaft des Mittelalters*, edited by Cordula Nolte, 203–224. Korb: Didymos-Verlag, 2009.

———. "Archäologische Erkenntnisse zur Chirurgie und Prothetik in Mittelalter und Früher Neuzeit." In Nolte et al., *Dis/ability History*, 344–348.

Karcheski, Walter J. *Arms and Armor in the Art Institute of Chicago*. Chicago: Art Institute of Chicago, 1995.

Karpinski, Otto. *Studien über künstliche Glieder*. Berlin: Mittler, 1881.

Keating, Jessica. *Animating Empire: Automata, the Holy Roman Empire, and the Early Modern World*. University Park, Pennsylvania: Pennsylvania State University Press, 2018.

Keil, Baldur. "Eine Prothese aus einem fränkischen Grab von Griesheim, Kreis Darmstadt-Dieburg: Anthropologische und medizinhistorische Befunde." *Fundberichte aus Hessen* 17/18 (1980): 195–211.

Kinzelbach, Annemarie. "Zur Sozial- und Alltagsgeschichte eines Handwerks in der frühen Neuzeit: 'Wundärzte' und ihre Patienten in Ulm." *Ulm und Oberschwaben* 49 (1994): 111–144.

———. *Gesundbleiben, Krankwerden, Armsein in der frühneuzeitlichen Gesellschaft: Gesunde und Kranke in den Reichsstädten Überlingen und Ulm, 1500–1700*. Stuttgart: F. Steiner, 1995.

———. "Erudite and Honoured Artisans? Performers of Body Care and Surgery in Early Modern German Towns." *Social History of Medicine* 27:4 (2014): 668–688.

———. "Women and Healthcare in Early Modern German Towns." *Renaissance Studies* 28:4 (2014): 619–638.

———. *Chirurgen und Chirurgie-Praktiken: Wundärzte als Reichsstadtbürger 16. bis 18. Jahrhundert*. Mainz: Donata Kinzelbach, 2016.

Kirkup, John R. *The History of Limb Amputation*. London: Springer, 2007.

Klestinec, Cynthia. "Practical Experience in Anatomy." In *The Body as Object and Instrument of Knowledge: Embodied Empiricism in Early Modern Science*, edited by C. T. Wolfe and O. Gal, 33–57. Dordrecht: Springer, 2010.

———. *Theaters of Anatomy: Students, Teachers, and Traditions of Dissection in Renaissance Venice*. Baltimore: Johns Hopkins University Press, 2011.

———. "Renaissance Surgeons: Anatomy, Manual Skill and the Visual Arts." In *Early Modern Medicine and Natural Philosophy*, edited by Peter Distelzweig, Benjamin Goldberg, and Evan R. Ragland, 43–58. Dordrecht: Springer, 2016.

Knoche, Wilfried. *Prothesen der unteren Extremität: die Entwicklung vom Altertum bis 1930*. In collaboration with Stefan Bieringer and Beat Rüttimann. Dortmund: Bundesfachschule für Orthopädie-Technik, 2006.

Koeppe, Wolfram. "Setting the Standard: Forging a Culture of Magnificence." In *Making Marvels: Science and Splendor at the Courts of Europe*, edited by Wolfram Koeppe, 15–25. New Haven: Yale University Press, 2019.

Königer, Ernst. *Aus der Geschichte der Heilkunst. Von Ärzten, Badern und Chirurgen*. Munich: Prestel, 1958.

Kosmin, Jennifer. *Authority, Gender, and Midwifery in Early Modern Italy: Contested Deliveries*. New York: Routledge, 2020.

Krajbich, Joseph Ivan, Michael S. Pinzur, Benjamin K. Potter, and Phillip M. Stevens, eds. *Atlas of Amputations and Limb Deficiencies: Surgical, Prosthetic, and Rehabilitation Principles*. 3 vols. 4th ed. Rosemont: American Academy of Orthopaedic Surgeons, 2016.

Krebs, Robert E. *Groundbreaking Scientific Experiments, Inventions, and Discoveries of the Middle Ages and the Renaissance*. Westport: Greenwood, 2004.

Krötzl, Christian, Katariina Mustakallio, and Jenni Kuuliala, eds. *Infirmity in Antiquity and the Middle Ages: Social and Cultural Approaches to Health, Weakness and Care*. New York: Routledge, 2016.

Kudlick, Catherine. "Social History of Medicine and Disability History." In *The Oxford Handbook of Disability History*, edited by Michael Rembis, Catherine Kudlick, and Kim E. Nielsen, 105–124. New York: Oxford University Press, 2018.

La Rocca, Donald J. *How to Read European Armor*. New York: The Metropolitan Museum of Art, 2017.

Lachmund, Friedrich. *De Ave Diomedea Dissertatio: Cum Verâ ejus effigie aeri incisa, ex Muséo D. Friderici Lachmund Hildesheim* […]. Amsterdam, 1674.

Ladegaard Jakobsen, Anna-Lise. "A Cripple from the Late Middle Ages." *Ossa: International Journal of Skeletal Research* 5 (1978): 17–24.

Lamzweerde, Jan Baptist van. *Appendix, Variorum tam veterum, quam recenter inventorum Instrumentorum Ad Armamentarium Chirurgicum Joannis Schulteti* […]. Leiden, 1693.

Landes, David. *Revolution in Time: Clocks and the Making of the Modern World*. Cambridge, MA: Belknap Press, 1983.

Lanfrancus [Mediolanensis]. *Kleine Wundarzney* […]. Augsburg, 1528.

Lang, Carl. *Historischer Almanach für den deutschen Adel, und für Freunde der Geschichte desselben. 1793. Ritter Göz von Berlichingen, mit der eisernen Hand*. Frankfurt am Main: Fleischer, 1793.

———. *Historischer Almanach für den Deutschen Adel, und für Freunde der Geschichte desselben. 1794. Ritter Göz von Berlichingen, mit der eisernen Hand*. Frankfurt am Main: Guilhauman, 1794.

Lazenby, Richard A., and Susan K. Pfeiffer. "Effects of a Nineteenth Century Below-Knee Amputation and Prosthesis on Femoral Morphology." *International Journal of Osteoarchaeology* 3 (1993): 19–28.

Lefèvre, Wolfgang. "The Limits of Pictures: Cognitive Functions of Images in Practical Mechanics – 1400 to 1600." In *The Power of Images in Early Modern Science*, edited by Wolfgang Lefèvre, Jürgen Renn, and Urs Schoepflin, 69–88. Basel: Springer Basel AG, 2003.

Leong, Elaine. *Recipes and Everyday Knowledge: Medicine, Science, and the Household in Early Modern England*. Chicago: University of Chicago Press, 2018.

Leong, Elaine, and Alisha Rankin, eds. *Secrets and Knowledge in Medicine and Science, 1500–1800*. Farnham: Ashgate, 2011.

Lindemann, Mary. *Medicine and Society in Early Modern Europe*. 2nd ed. Cambridge: Cambridge University Press, 2010.

Linker, Beth. *War's Waste: Rehabilitation in World War I America*. Chicago: University of Chicago Press, 2011.

———. "On the Borderland of Medical and Disability History: A Survey of the Fields." *Bulletin of the History of Medicine* 87:4 (2013): 499–535.

Lis, Catharina, and Hugo Soly. "Subcontracting in Guild-Based Export Trades, Thirteenth–Eighteenth Centuries." In *Guilds, Innovation and the European Economy, 1400–1800*, edited by S. R. Epstein and Maarten Prak, 81–113. Cambridge: Cambridge University Press, 2008.

Löffler, Liebhard. "Götz von Berlichingen und seine Prothesen (Die beiden Jagsthäuser Hände)." *Orthopädie-Technik* 31:1 (1980): 11–15.

———. "Neues von alten Händen: Neuentdeckte und bisher kaum beachtete Arm- und Handprothesen." *Orthopädie-Technik* 5 (1981): 75–81.

———. *Der Ersatz für die obere Extremität: die Entwicklung von den ersten Zeugnissen bis heute*. Stuttgart: Enke, 1984.

———. "Die Braunschweiger Hand und Herzog Christian I. Altersbestimmung und Erbauerberufsgruppe." *Würzburger medizinhistorische Mitteilungen* 18 (1999): 65–74.

Long, Pamela O. "Power, Patronage, and the Authorship of *Ars*: From Mechanical Know-How to Mechanical Knowledge in the Last Scribal Age." *Isis* 88:1 (1997): 1–41.

———. *Openness, Secrecy, Authorship: Technical Arts and the Culture of Knowledge from Antiquity to the Renaissance*. Baltimore: Johns Hopkins University Press, 2001.

———. *Artisan/Practitioners and the Rise of the New Sciences, 1400–1600*. Corvallis: Oregon State University Press, 2011.

Lose, Laurentius, and Sebastian Greiff. *Chirurgisches Hand-Büchlein/ Oder Erneuerter Greif*. Meiningen, 1679.

Louis, Elan D., and George K. York. "Weir Mitchell's Observations on Sensory Localization and Their Influence on Jacksonian Neurology." *Neurology* 66:8 (2006): 1241–1244.

Lytton, D. G., and L. M. Resuhr. "Galen on Abnormal Swellings." *Journal of the History of Medicine and Allied Sciences* 33:4 (1978): 531–549.

Malgaigne, Joseph-François. *Surgery and Ambroise Paré*. Translated and edited by Wallace B. Hamby. Norman: University of Oklahoma Press, 1965.

Marchetti, Pietro de. *Seltzam- Außerlesen- Medicinisch-Chirurgische Observationes [...]*. Nuremberg, 1673.

Maurice, Klaus. *Die deutsche Räderuhr: Zur Kunst und Technik des mechanischen Zeitmessers im deutschen Sprachraum*. 2 vols. Munich: Beck, 1976.

———. "Jost Bürgi, or On Innovation." In Maurice and Mayr, *Clockwork Universe*, 87–102.

Maurice, Klaus, and Otto Mayr, eds. *The Clockwork Universe: German Clocks and Automata, 1550–1650*. New York: Neale Watson Academic Publications, 1980.

Mayer, Helmut. "Christian der Jüngere Herzog von Braunschweig-Lüneburg-Wolfenbüttel (1599–1626), Verwundung, Amputation und Tod—Ein Arm ohne Fleisch und Blut." *Braunschweigisches Jahrbuch für Landesgeschichte* 77 (1996): 181–201.

Mayr, Otto. *Authority, Liberty and Automatic Machinery in Early Modern Europe*. Baltimore: Johns Hopkins University Press, 1986.

Mays, S. A. "Healed Limb Amputations in Human Osteoarchaeology and their Causes: A Case Study from Ipswich, UK." *International Journal of Osteoarchaeology* 6 (1996): 101–113.

McVaugh, Michael. *Rational Surgery of the Middle Ages*. Florence: SISMEL edizioni del Galluzzo, 2006.

Mechel, Christian von. *Die eiserne Hand des tapfern deutschen Ritters Götz von Berlichingen, wie selbige noch bei seiner Familie in Franken aufbewahrt wird*. Berlin: Decker, 1815.

Mendelsohn, J. Andrew. "The World on a Page: Making a General Observation in the Eighteenth Century." In *Histories of Scientific Observation*, edited by Lorraine Daston and Elizabeth Lunbeck, 396–420. Chicago: University of Chicago Press, 2011.

Mendelsohn, J. Andrew, Annemarie Kinzelbach, and Ruth Schilling, eds. *Civic Medicine: Physician, Polity, and Pen in Early Modern Europe*. New York: Routledge, 2020.

Metzler, Irina. *Disability in Medieval Europe: Physical Impairment in the High Middle Ages, c.1100–c. 1400*. London: Routledge, 2006.

———. *A Social History of Disability in the Middle Ages*. New York: Routledge, 2013.

———. "The Social Model." In Nolte et al., *Dis/ability History*, 59–61.

Mihm, Stephen, Katherine Ott, and David Serlin, eds. *Artificial Parts, Practical Lives: Modern Histories of Prosthetics*. New York: New York University Press, 2002.

Mitchell, Piers D. *Medicine in the Crusades: Warfare, Wounds and the Medieval Surgeon*. Cambridge: Cambridge University Press, 2004.

Mondeville, Henri de. *Chirurgie de maître Henri de Mondevillie: composée de 1306 à 1320*. Translated by Edouard Nicaise. Paris: Félix Alcan, 1893.

Monter, E. William. *Studies in Genevan Government (1536–1605)*. Geneva: Librairie Droz, 1964.

Mukerji, Chandra. *Impossible Engineering: Technology and Territoriality on the Canal du Midi*. Princeton: Princeton University Press, 2009.

Munnicks, Johann. *Praxis Cheirurgica, Oder Wund-Artzney* […]. [Ulm]; Frankfurt, 1690.

Munt, Annette H. "The Impact of Dutch Cartesian Medical Reformers in Early Enlightenment German Culture (1680–1720)." Ph.D. dissertation. University College London, 2004.

Murphy, Hannah. *A New Order of Medicine: The Rise of Physicians in Reformation Nuremberg*. Pittsburgh: University of Pittsburgh Press, 2019.

Muys, Jan. *Neue Vernünfftige Praxis der Wund-Artzney* […]. Frankfurt an der Oder; Leipzig, 1688.

Niiranen, Susanna. "Sexual Incapacity in Medieval *Materia Medica*." In Krötzl et al., *Infirmity*, 223–240.

Nimwegen, Olaf van. "The Transformation of Army Organisation in Early-Modern Western Europe, *c*. 1500–1789." In *European Warfare, 1350–1750*, edited by Frank Tallett and D. J. B. Trim, 159–180. Cambridge: Cambridge University Press, 2010.

Nolte, Cordula, ed. *Phänomene der "Behinderung" im Alltag: Bausteine zu einer Disability History der Vormoderne*. Affalterbach: Didymos-Verlag, 2013.

Nolte, Cordula, Bianca Frohne, Uta Halle, and Sonja Kerth, eds. *Dis/ability History der Vormoderne: Ein Handbuch. Premodern Dis/ability History: A Companion*. Affalterbach: Didymos-Verlag, 2017.

Nutton, Vivian. "Humanist Surgery." In *The Medical Renaissance of the Sixteenth Century*, edited by A. Wear, R. K. French, and I. M. Lonie, 75–99. Cambridge: Cambridge University Press, 1985.

———. "Medicine in Medieval Western Europe, 1000–1500." In Conrad et al., *Western Medical Tradition*, 139–205.

Oakeshott, R. Ewart. *European Weapons and Armour from the Renaissance to the Industrial Revolution*. Woodbridge: Boydell, 2012.

Oettinger, Johann Peter. *A German Barber-Surgeon in the Atlantic Slave Trade: The Seventeenth-Century Journal of Johann Peter Oettinger*. Translated by Craig Koslofsky and Roberto Zaugg. Charlottesville: University of Virigina Press, 2020.
O'Malley, Michelle. "A Pair of Little Gilded Shoes: Commission, Cost, and Meaning in Renaissance Footwear." *Renaissance Quarterly* 63:1 (2010): 45–83.
Östling, Johan, David Larsson Heidenblad, Erling Sandmo, Anna Nilsson Hammar, and Kari Nordberg. "The History of Knowledge and the Circulation of Knowledge: An Introduction." In *Circulation of Knowledge: Explorations in the History of Knowledge*, edited by Johan Östling, David Larsson Heidenblad, Erling Sandmo, Anna Nilsson Hammar, and Kari Nordberg, 9–33. Lund: Nordic Academic Press, 2018.
Ott, Katherine. "The Sum of Its Parts: An Introduction to Modern Histories of Prosthetics." In Mihm et al. *Artificial Parts, Practical Lives*, 1–32.
———. "Disability Things: Material Culture and American Disability History, 1700–2010." In Burch and Rembis, *Disability Histories*, 119–135.
Otte, Andreas. "3D Computer-Aided Design Reconstructions and 3D Multi-material Polymer Replica Printings of the First 'Iron Hand' of Franconian Knight Gottfried (Götz) von Berlichingen (1480–1562): An Overview." *Prosthesis* 2 (2020): 304–312.
———. "Christian von Mechel's Reconstructive Drawings of the Second 'Iron Hand' of Franconian Knight Gottfried (Götz) von Berlichingen (1480–1562)." *Prosthesis* 3 (2021): 105–109.
Overcamp, Heydentryk. *Neues Gebäude der Chirurgie* [...]. Leipzig, 1689.
Pagel, Walter. *Paracelsus: An Introduction to Philosophical Medicine in the Era of the Renaissance*. 2nd ed. New York: Karger, 1982.
Pankofer, Heinrich. *Schlüssel und Schloss; Schönheit, Form und Technik im Wandel der Zeiten, aufgezeigt an der Sammlung Heinrich Pankofer*. Munich: G. D. W. Callwey, 1973/1974.
Panse, Melanie. *Hans von Gersdorffs "Feldbuch der Wundarznei"—Produktion, Präsentation und Rezeption von Wissen*. Wiesbaden: Reichert Verlag, 2012.
Pantin, Isabelle. "La traduction latine des Oeuvres d'Ambroise Paré." In Berriot-Salvadore and Mironneau, *Ambroise Paré*, 315–336.
———. "The Role of Translations in European Scientific Exchanges in the Sixteenth and Seventeenth Centuries." In *Cultural Translation in Early Modern Europe*, edited by Peter Burke and R. Po-chia Hsia, 163–179. Cambridge: Cambridge University Press, 2007.
Paracelsus. *Der grossen wundartzney/ Das ander Buch* [...]. Augsburg, 1536.
———. *Opus Chyrurgicum* [...]. Frankfurt am Main, 1565.
Paré, Ambroise. *Les Oeuvres* [...]. Paris, 1575.
———. *Les Oeuvres* [...]. Paris, 1579.
———. *Opera Ambrosii Parei* [...]. Paris, 1582.
———. *Les Oeuvres* [...]. Paris, 1585.
———. *De chirurgie* [...]. Dordrecht, 1592.
———. *Opera Chirurgica* [...]. Frankfurt am Main, 1594.
———. *Les Oeuvres* [...]. Paris, 1598.
———. *Wundt-Artzney oder Artzney-Spiegell* [...]. Frankfurt am Main, 1601.
———. *De chirurgie* [...]. Leiden, 1604.

——. *Opera Chirurgica* [...]. Frankfurt am Main, 1612.
——. *Les Oeuvres* [...]. Paris, 1614.
——. *The Workes* [...]. London, 1634.
——. *Wund-Artzney, oder Artzney spiegell* [...]. Frankfurt am Main, 1635.
——. *De chirurgie* [...]. Amsterdam, 1636.
——. *The Workes* [...]. London, 1649.
Park, Katharine. "The Imagination in Renaissance Psychology." M.Phil. thesis. University of London, 1974.
Parker, Geoffrey. *The Military Revolution: Military Innovation and the Rise of the West, 1500–1800*. 2nd ed. 19th print. Cambridge: Cambridge University Press, 2016.
Pelling, Margaret. *The Common Lot: Sickness, Medical Occupations, and the Urban Poor in Early Modern England*. London: Longman, 1998.
——. *Medical Conflicts in Early Modern London: Patronage, Physicians, and Irregular Practitioners, 1550–1640*. Oxford: Clarendon Press, 2003.
Perry, Heather R. *Recycling the Disabled: Army, Medicine, and Modernity in WWI Germany*. Manchester: Manchester University Press, 2014.
Petraeus, Heinrich. *Encheiridion Cheirurgicum* [...]. Nuremberg, 1625.
Pfaffenbiehler, Matthias. *Armourers*. Toronto: University of Toronto Press, 1992.
Poirier, Jean-Pierre. *Ambroise Paré: Un urgentiste au XVIe siècle*. Paris: Pygmalion, 2005.
Pomata, Gianna. "Menstruating Men: Similarity and Difference of the Sexes in Early Modern Medicine." In *Generation and Degeneration: Tropes of Reproduction in Literature and History from Antiquity to Early Modern Europe*, edited by Valeria Finucci and Kevin Brownlee, 109–152. Durham: Duke University Press, 2001.
——. "*Praxis Historialis*: The Uses of *Historia* in Early Modern Medicine." In *Historia: Empiricism and Erudition in Early Modern Europe*, edited by Gianna Pomata and Nancy G. Siraisi, 105–146. Cambridge, MA: MIT Press, 2005.
——. "Sharing Cases: The *Observationes* in Early Modern Medicine." *Early Science and Medicine* 15:3 (2010): 193–236.
Porter, Roy. *The Greatest Benefit to Mankind: A Medical History of Humanity*. New York: W. W. Norton, 1998.
Pouchelle, Marie-Christine. *The Body and Surgery in the Middle Ages*. Translated by Rosemary Morris. Cambridge: Polity Press, 1990.
Purmann, Matthäus Gottfried. *Der rechte und wahrhafftige Feldscher* [...]. Halberstadt, 1680.
——. *Neu herausgegebener Chirurgischer Lorbeer-Krantz, oder Wund-Artzney* [...]. Halberstadt, 1684.
——. *Kurtze, doch gründliche Anweisung* [...]. [S.l.], 1686.
——. *Fünff und zwantzig Sonder- und Wunderbare Schuß-Wunden Curen* [...]. Breslau, 1687.
——. *Grosser und gantz neugewundener Lorbeer-Krantz/ oder Wund-Artzney* [...]. Leipzig, 1692.
——. *Chirurgia curiosa* [...]. Leipzig, 1699.
Putti, Vittorio. *Historic Artificial Limbs*. New York: Paul B. Hoeber Inc., 1930.

Pyhrr, Stuart W. *Firearms from the Collections of the Prince of Liechtenstein*. New York: Metropolitan Museum of Art, 1985.

Pyhrr, Stuart W., and José-A. Godoy. *Heroic Armor of the Italian Renaissance: Filippo Negroli and His Contemporaries*. New York: The Metropolitan Museum of Art, 1998.

Quasigroch, Günther. "Die Handprothesen des fränkischen Reichsritters Götz von Berlichingen." *Waffen- und Kostümkunde* 1 (1982): 17–33.

Ragland, Evan. "Chymistry and Taste in the Seventeenth Century: Franciscus Dele Boë Sylvius as a Chymical Physician Between Galenism and Cartesianism." *Ambix* 56:1 (2012): 1–21.

———. "Experimental Clinical Medicine and Drug Action in Mid-Seventeenth-Century Leiden." *Bulletin of the History of Medicine* 91:2 (2017): 331–361.

Ramelli, Agostino. *Le diverse et artificiose machine [...]*. Paris, 1588.

Rang, Mercer, and George H. Thompson. "History of Amputations and Prostheses." In *Amputation Surgery and Rehabilitation: The Toronto Experience*, edited by J. P. Kostuik and R. Gillespie, 1–12. New York: Churchill Livingstone, 1981.

Rankin, Alisha. *Panaceia's Daughters: Noblewomen as Healers in Early Modern Germany*. Chicago: Chicago University Press, 2013.

Rather, L. J. "Thomas Fienus' (1567–1631) Dialectical Investigation of the Imagination as Cause and Cure of Bodily Disease." *Bulletin of the History of Medicine* 41:4 (1967): 349–367.

Reddig, Wolfgang F. *Bader, Medicus und Weise Frau. Wege und Erfolge der mittelalterlichen Heilkunst*. Munich: Battenberg, 2000.

Rehtmeyer, Philipp Julius. *Braunschweig-Lüneburgischen Chronica [...]*. Vol. 2. Braunschweig, 1722.

Rembis, Michael, Catherine Kudlick, and Kim E. Nielsen. "Introduction." In *The Oxford Handbook of Disability History*, edited by Michael Rembis, Catherine Kudlick, and Kim E. Nielsen, 1–18. New York: Oxford University Press, 2018.

Renner, Franz. *Ein [...] Handtbüchlein [...]*. Nuremberg, 1557.

———. *Ein [...] Handtbüchlein [...]*. Nuremberg, 1559.

———. *Ein köstlich und bewärtes Artzney-Büchlein [...]*. Amberg, 1609.

Roberts, Lissa, Simon Schaffer, and Peter Dear, eds. *The Mindful Hand: Inquiry and Invention from the Late Renaissance to Early Industrialisation*. Amsterdam: Koninklijke Nederlandse Akademie van Wetenschappen, 2007.

Roe, Thomas. *The Negotiations of Sir Thomas Roe [...] 1621 to 1628 [...]*. London, 1740.

Rogers, Clifford J., ed. *The Military Revolution Debate: Readings on the Military Transformation of Early Modern Europe*. Boulder: Westview Press, 1995.

Roodenburg, Herman. "The Senses." In *Early Modern Emotions: An Introduction*, edited by Susan Broomhall, 42–44. London: Routledge, 2017.

Roper, Lyndal. *The Holy Household: Women and Morals in Reformation Augsburg*. New York: Oxford University Press, 1989.

Rublack, Ulinka, and Pamela Selwyn. "Fluxes: The Early Modern Body and the Emotions." *History Workshop Journal* 53 (2002): 1–16.

Ryff, Walther Hermann. *Die groß Chirurgei [...]*. Frankfurt am Main, 1545.

———. *Letzte Theil der großen Teutschen Chirurgei [...]*. Frankfurt am Main, 1562.

Sachs, Hans. *A Sixteenth-Century Book of Trades: Das Ständebuch.* Translated by Theodore K. Rabb. Palo Alto: The Society for the Promotion of Science and Scholarship, 2009.

Sachs, Michael. "Matthäus Gottfried Purmann (1649–1711): Ein schlesischer Chirurg auf dem Weg von der mittelalterlichen Volksmedizin zur neuzeitlichen Chirurgie." *Würzburger medizinhistorische Mitteilungen* 12 (1994): 37–64.

———. *Geschichte der operativen Chirurgie.* 5 vols. Heidelberg: Kaden, 2000–2005.

Sander, Sabine. *Handwerkschirurgen. Sozialgeschichte einer verdrängten Berufsgruppe.* Göttingen: Vandenhoeck & Ruprecht, 1989.

Savage-Smith, Emilie. "The Exchange of Medical and Surgical Ideas Between Europe and Islam." In *The Diffusion of Greco-Roman Medicine into the Middle East and the Caucasus*, edited by John A. C. Greppin, Emilie Savage-Smith, and John L. Gueriguian, 27–55. Delmar: Caravan Books, 1999.

Savoia, Paolo. *Gaspare Tagliacozzi and Early Modern Surgery: Faces, Men, and Pain.* New York: Routledge, 2019.

Schadewaldt, H. "Padua und die Medizin." In *Soforttherapie Rehabilitation. Vorträge des XIII. Europäischen Fortbildungskongresses, veranstaltet vom Europaeum Medicum Collegium vom 13. bis 12. Mai 1970 in Salsomaggiore Terme (Italien)*, edited by G. W. Parade, 244–267. München-Gräfelfing: Werk-Verlag Dr. Edmund Banaschewski, 1971.

Scheutz, Martin, and Alfred S. Weiss. *Das Spital in der Frühen Neuzeit: Eine Spitallandschaft in Zentraleuropa.* Vienna: Böhlau Verlag, 2020.

Schilling, Ruth, and Kay Peter Jankrift. "Medical Practice in Context: Religion, Family, Politics and Scientific Networks." In *Medical Practice, 1600–1900: Physicians and Their Patients*, edited by Martin Dinges, Kay Peter Jankrift, Sabine Schlegelmilch, and Michael Stolberg, 131–148. Leiden: Brill Rodopi, 2016.

Schleiner, Winfried. *Medical Ethics in the Renaissance.* Washington, D.C.: Georgetown University Press, 1995.

Schlosser, Julius von. *Art and Curiosity Cabinets of the Late Renaissance: A Contribution to the History of Collecting.* Los Angeles: The Getty Research Institute, 2021.

Schmaltz, Tad M. *Early Modern Cartesianisms: Dutch and French Constructions.* New York: Oxford University Press, 2017.

Schmid, Joseph. *Examen chirurgicum* […]. Augsburg, 1644.

———. *Etliche kurtze und wohlbewehrte Artzneyen* […]. Augsburg, 1646.

———. *Spiegel der Anatomiae* […]. Augsburg, 1646.

———. *Kriegs-Arzney* […]. Frankfurt am Main, 1664.

———. *Kurtzer jedoch eigendlicher Bericht* […]. Augsburg, 1667.

———. *Speculum chirurgicum* […]. Augsburg, 1675.

———. *Instrumenta chirurgica* […]. Augsburg, 1697.

Scholz Williams, Gerhild, and Charles D. Gunnoe Jr., eds. *Paracelsian Moments: Science, Medicine and Astrology in Early Modern Europe.* Kirksville: Truman State University Press, 2002.

Schott, Heinz. "'Invisible Diseases'—Imagination and Magnetism: Paracelsus and the Consequences." In *Paracelsus: The Man and His Reputation, His Ideas and Their Transformation*, edited by Ole Peter Grell, 309–321. Leiden: Brill, 1998.

———. "Paracelsus and van Helmont on Imagination: Magnetism and Medicine before Mesmer." In Scholz Williams and Gunnoe Jr., *Paracelsian Moments*, 135–147.
Schotte, Margaret E. *Sailing School: Navigating Science and Skill, 1550–1800*. Baltimore: Johns Hopkins University Press, 2019.
Scultetus, Johannes. *Cheiroplotheke, seu [...] Armamentarium Chirurgicum [...]*. The Hague, 1656.
———. *Wund-Artzneyisches Zeug-Hauß [...]*. Frankfurt am Main, 1666.
———. *Wund-Artzneyisches Zeug-Hauß [...]*. Frankfurt, 1679.
———. *Armamentarium Chirurgicum [...]*. Leiden, 1693.
Seelig, Gero, Giulia Bartrum, and Marjolein Leesberg, eds. *Jost Amman: Book Illustrations*. 11 vols. Rotterdam: Sound & Vision Publishers, 2002.
Shaw, James, and Evelyn Welch. *Making and Marketing Medicine in Renaissance Florence*. New York: Rodopi, 2011.
Siraisi, Nancy. *Medieval and Early Renaissance Medicine: An Introduction to Knowledge and Practice*. Chicago: University of Chicago Press, 1990.
———. "How to Write a Latin Book on Surgery: Organizing Principles and Authorial Devices in Guglielmo da Saliceto and Dino del Garbo." In *Practical Medicine from Salerno to the Black Death*, edited by Luis García-Ballester, Roger French, Jon Arrizabalaga, and Andrew Cunningham, 88–109. Cambridge: Cambridge University Press, 1994.
———. "Medicine, 1450–1620, and the History of Science." *Isis* 103:3 (2012): 491–514.
Smith, Pamela H. *The Body of the Artisan: Art and Experience in the Scientific Revolution*. Chicago: University of Chicago Press, 2004.
———. "In a Sixteenth-Century Goldsmith's Workshop." In Roberts et al., *Mindful Hand*, 33–57.
———. "Making as Knowing: Craft as Natural Philosophy." In *Ways of Making and Knowing: The Material Culture of Empirical Knowledge*, edited by Pamela H. Smith, Amy R. W. Meyers, and Harold J. Cook, 17–47. Ann Arbor: University of Michigan Press, 2014.
———. "The Codification of Vernacular Theories of Metallic Generation in Sixteenth-Century European Mining and Metalworking." In Valleriani, *Structures of Practical Knowledge*, 371–392.
Société pour la conservation des monuments historiques d'Alsace. "Séance du 3 novembre 1856." In *Bulletin de la Société pour la conservation des monuments historiques d'Alsace*. Vol. 1, 243–251. Paris: Berger-Levrault, 1856.
Soliday, Gerald Lyman. *A Community in Conflict: Frankfurt Society in the Seventeenth and Early Eighteenth Centuries*. Hanover: Brandeis University Press, 1974.
Solingen, Cornelis. *Hand-Griffe der Wund-Artzney [...]*. Frankfurt an der Oder, 1693.
Soly, Hugo. "The Political Economy of European Craft Guilds: Power Relations and Economic Strategies of Merchants and Master Artisans in the Medieval and Early Modern Textile Industries." In *The Return of the Guilds*, edited by Jan Lucassen, Tine De Moor, and Jan Luiten van Zanden, 45–71. New York: Cambridge University Press, 2008.

Spehr, Ludwig Ferdinand. *Braunschweigischer Fürstensaal. Portraits der Fürsten und Fürstinnen aus dem Braunschweigischen Gesammthause von den ältesten bis auf die neueste Zeit*. Braunschweig: Trackert, 1840.

Stein, Claudia. *Negotiating the French Pox in Early Modern Germany*. Farnham: Ashgate, 2009.

Stolberg, Michael. *Experiencing Illness and the Sick Body in Early Modern Europe*. New York: Palgrave Macmillan, 2011.

———. "Bedside Teaching and the Acquisition of Practical Skills in Mid-Sixteenth-Century Padua." *Journal of the History of Medicine and Allied Sciences* 69:4 (2014): 633–661.

Stolz, Susanna. *Die Handwerke des Körpers. Bader, Barbier, Perückenmacher, Friseur: Folge und Ausdruck historischen Körperverständnisses*. Marburg: Jonas, 1992.

Strauss, Gerald. *Nuremberg in the Sixteenth Century*. New York: Wiley, 1966.

Strocchia, Sharon T. *Forgotten Healers: Women and the Pursuit of Health in Late Renaissance Italy*. Cambridge: Harvard University Press, 2019.

Stuart, H. S. M. Introduction to *The Autobiography of Götz von Berlichingen*. By Götz von Berlichingen. Edited by H. S. M. Stuart. London: Gerald Duckworth & Co. Ltd., 1956.

Stuart, Kathy. *Defiled Trades and Social Outcasts: Honor and Ritual Pollution in Early Modern Germany*. New York: Cambridge University Press, 1999.

[Sturm, Leonhard Christoph.] *Des geöffneten Ritter-Platzes Dritter Theil* [...]. Hamburg, 1705.

Swan, Claudia. "Eyes Wide Shut: Early Modern Imagination, Demonology, and the Visual Arts." *Zeitsprünge* 7:4 (2003): 560–581.

Tassin, Leonard. *Kurtze Kriegs-Wund-Artzney* [...]. Nuremberg, 1676.

Thurston, Alan J. "Paré and Prosthetics: The Early History of Artificial Limbs." *ANZ Journal of Surgery* 77:12 (2007): 1114–1119.

Topf, Jakob. *An Almain Armourer's Album: Selections from an Original MS. in Victoria and Albert Museum, South Kensington*. Edited by Harold Arthur Lee-Dillon Dillon. London: W. Griggs, 1905.

Tracy, Larissa, and Kelly DeVries, eds. *Wounds and Wound Repair in Medieval Culture*. Leiden: Brill, 2015.

Turnbull, David. "Traveling Knowledge: Narratives, Assemblage and Encounters." In *Instruments, Travel and Science: Itineraries of Precision from the Seventeenth to the Twentieth Century*, edited by Marie-Noëlle Bourguet, Christian Licoppe, and H. Otto Sibum, 273–294. London: Routledge, 2002.

Turner, Wendy J., and Tory Vandeventer Pearman, eds. *The Treatment of Disabled Persons in Medieval Europe: Examining Disability in the Historical, Legal, Literary, Medical, and Religious Discourses of the Middle Ages*. Lewiston: Edwin Mellen Press, 2010.

Uffenbach, Peter, ed. *Thesaurus chirurgiae* [...]. Frankfurt, 1610.

Ulmschneider, Helgard. *Götz von Berlichingen: Ein adeliges Leben der deutschen Renaissance*. Sigmaringen: Thorbecke, 1974.

Ulrich, Laurel Thatcher, Ivan Gaskell, Sara J. Schechner, and Sarah Anne Carter. *Tangible Things: Making History through Objects*. New York: Oxford University Press, 2015.

Ulrich-Bochsler, Susi, and R. Baumgartner. "Über drei Funde von Amputationen im Kanton Bern, Schweiz." *Anthropologischer Anzeiger* 46:4 (1988): 327–334.

Valeri, Mark. "Religion, Discipline, and the Economy in Calvin's Geneva." *The Sixteenth Century Journal* 28:1 (1997): 123–142.

Valeriani, Simona. "Grasping the Body: Physicians, Tailors, and Holy People." *Technology and Culture* 62:1 (2021): 467–493.

Valleriani, Matteo, ed. *The Structures of Practical Knowledge*. Cham: Springer, 2017.

———. "The Epistemology of Practical Knowledge." In Valleriani, *Structures of Practical Knowledge*, 1–19.

Van Cant, Marit. "Surviving Amputations: A Case of a Late-Medieval Femoral Amputation in the Rural Community of Moorsel (Belgium)." In *Trauma in Medieval Society*, edited by Wendy J. Turner and Christina Lee, 180–214. Boston: Brill, 2018.

Van 'T Land, Karine. "Sperm and Blood, Form and Food: Late Medieval Medical Notions of Male and Female in the Embryology of *Membra*." In *Blood, Sweat and Tears – The Changing Concepts of Physiology from Antiquity into Early Modern Europe*, edited by Manfred Horstmanshoff, Helen King, and Claus Zittel, 363–392. Boston: Brill, 2012.

Vekerdy, Lilla. "Paracelsus's *Great Wound Surgery*." In *Textual Healing: Essays on Medieval and Early Modern Medicine*, edited by Elizabeth Lane Furdell, 77–99. Leiden: Brill, 2005.

Verduyn, Pieter Adriaanszoon. *Neue Methode, die Glieder abzunehmen* […]. Amsterdam, 1697.

Vigo, Giovanni da. *Practica in chirurgia* […]. Lyon, 1516.

Virdi, Jaipreet. "Material Traces of Disability: Andrew Gawley's Steel Hands." *Nuncius* 35 (2020): 606–631.

Vollmuth, Ralf. *Traumatologie und Feldchirurgie an der Wende vom Mittelalter zur Neuzeit: Exemplarisch dargestellt anhand der "Großen Chirurgie" des Walther Hermann Ryff*. Stuttgart: F. Steiner, 2001.

Voragine, Jacobus. *The Golden Legend: Readings on the Saints*. Translated by William Granger Ryan. Princeton: Princeton University Press, 2012.

Voskuhl, Adelheid. *Androids in the Enlightenment: Mechanics, Artisans, and Cultures of the Self*. Chicago; London: The University of Chicago Press, 2013.

Wallis, Faith, ed. *Medieval Medicine: A Reader*. Toronto: University of Toronto Press, 2010.

Walther, Philipp Alexander Ferdinand. *Die Sammlungen von Gegenständen des Alterthums, der Kunst, der Völkerkunde und von Waffen im Grossherzoglichen Museum zu Darmstadt*. Darmstadt: Jonghaus, 1884.

Walz, Alfred. "Die Armprothese aus Metall des Herzog Anton Ulrich-Museums in Braunschweig." *Würzburger medizinhistorische Mitteilungen* 18 (1999): 55–63.

Wangensteen, Owen H., and Sarah D. Wangensteen. *The Rise of Surgery: From Empiric Craft to Scientific Discipline*. Minneapolis: University of Minnesota Press, 1978.

Wangensteen, Owen H., Jacqueline Smith, and Sarah D. Wangensteen. "Some Highlights in the History of Amputation Reflecting Lessons in Wound Healing." *Bulletin of the History of Medicine* 41:2 (1967): 97–131.

Wear, Andrew. "Medicine in Early Modern Europe, 1500–1700." In Conrad et al., *Western Medical Tradition*, 215–361.
Webster, Charles. *Paracelsus: Medicine, Magic and Mission at the End of Time*. New Haven: Yale University Press, 2008.
Welker, Manfred. *Historische Schlüssel und Schlösser im Germanischen Nationalmuseum*. Nuremberg: Germanisches Nationalmuseum, 2014.
Wetz, Hans Henning. "Zur Geschichte der Armprothetik." In *Geschichte operativer Verfahren an den Bewegungsorganen*, edited by Ludwig Zichner, 153–175. Darmstadt: Steinkopff, 2000.
Whaley, Leigh. *Women and the Practice of Medical Care in Early Modern Europe, 1400–1800*. Basingstoke: Palgrave Macmillan, 2011.
Williams, Alan. *The Knight and the Blast Furnace: A History of the Metallurgy of Armour in the Middle Ages & the Early Modern Period*. Leiden: Brill, 2003.
Williamson, Bess, and Elizabeth Guffey, eds. *Making Disability Modern: Design Histories*. London: Bloomsbury, 2020.
Wilson, Peter H. *The Thirty Years War: Europe's Tragedy*. Cambridge, MA: Belknap Press, 2009.
Wissell, Rudolf. *Des Alten Handwerks Recht und Gewohnheit*. 6 vols. 2nd ed. Edited by Ernst Schraepler. Berlin: Colloquium Verlag, 1971–1988.
Wittmann, Anneliese. *Kosmas und Damian: Kultausbreitung und Volksdevotion*. Berlin: Schmidt, 1967.
Woosnam-Savage, Robert C., and Kelly DeVries. "Battle Trauma in Medieval Warfare: Wounds, Weapons and Armor." In Tracy and DeVries, *Wounds and Wound Repair*, 27–56.
Wunderlich, Johann Jacob. *Paradoxa Sensatio, sive Dolor Membri Amputati [...]*. Tübingen, 1693.
Würtz, Felix. *Practica der Wundartzney [...]*. Basel, 1596.
———. *Practica der Wundartzney [...]*. Edited by Rudolph Würtz. Basel, 1612.
———. *Practica der Wund-Artzney [...]*. Edited by Rudolph Würtz. Lübeck, 1639.
Yonge, James. *Currus triumphalis [...]*. London, 1679.
Zimmerman, Kees, ed. *One Leg in the Grave Revisited: The Miracle of the Transplantation of the Black Leg by the Saints Cosmas and Damian*. Havertown: Barkhuis Publishing, 2013.
———. "Introduction." In Zimmerman, *One Leg in the Grave Revisited*, 11–21.

Index

Note: "n" after a page reference indicates the number of a note on that page; page numbers in *italic* refer to illustrations.

Albucasis 85
Amman, Jost 119
  woodcut 119–121, 133, 142, 146
amputation 2–6, 8, 12, 13, 15, 26, 60,
    64–74, 82–112, 119, 122–124, 128,
    142, 146, 196, 197, 201, 238–239,
    241
  decision to amputate 13, 51–53, 60,
      63–67, 69–70, 72–74, 93, 142–143,
      238–239, 241
    group consensus and 14, 51, 63,
        65–68, 70, 73–74, 239
    physicians and 14, 36, 51, 56, 63–66,
        67–70, 72, 90, 96, 122, 125, 128,
        130, 133, 143, 169
    spiritual approval and 70–72, 73,
        241
  future mobility and 70, 94, 96–98, 100,
      102–109, 133, 238–240
  ligatures and 93–94, 101–102, 104
  mortality rates 79n109, 82
  post-operative convalescence 119–125,
      127–129, 130–133, 143–145, 197,
      238–239
  punitive use of 87, 193
  regulations governing 67
  resulting stumps *see* stumps
  sites of 63, 82–86, 90, 93–96, 98–104,
      107–109, 111, 130, 141, 202
    digits 87–89, 93, 124, 129
    hands 1–2, 63, 66, 67, 87–89, 93, 127,
        132
    lower leg 68, 84, 93–107, 108–109,
        115n66, 238–239
    upper leg 63, 90

  upper limb 63, 93, 100, 142–145, 177,
      193, 196, 197, 198, 202
  "sleeping sponge" and 69, 127
  techniques 3–4, 6, 14, 63, 83–92, 93–96,
      98–104, 107–112, 130, 238–239,
      242–243
    "Botallo manner" 99
    flap amputation 104; *see also* Verduyn,
        Pieter Adriaanszoon
    "hand's-width method" 93–96, 98,
        103–104, 108–109, 111, 130
    mallet-and-wedge 87–89, 99
    "manner of Aquapendente" 100–102,
        104–105, 108, 110, 128
    rapid 87–92, 99
  women and 26, 58, 72–73, 167, 169
amputee-patrons 3–4, 8, 10–14, 43,
    144–145, 147, 155–156, 162, 169,
    192–202, 211, 227, 234, 239–243
amputees 3–5, 8, 10–14, 70, 79n109, 96–98,
    112, 119–125, 127–134, 141–147,
    155–156, 160, 162, 169, 191,
    192–202, 210–211, 238–243
  as patients 14, 119–125, 127–133,
      142–143
  as patrons *see* amputee-patrons
  popular stereotypes of 96–98, 200–201
  social status of 8, 96, 169, 195, 201, 217,
      241
  versus "disabled" 12, 192
Anaplerosis 36, 134
Aquapendente, Hieronymus Fabricius ab
    see Fabrizi, Girolamo
Arce, Francisco de 30, 86, 139
art cabinets 8, 11, 145, 162, 199–200

artificial limbs *see* prosthetic limbs
artisans 3–5, 8–15, 43, 137, 140, 146, 156, 160, 162, 170, 173, 184–185, 189–193, 195, 201–202, 210–214, 217, 221, 223–227, 231–234, 239–243
  armorers 3, 8, 10, 162, 179, 184–191, 215–216
  clockmakers 3, 5, 8, 10, 162, 173, 176–177, 179, 189, 191, 193, 195, 210, 214, 216, 221, 224–225, 227, 232, 241
    automata and 8, 177
  collaboration among 8, 14, 43, 177, 185, 189–191
  goldsmiths 8, 27, 40–43, 140, 173, 176–177, 185
  guilds and 7, 23–24, 32, 41, 67, 94, 136, 173, 188–191
  gunsmiths 173, 177, 179, 190, 193, 216, 227
  knowledge transfer and 9–10, 15, 211–214, 221–227, 233–234, 242
  leatherworkers 185, 188–190
  locksmiths 3, 5, 10, 40, 141, 162, 173, 176–177, 179, 184–185, 188–191, 193, 210–217, 221, 223–227, 231–234, 241
  master-apprentice system 7, 9, 13, 20, 22–33, 38, 71, 84, 94, 111, 185, 188–190, 214, 221, 223, 226–227, 242
  regulations and 24, 189–191
  ringmakers 173
  tailors 27, 40, 156
  weavers 27
  winch/windlass makers 173
  wives of 26
  woodworkers 5, 10, 162, 185, 188, 191

Balbronn Hand 156, *159*, 160, 162, 163, 166, 194–197
Barbette, Paul 31, 36, 53, 54, 59–61, 66, 91, 105, 111, 126, 140
  Chirurgische und anatomische Schrifften (1694) 54, 105
Bartisch, Georg 35
Battle of Fleurus 143–144
Bembo, Pietro 193
Berlichingen, Franziska von 166, 171
Berlichingen, Götz von 1–2, 5–6, 11, 127, 163, 166, 181, 188, 196, 239–240, 242
  amputation and 1–2, 6, 239
  autobiography 127, 188, 196, 239
  Ersthand and 163, 166, 181, 184
  prosthetic hand and 2, 181, 196
  Zweithand and 163, 166, 170, *172*, 196
Bohn, Johann 133
Botallo, Leonardo 30, 99
  Zwey Chirurgische Bücher (1676) 30
Braunschwieg-Wolfenbüttel, Friedrich Ulrich of 197
Braunschweig Hand 177–181, 192, 195–196, 198–200
Brunschwig, Hieronymus 20, 39, 86, 127
Burres, Lorenz 29

cabinets of curiosities 8, 145, 160, 199
Celsus, Aulus Cornelius 85, 91, 100
Chauliac, Guy de 41, 85
Christian the Younger (1599–1626), Duke of Braunschweig-Lüneburg 142–145, 177, 179, 189, 193, 197–198, 200
cold fire 3, 13, 51–61, 62–66, 69–70, 72, 74, 82–83, 86, 88, 90, 101, 103–105, 108, 111, 124, 128, 143–144, 169, 239
  causes of 56–59
  demonstration of 66–67, 73
  diagnosis of 13, 53, 55–56, 58–59, 62, 72
  treatment of 51–53, 59, 62–66, 69, 72–74, 82–83, 88, 90, 101–105, 108, 111, 124, 128, 143, 169
Colinet, Marie 26
Cosmas and Damian, miracle of 136–138
craftsmen *see* artisans
Cusin, Charles 195–196

d'Acquapendente, Girolamo Fabrizi d' *see* Fabrizi, Girolamo
Darmstadt Hand 181–184, 191, 194
Denisio, Jacob 128, 130
Descartes, René 110–111, 122–123, 133
  Principia philosophiae (1644) 111
design model of disability 162, 201
Dietz, Johann 27
disability, history of 3, 11–12, 121, 142, 162, 192, 201–202, 243
  cultural model of disability 12

Index 269

design model of disability 162, 201–202
social model of disability 11–12
Döring, Michael 122–125, 127–130, 132–133, 146
  correspondence with Fabry 122–133
  imagination and common sense 125, 129
Duffy, Elana 238–240

Eisfeld Hand 171, 174–176, 179, 184, 190–191, 194, 196
Ersthand 163–164, 166, 184, 194, 198

Fabrizi, Girolamo 28, 31, 32, 63, 81n121, 88, 100–105, 110, 116n80, 116n82
  "manner of Aquapendente" 100–102, 104–105, 108, 110, 128
false imaginations 125–126, 129–130, 132–133, 145–146, 241
  see also phantom limbs
flap grafts 134–135
Forrer, Robert 163, 166
French Disease 29, 57–58, 72, 169
French pox *see* French Disease
Fries, Joachim 177

Galen 35, 37, 54, 100, 110
  De tumoribus praeter naturam (1529) 54
Gangraena see hot fire
Geelmann, Georg 58
Gehema, Janus Abraham à 6, 32, 53, 58, 61, 67, 70, 122, 134–135, 137
  Der krancke Soldat (1690) 6
  Wolversehener Feld-Medicus (1684) 32, 53, 67
Gelb, Johann Wolfgang 176–177
Gersdorff, Hans von 20, 32, 39, 41, 69, 70, 72, 86, 94–98, 127, 136
  Feldbuch der Wundarznei (1517) 32, 93–97, 136
  Serratura woodcut 93–95
Goethe, Johann Wolfgang von 163, 166, 242
  Götz von Berlichingen mit der eisernen Hand (1773) 163
Greflinger, Georg 144
Greiff, Sebastian 29, 31, 54, 58, 62, 99–100
  Wolbewärte Wundarzney (1630) 54, 58
Griffon, Jean 25, 31, 56
Grüningen Hand 160–161, 166, 170, 181, 184, 194, 196, 198
gunpowder warfare 2–3, 6, 29, 57–58, 72, 86, 111, 143, 163, 169, 212–213
  contused injuries and 57–58, 72, 86, 169

Händel, Georg 27
heisse Brand, der: *see* hot fire
hemorrhaging 13, 85, 86, 90–94, 101–102, 104, 108, 127, 132–133
  exsanguination 63, 87, 90, 92, 101–102, 132, 143
hemostatic methods 90, 92
  cauterization 3–4, 62, 73, 90–92, 100–102, 107, 122, 127–128, 241
  cauterium actuale (actual cautery) 4, 62, 85, 90–92, 122, 127–128, 241
  cauterium potentiale (potential cautery) 4, 62, 90–92
  with cautery knife 90–91
  ligation 3, 13, 90–92, 212
  sutures 39
Hildanus, Guilelmus Fabricius *see* Hilden, Fabry von
Hilden, Fabry von 25–26, 29–32, 37, 39–42, 51–52, 54–58, 60–67, 70, 73–74, 86–88, 90–91, 94, 96, 98, 101–102, 105, 111, 122–133, 146–147, 167, 169, 213–214, 223, 240
  correspondence with Döring 122–133
  Gründlicher Bericht vom heissen und kalten Brand (1593) 54, 101, 131–132, 213–214
  Lithotomia Vesicae (1626) 73
  phantom limbs and 122–133, 146–147
  Wund-Artzney (1652) 40, 90
Hippocratic-Galenic Medicine 4, 6, 20–21, 56–57, 61, 64, 85, 94, 110–111, 126, 135
Hohenheim, Theophrastus von *see* Paracelsus
Hornstein, Marquand von 163, 166
Horch, Christoph 111
Horst, Georg 52
hot fire 13, 51–62, 69, 74, 124
  causes of 52, 56–58
  diagnosis of 51, 53–55, 58–59
  humoralism and 55–57, 59–61
  treatment of 51–53, 59–62

iatrochemicalism 110–111
iatrophysics 110–111
Ingolstadt Hand 167–171, 181, 191–192, 194–196, 198, 200
iron hands *see* mechanical limbs

Jessen, Johann von 30, 139–141
  Institutiones chirurgicae (1601) 30

Jousse, Mathurin 232
  La fidelle ouverture de l'art de serrurier (1627) 232

kalte Brand, der: see cold fire
Kassel Hand 171, 181, 184, 194, 196, 211, 218–222, 233
knowledge making 9, 15, 21, 38, 83, 107, 191–192, 212, 225, 241–243
  practical knowledge and 15, 107, 191–192, 212, 227, 241–243
Kunstbüchlein see recipe books
Kunstkammern see art cabinets

Lanfranc of Milan 85
le petit Lorrain 210, 212, 214, 218, 221, 223–227, 232–234
locking gauntlet 169
Lose, Laurentius 29, 53–54, 56
  Chirurgisches Hand-Büchlein (1679) 54
Ludwig X of Hessen-Darmstadt 181

malleable body 3–6, 9, 13, 15, 107, 112, 202, 211, 240–243
Marchetti, Pietro de 30, 128–129
material culture 3, 10–11, 155–156, 162, 166, 170–202
mechanical limbs 2–5, 8, 10–12, 15, 141, 155–202, 211–234, 239, 241–243
  adjustments and repairs 156, 190–191, 196–197, 242
  artifacts *see* Balbronn Hand; Braunschweig Hand; Darmstadt Hand; Eisfeld Hand; Ersthand; Grüningen Hand; Ingolstadt Hand; Kassel Hand; Nuremberg Hand; Ruppin Hand; Zweithand
  as composite products 184–192, 194–195
  attachment of 2, 99, 103–105, 160, 170, 196, 198, 216–217, 238–239
  commissioning of 4–5, 8, 11–12, 14, 162, 169, 184–185, 188–197, 200–202, 223–224, 226, 232–234, 239, 241
  cost of 179, 185, 188, 191, 193–196, 199, 201, 217
  degrees of complexity of 2, 14, 146, 166, 170–171, 194–197, 199, 221
  fit and finish of 2, 171, 179, 180–181, 184–185, 188, 190–191, 193–195, 198, 200–201

  historical accounts of 1–2, 11, 144–145, 162–163, 166–167, 169, 177, 179, 181, 184, 188–189
  intended uses of 163, 166–167, 169, 196–202
  material composition of 141, 144, 155–156, 160, 162–163, 167, 170, 173, 177, 184–185, 188, 193, 200–202
  mechanical elements 2, 167, 170, 179, 185, 188, 192, 194–196, 199, 214–222, 227–232
    finger blocks 156, 160, 170, 184, 194–196
    ratchets 170–173, 179, 192
    release levers 156, 158, 160, 167, 170–174, 179, 181, 184, 188, 194, 196, 215, 218, *220, 222*, 229, 231
    springs 156, 158, 167, 170–173, 176–177, 179, 188, 192, 194, 196, 212, 216, 218, *220, 222*, 226–229
  operation of 2, 156, 158, 160, 167, 169, 170–174, 179–185, 188, 191–192, 194–199, 214–222
  production of 14–15, 162, 170, 173, 176–177, 179, 184–185, 187–196, 201–202
    guilds and 173, 176, 188–191
    subcontracting and 189–191
  weight of 2, 93, 142, 156, 167, 181, 188, 196, 198, 221
Mechel, Christian von 171–172
  Die eiserne Hand des tapfern deutschen Ritters Götz von Berlichingen (1815) 172
Mercker, Johann 29, 58
Minadoi, Giovanni Tommaso 141
  De humani corporis turpitudinibus cognoscendis et curandis (1600) 141
Mitchell, Silas Weir 123
Mittelhausen, Hans von 156, 163, 197
Mondeville, Henri de 40–41, 85
Moulin, Johannes de 52
Muys, Jan 63–64, 91, 103, 109–111, 135, 141
  Neue Vernünfftige Praxis der Wund-Artzney (1688) 91

Noue, François de la 163
Nuremberg Hand 185–190, 192, 195, 198–200

Index

Padua, University of 7, 30–31, 44n18, 88, 90, 98, 100–102, 110, 128
patients 3–4, 6–7, 9–10, 12–14, 20, 24, 26–27, 29, 31, 37, 39–40, 42–43, 51–53, 55–74, 82–83, 85, 87–96, 98–109, 112, 119–147, 169, 214, 216–217, 223, 225, 232–233, 239–241
  emotional state of 1, 5, 108, 126–129, 133, 141, 146, 201
  see also amputees
Paracelsus 29–31, 56, 62, 98–101, 110, 119–120
  Amman woodcut and 119–120
  Der grossen wundartzney (1536) 110
  Opus Chyrurgicum (1565) 119
Paré, Ambroise 14, 28, 86, 92, 94, 96, 98, 104, 123, 126, 130–133, 135, 137, 141, 155, 189, 193, 210–218, 221, 223–234, 239, 243
  as an intermediary 213, 223, 226–228, 232–234
  book of artificial body parts 137, 210, 212, 221, 232–233
  le petit Lorrain and 210, 212, 214, 218, 221, 223–227, 232–234
  Les Oeuvres (1614) 210–218, 223–234
  phantom limbs and 123, 130–132
  woodcuts and 14, 210–218, 221, 223–234
  Wund-Artzney (1635) 211, 228
Pauw, Peter 25
Pfalzpaint, Heinrich von *see* Pfolspeundt, Heinrich von
Pfolspeundt, Heinrich von 69, 134
phantom limbs 3, 14, 122–133, 145–147, 239, 241
  debates over 14, 122–133, 145–147, 241
  phantom limb phenomenon (PLP) 123
  theories regarding 122–133, 145–147
physicians 7, 9–10, 13–14, 19–21, 23–25, 27, 29–32, 34, 36–37, 51–52, 56, 59, 61, 63–72, 74, 90, 96, 100, 111, 119, 121–122, 125, 128–130, 132–134, 143–145, 169, 195, 211
print shops 7–9, 13, 21, 28, 30, 32, 34, 43, 213, 224–226, 228, 230–231, 242
  see also surgical literature
prostheses 2–5, 8–14, 96–99, 102–106, 108–111, 133–134, 139–142, 144–147, 155–202, 210–234, 238–242
  arms 2–5, 10, 12, 140, 144–145, 155–202, 210–234, 242

  ears 139–140, 145, 213, 223
  eyes 139–140, 147, 155, 213, 223
  false restorations and 14, 134, 137, 139–143, 145–147
  hands 2, 4–5, 10, 12, 134, 155–202, 210–234, 242
  legs 93, 96–99, 102–106, 108–109, 140–141, 147, 156, 192–193, 200, 210, 213–214, 223, 225, 238–240
  lips and 134, 139
  noses 139, 155, 192, 213
  palates 139
  urination tubes 137, 147
  see also mechanical limbs
Purmann, Matthäus 19–21, 28–30, 32, 34, 70–71, 86, 96, 99, 105, 108, 111, 135
  Feldscher (1680) 29
  Wund-Artzney (1684) 19, 21, 105
putrefaction *see* hot fire; cold fire

recipe books 7, 24, 29, 83
Renner, Franz 29, 31, 34, 38, 139
  Handtbüchlein (1557) 34
Rehtmeyer, Philipp Julius 145
  Chronica (1722) 145
Ring, Philipp 189, 194
Ruppin Hand 156–158, 160, 162–163, 166, 170, 179, 181, 184, 193–194
Ryff, Walther Hermann 30, 54, 68–69, 73
  Die groß Chirurgei (1545) 54, 68
  Woodcut 68–69, 73

Sarasin, Jean-Antoine 56
Schmid, Balthasar 26
Schmid, Joseph 6, 26–28, 30–32, 34–38, 40, 42–43, 61, 71–72, 82–83, 101, 139
  Examen chirurgicum (1644) 26–28, 40, 71–72, 82–83, 101
  Kriegs-Arzney (1664) 28
  Instrumenta chirurgica (1697) 71
  Speculum chirurgicum (1675) 6, 27, 31, 34–37
  Spiegel der Anatomiae (1646) 26, 42–43
Schmidhammer, Jörg 173
Scultetus, Johannes 30–32, 34, 58, 64–65, 74, 86–91, 100, 102, 105, 110–111, 128–129
  Armamentarium Chirurgicum (1655) 31
  Wund-Artzneyisches Zeug-Hauß (1666) 65, 88–91, 102, 128–129

Slot, Cosmas 25, 31
Solingen, Cornelis 36, 39–40, 90–92, 103, 109, 132
  Hand-Griffe der Wund-Artzney (1693) 36
Sphacelus see cold fire
Spiegel, Adriaan van den 31, 88–89
St. Anthony's Fire 54, 72, 96–97
stumps 3–4, 79n109, 86–88, 90–94, 96–106, 108–112, 121–122, 124, 128–133, 137, 141–143, 156, 198, 225, 238–239, 241
  lengths of 4, 94–99, 101–107, 108–109, 111–112, 115n66, 198
  prosthetic technologies and 13, 93–94, 96–99, 101–107, 108–109, 110–112, 115n66, 141–142, 147, 156, 225, 238–239
Sturm, Leonhard Christoph 145
surgeons 1, 3–10, 12–15, 19–43, 51–74, 82–112, 119–147, 155, 169, 194, 196, 202, 210–211, 213–214, 217, 223–224, 232–234, 238–243
  draughtsmanship and 39
  guilds and 7, 23–24, 32, 67, 94
  habits and traits of 36–37, 39–40, 70–71, 74, 127–129
  human bodies and 3–4, 8–9, 12, 14, 41–43, 83, 100, 108–109, 112, 121–122, 133–134, 146–147, 202, 241–242
  instruments and 40, 59, 68–69, 71, 90–94, 100–101, 104, 109, 112, 122, 127
  physicians and 7, 9–10, 13–14, 19–21, 23–25, 27, 29–32, 34, 36–37, 51–52, 56, 59, 61, 63–70, 72, 74, 90, 96, 100, 111, 119–133, 143, 169, 194–195, 211
  prostheses and 14, 96, 98, 103–105, 137, 139–143, 147, 155, 196, 202, 210–211, 217, 242
  salaries of 24, 26, 167, 194–195
  surgical procedures and 3–4, 13, 38, 51–53, 56–58, 60–63, 65–69, 71, 82–96, 98–104, 107–108, 111, 122–124, 127, 134–136, 142–143
  training of 7–9, 20–21, 23–28, 32, 38, 71, 94
  types of
    barber-surgeons 6–7, 9, 22–24, 26–28, 30, 32–33, 35, 42, 55, 59, 61, 65, 67, 71, 82, 84, 87, 132, 139, 167, 211, 213, 223, 242
    field-surgeons 1, 6, 28–30, 32, 53, 67, 72, 82, 84, 107, 111, 122
    master surgeons 7, 9, 15, 20, 23–27, 32–33, 36–37, 39–41, 84, 111
    vernacular surgeons 13, 20–23, 33–39, 41–43, 84, 94, 111–112, 132, 211
    definition of 13, 33
  wives of 26, 72–73, 169
surgical knowledge 7, 9, 11, 20–21, 26–27, 29, 31–35, 38–40, 53, 59, 83–84, 92, 107, 121–122, 125, 146–147, 241, 243
  anatomy and 7, 23, 25–27, 32, 35, 40–42, 110, 213, 243
  craft traditions 25, 32, 40, 42
  humoralism and 26, 55–57, 59, 61, 64, 111, 135
  learned traditions 15, 21, 32, 34, 36, 38, 84, 94, 100, 103, 108, 111–112, 243
  transfer of 9, 21, 26–27, 35, 84
  vernacular knowledge 9, 15, 20, 33, 243
surgical literature 5–6, 8–10, 12–15, 20–23, 28–34, 36–40, 53–54, 59, 69–70, 72, 84–94, 96–105, 107–112, 119–147, 193, 202, 210–234, 239–243
  case histories and 6, 14, 29, 51–52, 56–59, 64–66, 69–70, 88–90, 110–111, 123–125, 128, 130–133, 135–136, 139, 141–142
  circulation of 8–9, 13, 20–21, 28–30, 84, 110, 211, 213–214, 221–234
  classical tradition and 21, 34–35, 38
  examination guides 27, 29, 72, 100–101
  field manuals 27–29
  German vernacular and 7–9, 13, 20–23, 28–30, 32, 84, 86, 90, 100, 104–105, 110–111, 129–130, 134, 141, 211, 213–214, 224–225, 230–232
  Latin and 7–9, 13, 20–23, 28–30, 32, 35–36, 43, 105, 133, 213, 223–226, 230–231
  religion and 34, 36–37, 41, 43, 70–73, 84, 90, 119, 130, 136, 197
  surgical observations and 27, 29, 31, 33, 58, 69, 88, 90, 122, 125, 134–135, 137, 167–168
  see also print shops
Sylvius, Francois de le Boë 111

Tagliacozzi, Gaspare 134
Tassin, Leonard 30
Tauber, Johann 30

Index

technical knowledge transfer 210–234
Thirty Years' War 7, 98, 143–144, 181, 189, 200
Toppinus, Stephan 51–52, 70, 72
Torriano, Gianello 177
tourniquets 104

Uffenbach, Peter 28, 224
  Thesaurus chirurgiae (1610) 28
Ulrich, Duke Anton 145
Urstisius, Emanuel 52

Van Horne, Johannes 30
Verduyn, Pieter Adriaanszoon 104–106, 109, 141
  Dissertatio epistolaris de nova artuum decurtandorum ratione / Neue Methode, die Glieder abzunehmen (1696/1697) 104, 141
  flap amputation and 104–105

vernacular surgeons *see* surgeons
Vesalius, Andreas 25, 35
  De humani corporis fabrica (1543) 35
Voragine, Jacob de 136
  Legenda aurea (c. 1260) 136

Wagner, Ulrich 189
Welser, Ulrich 26, 167
wheellocks 179, 195
Wunderkammern see cabinets of curiosities
Würtz, Felix 31–32, 35, 38–39, 140
  Practica der Wundartzney (1596) 35
Würtz, Rudolph 35
Wyss, Ulrich 163

Yonge, James 96n117

Zweithand 163, 165–166, 170–172, 177, 184, 192, 194, 196

EU authorised representative for GPSR:
Easy Access System Europe, Mustamäe tee 50,
10621 Tallinn, Estonia
gpsr.requests@easproject.com

www.ingramcontent.com/pod-product-compliance
Lightning Source LLC
Chambersburg PA
CBHW051605230426
43668CB00013B/1988